Foundations for Practice in Occupational Therapy

Commissioning Editor: Rita Demetriou-Swanwick
Development Editor: Catherine Jackson
Project Manager: Priya Dauntess
Designer/Design Direction: Kirsteen Wright
Illustration Manager: Gillian Richards

Foundations for Practice in Occupational Therapy

FIFTH EDITION

Edited by

Edward A.S. Duncan PhD BSc(Hons) DipCBT

Senior Research Fellow, Nursing, Midwifery and Allied Health Professions
Research Unit, University of Stirling, Scotland UK

Foreword by

Elizabeth Townsend PhD OT(C) RegNS FCAOT

Professor Emerita, School of Occupational Therapy, Dalhousie University, Nova Scotia, Canada

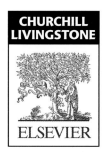

CHURCHILL LIVINGSTONE

ELSEVIER

Edinburgh   London   New York   Oxford   Philadelphia   St Louis   Sydney   Toronto   2011

CHURCHILL
LIVINGSTONE
ELSEVIER

First edition 1992
Second edition 1997
Third edition 2001
Fourth Edition 2006
Fifth Edition 2012
  Reprinted 2013 (twice)

ISBN 978 0 7020 5312 2

British Library Cataloguing in Publication Data
A catalogue record for this book is available from the British Library

Library of Congress Cataloging in Publication Data
A catalog record for this book is available from the Library of Congress

Notices
Knowledge and best practice in this field are constantly changing. As new research and experience broaden our understanding, changes in research methods, professional practices, or medical treatment may become necessary.

Practitioners and researchers must always rely on their own experience and knowledge in evaluating and using any information, methods, compounds, or experiments described herein. In using such information or methods they should be mindful of their own safety and the safety of others, including parties for whom they have a professional responsibility.

With respect to any drug or pharmaceutical products identified, readers are advised to check the most current information provided (i) on procedures featured or (ii) by the manufacturer of each product to be administered, to verify the recommended dose or formula, the method and duration of administration, and contraindications. It is the responsibility of practitioners, relying on their own experience and knowledge of their patients, to make diagnoses, to determine dosages and the best treatment for each individual patient, and to take all appropriate safety precautions.

To the fullest extent of the law, neither the Publisher nor the authors, contributors, or editors, assume any liability for any injury and/or damage to persons or property as a matter of products liability, negligence or otherwise, or from any use or operation of any methods, products, instructions, or ideas contained in the material herein.

Dedication

In memory of Dr Gary Wayne Kielhofner (1949–2010). Gary was a visionary, an exceptional scholar, a modern day father of occupational therapy, and a highly valued colleague. His work changed the life of countless people with disabilities, and formed generations of occupational therapists throughout the world. He will be greatly missed.

Contents

Foreword

As I write this Foreword, I am reflecting on the advances made in **Foundations for Practice in Occupational Therapy** which is the latest edition of Rosemary Hagedorn's classic occupational therapy text. Edited and partly authored by Dr. Edward Duncan of Scotland, **Foundations for Practice in Occupational Therapy** displays a new milestone in occupational therapists' abilities and insights to articulate what occupational therapists do. Here you will discover the latest views on occupational therapy's complex philosophy, models, frames of reference, and practice possibilities to make a difference in the world. As Dr. Duncan states in Chapter 1: "Occupational therapy practice appears deceptively simple…[yet]…Occupational therapy's theoretical and evidence base is rapidly developing and the profession has entered an exciting new era as therapists become increasingly research-active in a variety of ways—from collaborating in clinical data collection to acting as a principal investigator".

I am impressed with the comprehensiveness and thoughtfulness of **Foundations for Practice in Occupational Therapy**. In one compact text, occupational therapy practitioners and others can access the essence of mainstream occupational therapy knowledge and its application in recognizable areas of practice for the 21st century. I liked the tone of Section I's introductory chapters that invite occupational therapists to embrace theory to explain and guide diverse practice applications. The invitation is enriched with reflective notes on the importance of theory and historical insights on external and internal influences that have shaped occupational therapy. I imagine that Section II will be particularly appealing to occupational therapists with chapters that summarize five well known Conceptual Models: The Model of Human Occupation (MOHO); The Canadian Model of Occupational Performance (CMOP); The Person-Environment-Occupational Performance Model (PEOP); The Information Processing Model; and the Kawa (River) Model. The appeal of Sections III and IV will be the concise overviews of five, well-known Frames of Reference and three important, evolving areas of knowledge: clinical reasoning, community-based rehabilitation, and occupational science.

Features that I find helpful in **Foundations for Practice in Occupational Therapy** are the clear use of language, case studies, examples, figures and tables. This will be a book that can be used over and over again to stimulate discussions and to check for theoretical guidance in the midst of a busy practice. *Key Points* provided at the beginning of most chapters will help to focus the reader; *Reflective Learning* questions at the end of chapters will help to engage the reader. I highly recommend this as a concise text that explains occupational therapy to newcomers such as students and to those who know the profession well.

Elizabeth Townsend
2010

Introduction

Theoretical concepts in occupational therapy provide the cornerstone to practice. Such a position, however, may not be widely held by all members of the profession. As a student, I remember being inspired by the lectures and tutorials that surrounded the theory of occupational therapy. Whilst many of the concepts were not the easiest to grasp, I slowly realized that these theoretical foundations provided rich explanations and frameworks for practice. I found the philosophical basis and conceptual development of occupational therapy inspiring. Practice placements were (mostly) equally inspiring. It was through these experiences that I saw, at first hand, the vital importance of occupation in human life. Theory and practice — both inspiring and rich experiences and ones that I continue to treasure as important components of my professional development. Perhaps because of my positive experiences, both academic and practical, I was equally struck by how rarely these concepts connected. I and several of my student peers would often be told, 'Forget what they tell you in college, this [practice placement] is where you will learn what occupational therapy is *really* about', or variations on a similar theme. Such experiences were very disheartening, both for us as students and, I'm sure, for our lecturers, who strove to provide an excellent and relevant educational experience. Sadly, this experience was not simply a sign of its times and 20 years on, despite significant theoretical developments with increasingly obvious relevance to practice, and new generations of therapists educated since my time, students continue, at times, to meet the same barriers when they attempt to integrate theory in practice.

About me

The richness of my undergraduate academic experience impacted upon my early development as an occupational therapist and I searched for ways in which to integrate theory into practice. Working initially within community mental health teams in Glasgow, I was acutely aware of the challenge this involved. During this period I became increasingly interested in cognitive behavioural therapy (CBT). I was impressed by CBT's recognized evidence base, everyday clinical utility and resonance with occupational therapy practice. Through further study I gained a postgraduate diploma in CBT and recognized its strengths, both as a form of psychotherapy and as an approach that has much to offer occupational therapy.

After a few years working in the community, I had the fortunate experience of being part of a new occupational therapy department in a high-security forensic hospital. This was an exciting clinical experience. The department was initially small, but staffed with enthusiastic and committed clinicians and supported by visionary management. An early decision was made that the department would select an occupational therapy conceptual model to be the first (but not the only) informing body of knowledge; it was unanimously agreed that the Model of Human Occupation (MOHO) most appropriately met our patients' and environment's needs. Explicitly embracing a conceptual model of practice was a very challenging, fulfilling and effective experience. This, once again, convinced me of the importance of practising occupational therapy from a sound theoretical perspective.

Another crucial seed sown during my undergraduate studies was the importance of clinical research. The development and implementation of clinical research now defines my professional vision. Theoretical concepts, whilst initially forming in a person's or persons' head, must swiftly be turned into research questions that test and refine the theory, building on ideas with evidence. My research career has developed through a series of stages, from clinical collaborator to principal investigator, leading to my present academic appointment. I view research as an essential component of practice. All clinicians must at least be able to make sense of the evidence. Others, in undertaking clinical research, contribute to a vital process of building theory to inform practice.

About the book

Foundations for Practice in Occupational Therapy is a well-known textbook. Its first edition was published during my undergraduate studies and was rarely far from my desk. Successive generations of therapists gratefully learnt from Rosemary Hagedorn's (author of the first three editions) perspective of occupational therapy. Editing the 4th edition of *Foundations for Practice* was not a task that I undertook lightly. Rosemary prefaced the third edition by stating that it was built upon 30 years of professional practice. Viewed in such terms, I had only a third of that experience to offer, but my experience was different. My vision for the text also differed. It was time, as Rosemary generously acknowledged in her Foreword to the 4th edition, for a new perspective. The 4th edition did not rely on my thoughts alone and indeed was greatly enriched by the inclusion of clinicians and academics from the UK, USA, Canada, Australia and Japan. The 4th edition of *Foundations for Practice* aimed to have an ever-greater integration of evidence-based theories and practice, as well as greater collaboration between academics (for want of a better word) and clinicians. Health policies vary internationally; however, each demands that the profession delivers the highest level of clinically relevant evidence-based practice. These demands shaped the last edition of this book. A conscious decision was taken to move away from personal perspectives of practice towards more theoretically driven, evidence-based practice. The aim was to provide a text that presented the fundamentals of occupational therapy's theoretical foundations in an accessible way and developed these to enable the book to be a useful text for students throughout their studies and for clinicians in practice. Given its prior success and prestige, it was with more than a slight degree of apprehension that I took over at the 'helm'. The overwhelmingly positive feedback to the 4th Edition has therefore been very gratifying, and is due in no small part to the excellent input from all the contributors.

This 5th edition of *Foundations for Practice in Occupational Therapy* builds on the preceding edition. All chapters have been revised and updated, new chapters have been written and some pre-existing chapters have new authors. A new structure has been placed on the main chapters of the book, with *Key points* to indicate the key themes and issues of each chapter, and useful *Reflective learning* questions to help the reader reflect on the issues raised in the chapter they have just read.

I hope this book continues to be valuable to a range of occupational therapists and in its own way continues to help to address the gaps between theory and practice. As always, I appreciate constructive appraisal and look forward to hearing suggestions for ways that future editions could be improved.

Edward Duncan
2011

For more information on the work of Dr Edward Duncan visit:
http://stir.academia.edu/EdwardDuncan

Twitter: @easduncan

Acknowledgements

This book would not have been possible without the dedicated input of a range of individuals.

The contributors

As with the last edition, I have been extremely privileged to work with a range of outstanding occupational therapists. I have known a few of the contributors since my earliest student days; their influence on me is greater than they could imagine. Others I have come to know over the last 20 years and they too have shaped my development. A few I have gratefully come to know through the development of this latest edition. In various ways they have all helped shape this book. Each of them has my greatest respect and thanks for their contribution to this text, their work in the development of occupational therapy theory and practice, and their genuine care and compassion for the people they meet through their work.

The publishers

Elsevier have been incredibly supportive throughout the development and production of this book.

Particular thanks must be given to Catherine Jackson, who has guided me with great patience and wisdom.

Nursing Midwifery and Allied Health Professions Research Unit

I am very fortunate to work in a highly respected interdisciplinary research unit. Whilst not contributing directly to the text, my colleagues continually inspire and challenge me to find ways to implement research in practice and 'bridge' the theory–practice divide. Whilst not immediately apparent, our discussions and work have left an imprint throughout this text.

My family

Anne, Catherine, Eleanor and Joseph bring immense love and laughter to my life. Each of them, and all of them together, enrich me and support me in so many ways. This work would not have been achieved without them.

Cover painting by Michel Pochet

Selecting appropriate artwork for *Foundations for Practice in Occupational Therapy* was not easy. I hope that the image selected is, to some extent, an effective representation of the book's vision. The picture is of the Forth Bridge. This bridge, a highly complex structure, links two sides of the same thing. It has, therefore, many similarities to the new edition of this book, which highlights the intricacy of occupational therapy and brings together its two sides — theory and practice. The Scottish significance is also close to my heart! The picture is the creation of Michel Pochet, a good friend, to whom I am grateful for granting permission for its use.

Michel Pochet, a Parisian born in Provence in 1940, spent his childhood under the hot sun and unique light of Corsica. At the age of 13 he wanted to become a painter, and to help nurture his talent his mother returned to painting herself. She was a perceptive and unaffected watercolourist, and Pochet learned his technique, which is still evident in his work, from her.

At 17, Pochet moved to Paris to study architecture at the School of Fine Arts, the best school of its kind in France. He continued to paint, sculpt, and write poetry, novels and essays, his main subject being the relationship between God and beauty. Several of his books have been translated into Italian, Flemish, German, Portuguese, English and Spanish.

Michel Pochet lives and works in Rome, where he founded an international artistic centre, the Centro Maria, to promote art 'in communication with God'. Details of the Centro Maria and Michel Pochet's work can be found at: http://www.flars.net/centromaria.

Edward A.S. Duncan

Contributors

Julie Bass PhD OTR/L FAOTA
Professor, Henrietta Schmoll School of Health,
St Catherine University, St Paul, Minnesota, USA

Carolyn M. Baum PhD OTR
Professor of Occupational Therapy and Neurology, and
Elias Michael Director, Programme in Occupational
Therapy, Washington University School of Medicine,
Saint Louis, MO, USA

Sheena E.E. Blair DipCOT MEd EdD FHEA FCOT
Formerly Head of Division of Occupational Therapy and
Programme Leader for Professional Doctorate, Glasgow
Caledonian University, Glasgow, UK

Charles Christiansen EdD OTR OT(C) FAOTA
Executive Director, American Occupational Therapy
Foundation, Bethesda, MD, USA

Margaret A. Daniel MA BSc DipCOT MBACP(Snr Accred)
UKRC
Clinical Specialist Occupational Therapist in
Psychotherapy, Glasgow, Scotland

Edward A.S. Duncan
Senior Research Fellow, Nursing, Midwifery and Allied
Health Professions Research Unit, University of Stirling,
Scotland UK

Leisle Ezekiel
Senior Lecturer, Occupational Therapy, Oxford Brookes
University, Oxford, UK

Sally Feaver MA BA(Hons) DipCOT
Principal Lecturer, Occupational Therapy, Oxford Brookes
University, Oxford, UK

Kirsty Forsyth
Professor, Subject of Occupational Therapy and Arts
Therapies, School of Health Sciences, Queen Margaret
University, Edinburgh, UK

Michèle Hébert PhD OT (Aut On)
Associate Professor, Occupational Therapy Programme,
Health Sciences Faculty, University of Ottawa, Ottawa,
Ontario, Canada

Sheila Heinicke BSc MEd
Occupational therapist working in community based
mental health in St. Thomas, Ontario, Canada

Michael K. Iwama PhD OT(C) MSc BScOT BSc
Associate Professor, Department of Occupational Science
and Occupational Therapy and Graduate Department of
Rehabilitation Science, Faculty of Medicine,
University of Toronto, Toronto, Canada

Gary Kielhofner DrPH OTR
Formerly Professor, Department of Occupational Therapy,
University of Illinois at Chicago, Chicago, Illinois, USA

Kee Hean Lim MSc DipCOT
Lecturer in Occupational Therapy, Brunel University,
Middlesex, UK

Ian R. McMillan MEd PgDipEdRes DipCOT CertEd
Head of Subject: Occupational Therapy and Arts
Therapies, School of Health Sciences, Queen Margaret
University, Edinburgh, UK

Matthew Molineux BOccThy MSc PhD
Associate Professor, School of Occupational Therapy
and Social Work, and Centre for Research into
Disability and Society with Curtin Health Innovation
Research Institute, Curtin University of Technology,
Perth, Australia

Davina M. Parker DipCOT MSc
Head of Occupational Therapy, University Hospital
Birmingham NHS Foundation Trust, UK

Jackie Pool DipCOT
Managing Director, Jackie Pool Associates Limited,
Hampshire, UK

Thelma Sumsion PhD OT Reg (Ont)
Formerly Associate Professor, University of Western
Ontario, School of Occupational Therapy, Elborn College,
London, Ontario, Canada

Rachel Thibeault PhD OT(C)
Professor, Occupational Therapy Programme, University of
Ottawa, Ottawa, Ontario, Canada

Lesley Tischler-Draper MSc. O.T. O.T. Reg. (Ont.)
Occupational therapist working in Ambulatory Care in
London, Ontario, Canada

Carolyn A. Unsworth PhD OTR AccOT
Associate Professor, Research and Higher Degrees
Co-ordinator, School of Occupational Therapy,
La Trobe University, Melbourne, Victoria, Australia

Gail E. Whiteford BAppSc
Head, Albury–Wodonga Campus Professor and Chair,
Occupational Therapy, Charles Sturt University, Albury,
New South Wales, Australia

Section 1

Introduction to the philosophy, principles and practice of occupational therapy

Introduction

Edward A.S. Duncan

Foundations for Practice

Foundations for Practice was originally published in 1992. In it Rosemary Hagedorn presented the first comprehensive British introduction to the theoretical foundations of occupational therapy. The book was an instant success. Nineteen years and four editions later, *Foundations for Practice* remains a popular text. The profession remains greatly indebted to Rosemary Hagedorn for her work, as successive cohorts of occupational therapy students have used her *Foundations for Practice* to guide their theoretical knowledge development. In 1995, Rosemary's achievements were rightly acknowledged when she was selected to deliver the prestigious Casson Memorial Lecture at the College of Occupational Therapists' Annual Conference. In 1998 the honour of becoming a Fellow of the College of Occupational Therapists was conferred on her.

The first three editions of *Foundations for Practice* were shaped by Rosemary's personal perspective and based on her lifetime career and experience as an occupational therapist. The 4th edition, whilst maintaining the general aim and shape of previous editions, necessarily took a 'new' perspective. It provided an evidence-based introduction to the foundations of occupational therapy, linking theory ever more closely to practice, with the aspiration that practice will become increasingly based on sound theory and evidence. To achieve this, national and international expertise from clinical and academic environments was drawn upon, and the text evolved into an edited international publication. This 5th edition represents another step forward for the text and for the profession.

The purpose of this book

This book is intended for use as an introduction to the theoretical foundations of occupational therapy. Each chapter has been written to provide a comprehensive introduction to its topic, highlighting key contemporary issues and focusing on its specific relevance to practice. Of obvious use to students, the book's expanded and revised content will also make it a valuable resource for clinicians who wish to practise from a sound theoretical and evidence base. It may also assist non-occupational therapists to achieve a better understanding of the scope and practice of the profession.

The contents of this book

This current edition is revised, updated and expanded. It is arranged in four sections.

Section 1 introduces the philosophy, principles and practice of occupational therapy. Key concepts concerning the philosophical and theoretical basis of the profession are defined and summarized. The section outlines some of the main external influences on the profession and places particular emphasis upon the various shifts that have occurred within occupational therapy's theoretical foundations over time. In order to understand the external influences that continue to shape occupational therapy clearly, this section explores the impact that various philosophical systems have had on its theory and practice.

The section then continues by focusing on the historical and contemporary internal influences that have affected the development of occupational therapy. It provides an overview of occupational therapy definitions, and outlines the practice and skills required of an occupational therapist. This section presents a description of the processes through which occupational therapy is carried out and concludes by introducing frames of reference and conceptual models of practice, outlining their roles and mutually dependent relationships in practice.

Section 2 provides an introduction to conceptual models of practice. Five conceptual models of practice are presented. They do not represent all the available models; a conscious decision was taken to present conceptual models that are evidence-based, reflect popular usage in practice, or are topical. They include the Model of Human Occupation (Chapter 6), the Canadian Model of Occupational Performance (Chapter 7), the Person–Environment–Occupational Performance Model (Chapter 8), the Functional Information-processing Model (Chapter 9) and the *Kawa* (River) Model (Chapter 10).

Section 3 introduces five frames of reference in occupational therapy practice. Each chapter is written by occupational therapists experienced in their theory and direct reference is made to their application in practice. Chapters are presented on the client-centred frame of reference (Chapter 11), the cognitive behavioural frame of reference (Chapter 12), the psychodynamic frame of reference (Chapter 13), the biomechanical frame of reference (Chapter 14), and the theoretical approaches to motor control and cognitive–perceptual function (Chapter 15).

Section 4 provides an introduction to other important areas of theory. Clinical reasoning is in many ways the 'glue' that holds together theoretical reasoning and flexibly responsive practice; Chapter 16 presents a new and engaging overview of clinical reasoning research and practice in occupational therapy. Community-based rehabilitation is a generic theoretical approach that aims to enhance the quality of life of people who have disabilities, by meeting their basic needs and working for inclusion and participation. Whilst this approach is not unique to occupational therapy, the profession is playing an emerging role as it works in this way in communities where the need is greatest; Chapter 17 therefore presents community-based rehabilitation and its relationship with occupational therapy practice. Occupational science has been a prolific focus of research and debate in occupational therapy over the last 20 years; it has been met with both enthusiasm and consternation. Chapter 18 provides an excellent introduction to the field and explores the breadth of occupational science, without shirking from the controversy surrounding it.

Advice to readers

There are several ways in which this book can be read. For those who are particularly new to the area or who have not read about theoretical constructs in occupational therapy for some time, it is strongly advisable to work through Section 1 before moving on to other chapters. However, you may feel familiar enough with these concepts and wish to focus on a particular topic. In this situation it is possible to go directly to the chapter(s) of interest. Do not, however, assume that all your answers will always be covered in one chapter. In order to understand fully what each author is saying, it is often necessary to take a step away from any professional biases one may have and enter fully into the perspective of other contributors: a task that may often prove more challenging in practice than in principle. It is therefore advisable to read across chapters and evaluate differing perspectives. Throughout this process it is important to take a critically evaluative approach to the material presented.

Understanding occupational therapy

Occupational therapy has a broad knowledge base, derived from medical and social sciences, as well as the moral treatment and arts and crafts movements. Therapists work with all age groups and assist with a wide range of medical, social and environmental problems. Occupational therapy practice appears deceptively simple. Its focus is the doing of everyday activites; its 'complexity' is in understanding the factors that influence and shape these activities and in constructing interventions that will enable each client to achieve their goals.

The principal concerns of occupational therapy

Each person wants to participate effectively in a meaningful life, and to remain healthy and happy. To achieve these goals, it is argued, a person needs a degree of personal competence in a range of culturally accepted, useful and meaningful occupations. What these occupations are will differ from person to person according to individual and collective needs and circumstances.

Occupational therapy

- Is concerned with the key elements of occupational performance and identity: how a person identifies themselves and their future aspirations, their roles and their relationships, together with their personal capacity for fulfilling these within their physical and social environment.
- Aims to enable and empower people to be competent and confident in their daily lives, and thereby to enhance well-being and minimize the effects of dysfunction or environmental barriers.

Occupational therapists

- Use everyday occupations and tasks creatively and therapeutically to achieve goals that are meaningful to people and relevant to their daily life.
- Encourage people to collaborate in the therapeutic process in order to become partners in the design and direction of therapy and the (re)enabling of their life.

Competence and dysfunction

Occupational therapists believe that *occupational competency* in everyday activities depends on a complex interaction between the individual, the things they do, and their environment. An individual's well-being is directly related to the quality of this interaction. When a person is performing, they are able to meet the demands of each task, to respond adaptively to the demands of each environment, and to use the skills and knowledge they have learnt in order to act, interact and react appropriately in all the everyday situations that they encounter.

The opposite to occupational competence is *occupational dysfunction*. This is a temporary or enduring inability to engage in the roles, relationships and occupations expected of a person of comparable age and sex within a particular culture. Occupational dysfunction becomes apparent when a person is unable to do the ordinary everyday things they want

or need to do. It is often when a person experiences occupational dysfunction that they are referred to an occupational therapist. The reasons for dysfunction are very variable and range from the simple to the extremely complex.

The occupational therapy perspective

Occupational therapists endeavour to understand the nature of a client's *occupational identity* (who they are and who they would like to be), as well as their *occupational performance* (what their physical, cognitive and social abilities are). Frequently employing a conceptual model of practice and or an appropriate frame of reference, within the context of the process of care (see Chapter 4 for further information), action is taken to reduce the impact of a client's condition (or the effect of the environment in relation to their condition) and maximize each client's ability to engage in valued daily activities.

Occupational therapists are not, however, limited to considering the impact of health problems on a client's life, important though these may be. Occupational dysfunction is frequently associated with a failure to adapt to a changing set of circumstances that can overload one's personal capacity to respond. A client may have lost skills or never have learnt them. They may have some negative emotional reaction connected with a task. The physical environment may be badly designed, too demanding or not demanding enough. The social environment may be too stressful or insufficiently supportive. The task may be too difficult or the tools used inappropriate. The role of the occupational therapist is to intervene to help each individual to balance these factors, regain competence and (re)develop meaning and purpose in life.

Most people become dysfunctional to some extent when faced with an unfamiliar or difficult situation or when confronted by a very stressful life event. Such dysfunction is usually transient and either resolves when the stress is removed, responds to minimal advice or assistance, or disappears once the person has learned how to cope. This type of dysfunction may also occur as a result of external factors when there is no personal impairment or health condition. One way of looking at occupational dysfunction is to describe it as a lack of balance or 'fit' between the skills of a client, the challenges of their environment and the difficulties of their required occupation. Occupational therapists address occupational dysfunction using a range of interventions that often include adapting the demands of an everyday activity, altering the physical or social environment, teaching a client a new repertoire of skills or helping them to re-establish ones they have lost. Frequently, the kind of complex occupational dysfunction that requires intervention from an occupational therapist is persistent and will often affect many aspects of clients' lives. Unfortunately, to date, negligible research exists, in several areas of occupational therapy (e.g. mental health), making it difficult to distinguish those individuals who are likely to experience persistent occupational dysfunction from those who are not. Consequently, it is possible that therapists are missing valuable opportunities for early intervention with clients who do not initially appear as if they will have enduring occupational dysfunction. Further predictive research is required, in areas of complexity, in order for occupational therapists to become more targeted and effective in their interventions.

Acknowledging competing ideas

From source to outlet, rivers follow the path of least resistance; in wrestling with occupational theory it is tempting for therapists to do the same. This book offers no simple solutions to the use of theory in practice. However, therapists are encouraged to choose the best theories to drive practice, not simply the easiest. Occupational therapy's theoretical and evidence base is rapidly developing and the profession has entered an exciting new era as therapists become increasingly research-active in a variety of ways — from collaborating in clinical data collection to acting as a principal investigator. Consequently, idiosyncratic perspectives of practice are increasingly challenged, well-known conceptual models of practice and frames of reference are increasingly evaluated, and new theoretical perspectives and questions have arisen.

Several contrasting theoretical perspectives are presented within this book. Examples of such perspectives include theorists' understanding of conceptual models of practice (see Chapter 5), their understanding of complexity (see Chapters 3, 12, 13 and 18) and culture (see Chapters 6 and 10), and the manner in which professional knowledge is developed (see Chapters 3, 6, 16 and 18). The debate caused by such contrasting perspectives should be

embraced and not shunned, as they illustrate the challenges of developing the profession's theoretical and evidence base. Readers are encouraged to use the index and cross-references within each chapter in order to understand these issues in greater depth.

These competing ideas will, amongst others, shape the future of occupational therapy theoretical research. Through the crucible of reflection and research, clinically relevant theories will be questioned, challenged and refined. From them, practice will become ever more evidence-based, and, consequently, clients will receive a more effective and meaningful service.

A look to the future

Delivery of effective occupational therapy is an ethical and professional imperative. Practice should be consistently effective. To reach this goal, practice needs to become increasingly evidence-based and to be delivered in a flexibly responsive manner to meet the needs of individual patients. Each client should receive a similarly high-quality service, regardless of their location or the therapist with whom they are working. Such consistency is difficult to achieve.

It is well recognized that therapists' individual judgements, regardless of expertise, are affected by a wide range of biases and *heuristics* (mental shortcuts) (Grove & Meehl 1996, Grove et al 2000). Therapists, using personal judgement alone, are often much less effective than they believe. The embracing of evidence-based conceptual models of practice and frames of reference supports therapists in giving consideration to a wide range of factors and should increase therapists' consistency and agreement. Used in this way, theoretical frameworks enable therapists to provide comprehensive interventions with clearly definable and measurable outcomes. Some therapists may react against this suggestion and feel that using such theories places undue constraints on their practice. Perhaps they will suggest that this perspective appears to make practice fit theory instead of theory fitting practice, and is therefore not client-centred. This, however, is a fallacy, a false dilemma. Such a position distracts attention from the known biases of individual therapist judgements by suggesting that conceptual models and frames of reference lack perfection and this is a reason for their rejection. Whilst existing theoretical frameworks undoubtably need to be enhanced, this does not justify practising from a perspective of individual judgement that is known to be flawed. Theoretically driven and evidence-based occupational therapy must be embraced in practice. Our clients deserve no less.

Summary

This chapter has provided some background to previous editions of the book. This edition continues to build on its predecessors. The book has been thoroughly updated and new chapters are included from leading academics in the field. The theoretical basis of occupational therapy has developed over several years and has reached a very exciting stage. Several contributors to this text offer conflicting opinions about theoretical issues. Such a divergence of opinion is useful. It will, through academic debate and research, strengthen the profession and provide it with an ever more robust theoretical evidence base. Engage in the issues presented and think critically about what you read.

References

Grove, W.M., Meehl, P.E., 1996. Comparative efficiency of informal (subjective, impressionistic) and formal (mechanical, algorithmic) prediction procedures: the clinical/statistical controversy. Psychology, Public Policy, and Law 2, 1–31.

Grove, W.M., Zald, D.H., Boyd, S.L., et al, 2000. Clinical versus mechanical prediction: a meta-analysis. Psychological Assessment 12 (1), 19–30.

Theoretical foundations of occupational therapy: external influences

2

Edward A.S. Duncan

OVERVIEW

This chapter outlines the main external influences on occupational therapy's theoretical foundation. *Philosophy* may appear to be a somewhat unrelated subject to the applied nature of occupational therapy; however, in order to gain a comprehensive understanding of occupational therapy theory, it is necessary to gain a conceptual understanding of the impact that various philosophical systems have had upon healthcare in general and occupational therapy in particular. This chapter commences with an overview of what theory is and the main factors that have influenced theoretical developments within occupational therapy. A particular emphasis is placed upon the various shifts that have occurred within occupational therapy's theoretical foundations over time. In order to understand clearly the various external influences that have shaped and continue to shape the theoretical foundations of occupational therapy, this chapter dedicates a significant proportion of space to understanding the impact that various philosophical systems have had on theory and practice.

Key points

- Occupational therapy's development has been shaped by the influence of a variety of external philosophical influences.
- This chapter provides an overview of key external influences and how they have shaped the profession.
- The Enlightenment and its consequent influence have led to the development of the evidence-based practice movement.
- Despite its critics, evidence-based practice will remain the dominant force in occupational therapy development over the forthcoming decade and beyond.

What is theory?

The *Chambers Dictionary* (Schwartz 1994) defines theory as 'an explanation or system of anything; an exposition of the abstract principles of a science or art' (p.1795). Despite calls to the contrary (e.g. Ryan 2001), theories, within occupational therapy, are often viewed as being detached from practice. Indeed, until recently, there has been a prevailing tendency to view theories as the activities that a student undertakes whilst in university, whilst practice experience is gained on fieldwork education. Implicit within this split understanding of theory and practice is the idea that theory is unimportant to practice and vice versa. This has led to a theory–practice gap within occupational therapy and other allied health professions (Ryan 2001). This gap is most evident in the difficulties that clinicians have in embedding research in practice (McCluskey & Lovarini 2005). Metcalfe et al (2001) undertook a postal questionnaire study among four allied health professional groups (dietitians, occupational therapists, physiotherapists, and speech and language therapists) within a single English National Health Service (NHS) region; 80% (n=573) of the sample responded. Whilst each group agreed that research (from which sound theory develops) was important, they also highlighted barriers to using such knowledge. These barriers included understanding the literature, insufficient time, inadequate facilities, professional isolation and resistance from colleagues. It is apparent, therefore, that when theory is viewed as a distinct reality from practice, real barriers to their use develop. Such barriers are not simple to overcome. In order to address this issue, theory should grow in and from practice, and be viewed as central to all that it means to be an occupational therapist. It is precisely for this reason that this book places particular emphasis on the clinical application of theories in practice. Each chapter achieves this in a different manner.

Within occupational therapy, the term 'theory' has wide usage and meaning. It has been used broadly to discuss theoretical understandings of the profession in general, to refer to broad theories that are not profession-specific (e.g. Freud's understanding of development), and finally as a term used to identify developments in understanding that are particular to occupational therapy. Kielhofner (2002) states that theory should be viewed as 'a network of explanations that label and describe phenomena and propositions that specify relationships between concepts. It is important to differentiate theoretical explanations that give a plausible account for how something works from mere description of statements of beliefs or values' (p.4).

Where do theories come from?

All professions are formed and informed by ideas, explanations and systems that assist individuals and services in understanding and guiding what they are or should be doing. Theoretical ideas develop from a variety of principles, which can include the research and knowledge available at the time, the values, attitudes and ethical basis of the individual(s), and their practical experience of the phenomenon under question. All of these factors can be strongly influenced by the prevailing environmental influences.

Environmental influences on theory development

Professions do not exist in isolation and are therefore open to influence from the pressures and prevailing norms of other professional groups and the environment in which they exist. Occupational therapy, existing predominantly within the health and social fields of society, has been observably influenced by the environmental influences within these settings and the prevailing pressures on professional groupings within these fields. In order to understand the environmental influences that have shaped occupational therapy throughout the ages, it is necessary to take a

historical viewpoint of the development of the profession. One may ask how history relates to theory; however, when history is read, it becomes apparent that it is interesting not only for its own sake, but also because it 'facilitates understanding of contemporary roles and relationships. Just as our sense of personal identity demands roots in the past from family history, our professional identity and understanding of the contexts in which we work are enhanced by knowledge of their development' (Paterson 1997). Such history, Paterson (1997) continues, illustrates that, whilst early occupational therapy intervention held a humanistic concern for individuals' well-being, it was consistently accompanied by efforts to build a theoretical understanding about the various processes involved in their work.

When examining the history of occupational therapy, or at least the effect of occupation on health, it is possible to go back as far as biblical and classical periods, where the remedial and health promotional effects of occupation can easily be seen (Wilcock 2001b). Occupation came to the fore of care again in the 19th century, with the development of 'moral treatment', although the focus of occupation during this period was perhaps more for economic than therapeutic gain (Wilcock 2001a). Whilst this appears to be a less than positive image of occupational therapy, it is perhaps in the 'moral treatment' movement and the vision of William Tuke, a Quaker and key proponent of 'moral treatment', that the enduring patient-centred philosophy of occupational therapy can find its roots (Tuke 1813). With the onset of the 20th century and the formal establishment of occupational therapy training within the UK, the environmental effects of medicine and other disciplines upon occupational therapists can be seen more clearly. Such influential effects on theoretical and practice development have been described as 'paradigmatic shifts' in the profession's understanding of the who, what and why of its existence (Kielhofner 2009) (see Chapter 3 for further information).

The influence of philosophy

Further to the external environmental influences that have directly shaped occupational theory and practice, it is also important to note the influence of philosophical perceptions of 'reality' and their impact on the development of occupational theory and practice. Philosophy is 'the pursuit of wisdom or knowledge . . . the principles underlying any sphere of knowledge' (Schwartz 1994, p.1280). A basic understanding of the philosophical principles relating to 'truth' is important for occupational therapists to attain, as it is from these that the foundational concepts for future theoretical developments discussed in this book emanate. Fundamentally, two concepts exist within the various philosophies that are central to all theoretical understanding: *ontology* and *epistemology*. Ontology can be most easily understood as the nature of knowledge, whilst epistemology is the approach taken to knowledge (Hill Bailey 1997). Both are complex. Two fundamental views of nature exist that are important to understand when considering occupational therapy's theoretical developments: *positivism* and *anti-positivism*.

Positivistic and post-positivistic paradigms

Positivism contends that there is an absolute reality, which can be measured, studied and understood, whilst post-positivism has been described as the perspective that an absolute reality can never be understood and may only be approximated (Denzin & Lincoln 2000). Positivism emerged from the thinking of the Enlightenment, an important period of philosophical development during the 17th century in Europe. Since its emergence, positivism has been very influential within medicine and healthcare in general. This influence has assisted in the discovery of cures for many diseases and has had a significant impact on people's lives (Creek 1997).

Influence of positivist thinking on healthcare and occupational therapy

As discussed above, positivism and the scientific approach are believed to have directly influenced occupational therapy's willing acceptance of the reductionist period, during which occupational therapists attempted to gain professional credibility through employing medical-type interventions and theoretical concepts that were not necessarily understood through an occupational framework (Pols 2002). Whilst the profession has moved on within itself, it continues to be externally influenced by the positivistic tendencies of healthcare in general. Most recently, this influence can be witnessed through its acceptance of evidence-based practice (EBP).

Evidence-based medicine (as the term was originally known) emerged from the McMaster medical school in Canada during the 1980s (Taylor 2000). However, the origins of the concept can be traced to the mid-19th century and Paris, and to Charles Alexandre Louis, considered a founding father of modern medical statistics (Hadjiliadis 2004). Sackett et al (1996) defined evidence-based medicine as 'the conscientious, explicit and judicious use of current best evidence in making decisions about the care of individual patients' (p.71). Best evidence, in this context, is information that has been researched using quantitative methods such as randomized control trials and meta-analysis, both procedures that embrace the objective/positivistic nature of knowledge. EBP is not, however, a purely objective pursuit. Sackett et al (1996) emphasized that EBP is only part of the clinical decision-making process. Taylor (2000) reinforces this, stating, 'Evidence is gathered conscientiously but is used judiciously so that the experience of the OT, the needs of the patients/client, the demands of the system and the up to date best evidence are weighed together in order that the best care is given' (pp.2–3). EBP has proven to be more than a passing trend and its influence is embedded within government healthcare policy and the College of Occupational Therapists' *Code of Ethics* (Taylor & Savin-Baden 2001). Despite the original emphasis on individual experience, as outlined in the above quotation from Sackett et al (1996), EBP has well-developed hierarchies of evidence that place greatest importance on objective studies such as meta-analysis and randomized control trials, with least emphasis given to clinical experience. Such studies are not universally accepted as appropriate methods to be used within occupational therapy and their use or potential use has been the subject of great debate within British occupational therapy literature (Bannigan 2002, Copley 2002, Hyde 2002, 2004, Legg & Walker 2002, MacLean & Jones 2002, Bryant 2004, Eva & Paley 2004). These authors have expressed strong views about the nature of evidence and its potential use or misuse in guiding practitioners' practice.

Such is the impact of EBP for occupational therapists that it has been described as 'a contemporary preoccupation' (Whalley-Hammell 2001). Despite research indicating that the majority of occupational therapists within one particular region of England (South and West) were overwhelmingly in favour of EBP (Curtin 2001), the realization of a fundamentally positivistic philosophy continues to be criticized by some within occupational therapy literature as incongruent with the profession's values and beliefs (Ballinger & Wiles 2004).

Anti-positivistic paradigms

Not everybody agrees with the suppositions of positivistic and post-positivistic thinking. Many theorists view such structures as fundamentally restrictive and ignorant of alternative perspectives. This has led to the development of, amongst others, constructivist, interpretive and critical theory paradigms of nature. The fundamental basis of such approaches is that they propose multiple constructed realities, as different people are likely to experience the world in differing ways. This, in turn, leads to 'radical scepticism' regarding the possibilities for knowledge and a belief that research, and consequently theoretical developments, is only an interpretation of multiple realities (Henwood & Nicholson 1996). Anti-positivism is not, therefore, a single set of beliefs, but a set of approaches, each of which places a particular emphasis on the way that people may experience and understand the world. Such theories often appear initially attractive for occupational therapy, as the profession has frequently tried to define itself separately from the more traditional medical positivistic approach to healthcare. However, these philosophical approaches, whilst useful in delivering an alternative perspective of reality, are often unhelpful in a health economic era where finances are often restricted and scarce resources are dedicated to interventions that have a known efficacy (Duncan 2004). There are too many anti-positivistic philosophies to describe in this text and it is suggested that the interested reader should consult the bibliography and beyond for further information. Some anti-positivistic theories are, however, of particular importance or have been increasingly used in occupational therapy research; three of these theories are introduced below as a primer for further reading.

Phenomenology

Developed by the German philosopher Edmund Husserl (1859–1938), phenomenology focuses on describing personal experiences and interpreting these experiences for individuals without developing overarching theories of truth (Schwartz 1994). The fundamental theory that forms phenomenology is

that 'meaning can only be understood by those who experience it' (DePoy & Gitlin 1998). As we each experience life in differing ways, we will each therefore also make sense and find meaning in differing ways. Occupational therapy literature is increasingly influenced by phenomenological thought. This influence stems from its roots in 'moral treatment' and the arts and craft movement (Mattingly & Fleming 1994).

From a phenomenological perspective, illness or disease is not viewed simply as a matter of physiological dysfunction, but is understood through the impact that it has on the broader social impact of the person in society (Mattingly & Fleming 1994). Several occupational therapy studies have explicitly used a phenomenological approach in their research (e.g. Grisbrooke 2003, Henare et al 2003, Reynolds 2003, Paddy et al 2004).

As occupational therapists are often interested in viewing a person *holistically*, it is easy to see where phenomenological thought resonates with occupational theory and practice. An interest in the phenomenological approach to engaging with clients naturally leads occupational therapists to encourage clients to discuss their experiences of illness or disability and to develop meaningful life stories. This technique is known as using a narrative approach. A specific occupational therapy assessment has also been developed from this perspective (Kielhofner et al 1998).

Feminism

Feminism is a global term referring to the advocacy of women's rights. Fundamentally, feminism can be explored through three perspectives: liberal feminism, which focuses on the impact of socialization into gender roles; radical feminism, which posits that existence within a patriarchal society subordinates women; and Marxist feminism, which focuses on the exploitation of the capitalist class and its consequential effects on women (Hartery & Jones 1998). Occupational therapy's gender imbalance is believed to have had a considerable impact upon its development and position in society. Wilcock (2001a, 2001b) acknowledges the overwhelming dominance of female occupational therapists during the early years. Whilst this appears to have been initially unquestioned and indeed related to caring roles previously associated with females (e.g. nursing and infant teaching), its potentially negative impact has more recently been considered. Taylor (1995) used a feminist approach to reflect on the impact of being a predominantly female profession. She highlights how occupational therapy has developed under the mantle of medicine, a profession that is dominated by men and is said to espouse the patriarchal values of society (Hugman 1991). Taylor (1995) relates this relationship to the distancing of the profession from its original connections with the arts and crafts movements and consequential move towards objective science. MacWhannell and Blair (1998) continue this theme, stating that:

> a recurring issue within occupational therapy literature is a concern with the development of standardised assessment [a consequence of the patriarchal influence]. If the features that draw people to the profession are associated with engaging people in a process that moves towards growth and personal change and are not measurable or directly open to standardised outcome measures, the profession is in a conceptual conundrum. It is torn between one set of values and another. (p.64)

The impact of the profession's gender imbalance upon occupational therapy's development is unquestionable; it has affected both the profession's value base and its position within society. Taking a single stance on the impact of gender on the profession is, however, unlikely to be beneficial in the long term and leaves one open to bias. A non-occupational therapy example of how such bias can affect the theoretical and research basis of a subject is evident in two studies of therapeutic interventions with women who self-harm and are resident in secure units in England. Liebling and Chipchase (1996) describe a therapeutic group intervention for women who self-harm. Instead of taking a cognitive behavioural approach (see Chapter 12), which is widely used with this client group, Liebling and Chipchase (1996) employed feminist group therapy (Burstow 1992). The authors initially used a range of outcome measures, but these were abandoned, apparently because of resistance. Taking a feminist theory perspective, the authors interpreted this as a rejection of control. Low et al (2001), working with the same client group in a similar environment, carried out a similar study using a broadly cognitive behavioural approach. Unlike Liebling and Chipchase (1996), Low et al (2001) employed a range of psychometric assessments without apparent detrimental impact. This example of differing outcomes based on opposing philosophical foundations highlights the dangers of adhering to one perspective and the impact that this can have on research and practice, without considering one's own personal biases in influencing the interpretation or outcome of an event.

Kelly (1996), a male occupational therapist, recognized the continuing existence of the feminist principle within occupational therapy, but suggested that 'any system based upon the feminine principle or the masculine principle alone will not be sufficient; they must merge and actualise in the practice of occupational therapy' (p.6).

Postmodernism

Postmodernism is not an easy concept to grasp. It is a concept that has affected a wide range of disciplines, from the arts to the sciences, and architecture to technology. It is not, therefore, surprising that occupational therapy has also been evaluated from a postmodernist perspective. Before considering postmodernism, it is perhaps useful to define modernism. Modernism arose from the visual arts movements and comprised a revolt against the perceived constraints of the Victorian era. Modernism focuses on subjectivity and multiple realities. Phenomenology arose during the modernist era (1945–1970s).

Postmodernism arose from a rejection of thinking founded during the Enlightenment, in which it was believed that the objective truth of a situation could be discovered (Creek 1997). Webber (1995), in explaining the postmodernistic rejection of objectivity, states that 'there is nothing to be gained from past "explanatory systems" but that there is a real danger in generalising or universalising since each individual or event is unique' (p.439). Postmodernism, therefore, directly challenges the concept of objectivity and suggests that, if reality can be described at all, it is as a process of continual change that focuses on the local rather than the universal. Such concepts are attractive to occupational theorists and practitioners, as they appear to validate professional values of the worth of an individual and the uniqueness of each moment and activity.

Within occupational therapy's theory development, both Webber (1995) and Creek (1997) align themselves with postmodernism in their rejection of scientific objectivity and the use of standardized assessments and outcome measurements in practice. Many occupational therapists' rejections of objectivity, universal models and standardized assessments can find a philosophical advocate within postmodernistic thinking.

The limitations of positivistic thinking within occupational therapy practice are evident. However, outright rejection of objective theories and philosophical foundations requires careful consideration. Occupational therapists work in predominantly positivistic systems (such as healthcare) and are required to demonstrate their worth within such environments. It is unlikely, therefore, that a purely postmodernistic stance will greatly affect the philosophical basis of healthcare and may in fact lead to great professional isolation for occupational therapists in an increasingly evidence-based context. However, healthcare environments are evolving and moving from a purely positivistic understanding of reality. This is perhaps most starkly evident in the prominence given to service users' experiences within healthcare today. What, then, is the way forward for occupational therapy and theory development?

Traditionally, positivism and anti-positivism have been viewed as too conceptually conflicting to merge in any meaningful manner. However, the complex nature of developing meaningful and transferable theories upon which to enhance individuals' level of care and intervention requires the employment of a variety of approaches.

Miller and Crabtree (2000) succinctly describe how such a merger of thought could exist. Discussing healthcare research, they suggest that researchers (and theorists) should, 'see with three eyes — the biomedical eye [of objectivity], the inward searching eye of reflexivity [the therapists'/theorists' personal reflections] and a third eye that looks for the multiple nested contexts [embracing postmodernistic thought]' (p.611). Combining such philosophical foundations is a strongly contested arena and has been described in research terms as the separatist versus combinist debate (Duffy 1987). The integration of such opposing perspectives has been criticized as an ontological impossibility, as each is based on diametrically opposing assumptions (Hill Bailey 1997). These assumptions can be summarized into two principles:

- scientific realism — the belief that the world has an existence independent of our perception of it
- scientific idealism — the belief that the external world consists of representations and is a creation of the mind (Williams & May 1996, Pope & Mays 2000).

Scientific realism has been dismissed as naïve (Lincoln & Guba 1985). Instead, Lincoln and Guba (1985) suggest that the truth is most clearly understood as the best-informed and most sophisticated construction on which there is a consensus. Postmodernists reject this proposal and hold that all perspectives are unique and equally valid.

A further philosophical perspective, known as 'subtle realism', has also been offered that attempts to integrate the realist and idealist perspectives (Duncan & Nicol 2004). Its proponents state that all knowledge involves subjective perceptions and observations, and concede that various individuals will produce different pictures of the reality under study. However, such a stance is not taken to the extent of extreme realists (Schutz 1967). Hammersley (1990) and Kirk and Miller (1986) propose that subjective perceptions and observations do not preclude the existence of independent phenomena, and that objects, relationships and experiences can be studied and understood. The subtle realist understands that there is no manner in which an individual can claim to have absolute certainty regarding a phenomenon. Rather, 'the objective should be the search for knowledge about which we can be reasonably confident. Such confidence will be based upon judgements about the credibility and plausibility of knowledge claims' (Murphy et al 1998) (p.69). This concept has been criticized as having no true ontological basis (Seale 1999). However, others (Smith & Heshusius 1986) argue that subtle realism is a post-positivist/realist approach. Despite such criticisms, the subtle realist approach is increasingly being embraced in healthcare and supported as a positive advancement for theoretical and research development in healthcare (Murphy et al 1998). The challenges in developing occupational therapy theory 'reach to the ontological and epistemological roots of knowledge' (Duncan 2004). Subtle realism offers a philosophical foundation that embraces the complexity of knowledge and of occupational therapy, within the intricacies and realities of its working environments, and provides a useful alternative perspective for future research and theoretical development.

Marxism

Marxist thought is undoubtedly best known for its impact upon politics and sociology during the 20th century. Most people, on hearing the word Marxist, think of the historical communist regime of the

Eastern Bloc (Wilcock 2001a). Such was the impact of Marx's political thinking that his founding philosophies of the centrality of occupation remain relatively unknown. This is, in part, due to the fact that the majority of his early writings were not published in English until the mid-20th century (Wilcock 2001a). The inclusion of a section on Marx may surprise some readers, yet he could be described as an early occupational scientist (Wilcock 2001a) (see Chapter 18 for an introduction to occupational science). Fundamentally, Marx (1964) developed the concept of 'alienated labour', which he viewed as an inevitable consequence of capitalist societies. Whilst Marx believed that occupations should be uplifting and socially involving, he also believed that, in general, individuals' productive occupations were developed to produce commodities (Corrigan 2001). In essence, Marx argued for a more socially just way of living: one that recognized that individuals require satisfaction in what they do, as well as adequately meeting life's requirements. Marx viewed the difficulties that faced individuals in life as largely being a result of the imposition of social organization rather than naturally occurring (Hartery & Jones 1998). Such a vision of occupation suggests that occupational therapists should focus on being agents of social change rather than a part of the process that maintains social conformity. Indeed, Corrigan (2001) suggests that 'the profession's need to maintain credibility within other discourses inadvertently diminishes its capacity to act socially' (p.204). In other words, it could be suggested that in occupational therapy's determination to become accepted within the systems in which it works it has, to a certain extent, limited its potential to become a social agent for change. Increased recognition of the impact of society on the individual's occupational potential has, however, redressed this balance to a certain extent, and occupational therapists are increasingly adding their voice as agents of social change. The Person–Environment–Occupation model of practice has embraced occupational therapy as an agent of social change (see Chapter 8) and this too has been enhanced through occupational therapy's involvement in community-based rehabilitation (see Chapter 17).

Culture

The nature of culture is complex and is not easily defined. Culture refers to shared meanings through which individuals interact and the specific beliefs, values and norms that shape the everyday behaviour of individuals and groups of people. The breadth of occupational therapy practice is now international, and multicultural societies are commonplace within Western societies (Dyck 1998). It is appropriate, therefore, to question whether the philosophical foundations of the profession and the professional frames of reference and models of practice that have developed from them (which have been developed in Western society) are relevant to substantial populations with whom occupational therapists interact. Occupational therapy is recognized as a profession that embraces Western values (e.g. independence) and the maintenance of a 'healthy' life role balance between work, leisure and self-care. Such concepts may, however, be of less importance to people of other cultures. These issues have led to the presentation of alternative philosophical constructs of occupational therapy that are based on Eastern philosophies (Jang 1993, Dawson 2000) (see Chapter 16 for information about an emerging alternative model of practice from Japan). However, cultural incompatibility of Western-based occupational therapy models should not be assumed, as evidence of cultural incongruity is lacking. Indeed, evidence for the compatibility of Western-based models of practice (such as the Model of Human Occupation (see Chapter 14)) with culturally diverse environments, such as African traditional healers (Kelly 1995) and other cultures, suggests that such approaches can find resonance in culturally diverse populations.

Consideration of the societal culture in which occupational therapy is practised and the cultural groupings of an individual within any given environment are of the utmost importance to occupational therapy practice. An individual's cultural background, whether at a macro level (e.g. country or religion) or at a micro level (e.g. an individual's family, work and social background), will undoubtedly affect their belief in self, habits and routines and the social and physical environment in which they exist. This should, in turn, affect the manner in which the occupational therapist relates to an individual and the nature of their collaboration. The precise impact of employing a Western-based cultural model of practice on individuals from other cultural backgrounds, however, remains uncertain. Undoubtedly, the relationship of culture to occupational therapy theory and practice will remain a topical theme in the future.

Summary

Occupational therapy has been shaped by a wide variety of philosophies throughout the course of its history to the present day. These theories form the foundation of the profession's current theoretical developments. It is possible to see how each of the philosophies has moulded the profession through its paradigmatic shifts and how each of them provides lenses though which the profession and an individual's professional practice can be understood today. Each reader is invited to reflect on the discussions presented in this chapter and to consider where their philosophical life perspectives place them and what impact this has on their practice as an occupational therapist.

Reflective learning

- What philosophical perspectives influence how you live your life and what your values are?
- How do these perspectives affect your practice?
- Do you have any philosophical beliefs or values that may ethically affect your practice? If yes, how do you avoid this occurring? If no, what sort of philosophical beliefs could affect your practice?
- What role do you think culture has in how occupational therapists practise?

References

Ballinger, C., Wiles, R., 2004. A critical look at evidence based practice. British Journal of Occupational Therapy 64 (5), 253–255.

Bannigan, K., 2002. EBP, RCTs and a climate for mutual respect. British Journal of Occupational Therapy 65 (8), 391–392.

Bryant, W., 2004. Numbers in evidence. British Journal of Occupational Therapy 6 (2), 99–100.

Burstow, B., 1992. Radical Feminist Therapy. Sage, Newbury Park.

Copley, J., 2002. RCTs: continuing the debate. British Journal of Occupational Therapy 65 (7), 346–347.

Corrigan, K., 2001. Doing time in mental health: discipline at the end of medicine. British Journal of Occupational Therapy 64 (4), 203–205.

Creek, J., 1997. . . . the truth is no longer out there. British Journal of Occupational Therapy 60 (2), 50.

Curtin, M., 2001. Occupational therapists' views and perceptions of evidence-based practice. British Journal of Occupational Therapy 64 (5), 214–222.

Dawson, F., 2000. The three-dimensional model of self: a Japanese model of practice. British Journal of Occupational Therapy 63 (7), 340–342.

Denzin, N.K., Lincoln, Y.S., 2000. Introduction: the discipline and practice of qualitative research. In:

Denzin, N.K., Lincoln, Y.S. (Eds.), Handbook of Qualitative Research. Sage, Thousand Oaks.

DePoy, E., Gitlin, L.N., 1998. Introduction to Research, second ed. Mosby, St Louis.

Duffy, M., 1987. Methodological triangulation: a vehicle for merging quantitative and qualitative research methods. Journal of Nursing Scholarship 19, 130–133.

Duncan, E.A.S., Nicol, M., 2004. Subtle Reasoning and Occupational Therapy: An Alternative Approach to Knowledge Generation and Evaluation. The British Journal of Occupational Therapy 67 (10), 453–456.

Dyck, I., 1998. Multicultural society. In: Jones, D., et al (Eds.), Sociology and Occupational Therapy: An Integrated Approach. Churchill Livingstone, Edinburgh.

Eva, G., Paley, J., 2004. Numbers in evidence. British Journal of Occupational Therapy 67 (1), 47–50.

Grisbrooke, J., 2003. Living with lifts: a study of users' experiences. British Journal of Therapy and Rehabilitation 10 (2), 76–81.

Hadjiliadis, D., 2004. Early clinical statistics. Internet web presentation.

Hammersley, M., 1990. Reading Ethnographic Research. Longman, New York.

Hartery, T., Jones, D., 1998. What is sociology? In: Jones, D., et al (Eds.), Sociology and Occupational Therapy:

An Integrated Approach. Churchill Livingstone, Edinburgh.

Henare, D., Hocking, C., Smythe, L., 2003. Chronic pain: gaining understanding through the use of art. British Journal of Occupational Therapy 66 (11), 511–518.

Henwood, K., Nicholson, P., 1996. Qualitative research. The Psychologist 3, 109–110.

Hill Bailey, P., 1997 Finding your way around qualitative methods. Journal of Advanced Nursing 25, 18–22.

Hugman, R., 1991. Power in Caring Professions. MacMillan, London.

Hyde, P., 2002. RCTs: legitimate research tool or fancy mathematics? British Journal of Occupational Therapy 67 (2), 89–93.

Hyde, P., 2004. Fool's gold: examining the use of gold standards in the production of research evidence. British Journal of Occupational Therapy 67 (2), 89–93.

Jang, Y., 1993. Chinese culture and occupational therapy. Journal of the Occupational Therapy Association of the Republic of China 11, 95–104.

Kelly, G., 1996. Feminist or feminine? A feminine age . . . British Journal of Occupational Therapy 59 (7), 345.

Kelly, L., 1995. What occupational therapists can learn from traditional healers. British Journal of Occupational Therapy 58 (3), 111–114.

Kielhofner, G., 2002. Model of Human Occupation, third ed. Lippincott Williams & Wilkins, Baltimore.

Kielhofner, G., 2009. Conceptual Foundations of Occupational Therapy, fourth ed. FA Davis, Philadelphia.

Kielhofner, G., Malisson, T., Crawford, C., et al, 1998. A User's Manual for the Occupational Performance History Interview (V2) (OPHI II). University of Illinois, Chicago.

Kirk, J., Miller, M., 1986. Reliability and Validity in Qualitative Research. Sage, Newbury Park.

Legg, L., Walker, M., 2002. Let us use randomized control trials. British Journal of Occupational Therapy 65 (3), 149.

Liebling, H., Chipchase, H., 1996. Feminist group therapy for women who self harm: an initial evaluation. Issues in Criminological & Legal Psychology 25, 24–29.

Lincoln, Y.S., Guba, E.G., 1985. Naturalistic Inquiry. Sage, Newbury Park.

Low, G., Jones, D., Duggan, C., 2001. The treatment of deliberate self harm in borderline personality disorder using dialectical behaviour therapy: a pilot study in a high security hospital. Behavioural and Cognitive Psychotherapy 29, 85–92.

MacLean, F., Jones, D., 2002. RCTs: need for wider debate. British Journal of Occupational Therapy 65 (6), 294–295.

MacWhannell, D., Blair, S.E.E., 1998. Sex, gender and feminism. In: Jones, D., et al (Eds.), Sociology and Occupational Therapy: An Integrated Approach. Churchill Livingstone, Edinburgh.

Mattingly, C., Fleming, M.H., 1994. Clinical Reasoning: Forms of Inquiry in a Therapeutic Practice. FA Davis, Philadelphia.

McClusky, A., Lovarini, M., 2005. Providing education on evidence-based practice improved knowledge but did not change behaviour: a before and after study. BMC Medical Education 5, 40. Available from http://www.biomedcentral.com/1472-6920/5/40 (accessed 18.03.10).

Metcalfe, C., Lewin, R., Wisher, S., et al, 2001. Barriers to implementing the evidence base in four NHS therapies: dieticians, occupational therapists, physiotherapists, speech and language therapists. Physiotherapy 89 (8), 433–441.

Miller, W.L., Crabtree, B.F., 2000. Clinical research. In: Denzin, N.K., Lincoln, Y.S. (Eds.), Handbook of Qualitative Research. Sage, Thousand Oaks, CA.

Murphy, M.K., Black, N.A., Lampling, D.L., et al, 1998. Consensus development methods and their use in clinical guidelines development. Health Technology Assessment 2 (3), 1–88.

Paddy, A., Wright-St Clair, V., Smythe, L., 2004. Aspects of the relationship following face-to-face encounters in occupational therapy practice. New Zealand Journal of Occupational Therapy 49 (2), 14–20.

Paterson, C., 1997. An historical perspective of work practice services. In: Pratt, J., Jacobs, K. (Eds.), Work Practices: International Perspectives. Butterworth–Heinemann, Oxford.

Pols, V., 2002. The phoenix, staff and serpent. In: Wilcock, A. (Ed.), Occupation for Health. vol. 2. A Journey from Prescription to Self Health. College of Occupational Therapists, London.

Pope, C., Mays, N., 2000. Qualitative methods in health research. In: Pope, C., Mays, N. (Eds.), Qualitative Research in Health Care, second ed. British Medical Journal Group, London.

Reynolds, F., 2003. Explorin;g meanings of artistic occupation for women living with chronic illness: a comparison of template and interpretative phenomenological approaches to analysis. British Journal of Occupational Therapy 66 (12), 551–558.

Ryan, S., 2001. Breaking moulds — shifting thinking. British Journal of Occupational Therapy 64 (11), 252.

Sackett, D.L., Rosenberg, W.M.C., Gray, J.A.M., et al, 1996. Evidence-based medicine: what it is and what it isn't. British Medical Journal 312, 71–72.

Schutz, A., 1967. The Phenomenology of the Social World. North Western University Press, Evanston.

Schwartz, C., 1994. Chambers Dictionary. Chambers, Edinburgh.

Seale, C., 1999. Quality in qualitative research. Qualitative Inquiry 5, 465–478.

Smith, J., Heshusius, L., 1986. Closing down the conversation: the end of the quantitative-qualitative debate among educational enquirers. Educational Researcher 15, 4–12.

Taylor, J., 1995. A different voice in occupational therapy. British Journal of Occupational Therapy 58 (4), 170–174.

Taylor, M.C., 2000. Evidence-Based Practice for Occupational Therapists. Blackwell Science, Oxford.

Taylor, M.C., Savin-Baden, M., 2001. Whose 'evidence' are we applying? British Journal of Occupational Therapy 64 (5), 213.

Tuke, S., 1813. Description of the Retreat: An Institution near York for Insane Persons for the Society of Friends Containing an Account of its Origin and Progress, the Modes of Treatment and a Statement of Cases. W Alexander, York.

Webber, G., 1995. Occupational therapy: a postmodernist perspective. British Journal of Occupational Therapy 58 (10), 439–440.

Whalley-Hammell, K., 2001. Using qualitative research to inform the client-centred evidence-based practice of occupational therapy. British Journal of Occupational Therapy 64 (5), 228–234.

Wilcock, A.A., 2001a. Occupation for Health: A Journey from Prescription to Self-health. College of Occupational Therapists, London.

Wilcock, A.A., 2001b. Occupation for Health: A Journey from Self-health to Prescription. College of Occupational Therapists, London.

Williams, M., May, T., 1996. Introduction to the Philosophy of Social Research. UCL Press, London.

Theoretical foundations of occupational therapy: internal influences

3

Edward A.S. Duncan

OVERVIEW

The focus of this chapter is on the internal influences that shape the development of occupational therapy. The chapter commences with a historical overview of the foundations of occupational therapy. The wealth and importance of the historical foundations of occupational therapy are not always appreciated. Readers are encouraged not to skip this section (as can often be so tempting), but to read it and reflect on the relevance of the profession's pioneers for practice today. Having briefly reviewed the biographical and philosophical history of the profession, the chapter continues with an evaluation of the theoretical influences that have shaped the profession. The chapter then progresses to describe and evaluate contemporary approaches to knowledge development within the profession.

Key points

This chapter:
- provides a historical context to the development of occupational therapy
- gives a clear introduction to the central paradigm shifts that have occurred through the development of occupational therapy
- highlights the importance of using knowledge exchange mechanisms to ensure the rapid transfer of knowledge between research and practice
- provides an introduction to the concepts of complexity, complex interventions and complexity theory.

Historical perspectives

The only way of knowing where we are going is knowing where we have come from.

(Llobera 1998)

As discussed in Chapter 1, the historical basis for health through occupation can be traced back to the biblical times of the Old Testament and the Classical period of the Ancient Greeks and Romans (Wilcock 2001b). The focus of occupation in health came to the fore in Western society, however, during the development of Moral Treatment (p.74), which is recognized as providing a central philosophical basis for occupational therapy. The facts that occupational therapy has both a philosophical and a theoretical basis and that the philosophical basis came first place it in a unique position amongst health professionals (Schwartz 1994). Understanding this historical basis helps us to understand the tensions occupational therapists may perceive when they share their view of a person with other professionals, who view the person from a completely different philosophical perspective.

American founders

Occupational therapy, as we know it today, emerged at the beginning of the 20th century. Whilst occupation programmes are known to have been developed from the very beginning of the 20th century (Wilcock 2001a), it was in 1917 that the National Society for the Promotion of Occupational Therapy (which later became the American Occupational Therapy Association) was founded (Schwartz 1994). This group was formed by several individuals who came from various professional backgrounds:

- William Rush Dunton — a psychiatrist
- George Edward Barton and Thomas Bessell Kidner — architects
- Eleanor Clarke Slagle — social service background
- Susan Cox Johnson — a teacher of arts and crafts
- Susan Tracy — a nurse (Schwartz 1994).

The broad nature of the professional backgrounds is noteworthy. This group of individuals had a significant impact on the early conceptualization of occupational therapy. Their individual contributions to the field are not of particular interest in this text, however, and the interested reader is directed to other publications that have described this group in great depth (Schwartz 1994).

Another individual who had a significant impact on the transatlantic development of occupational therapy was Dr Adolf Meyer. Meyer (1866–1950) was born in Switzerland but spent the majority of his professional career in the USA, eventually as the director of the Johns Hopkins University Medical School. Meyer can be looked upon as the father of American psychiatry. Meyer visited the UK on several occasions and acknowledged the impact that these visits had on his development when he expressed 'a real personal indebtedness to British medicine and British Psychiatry', p.435. Perhaps one of the most influential of these visits was his first. Whilst on a travelling scholarship, Meyer attended a conference in Edinburgh at which he heard William James, the American pragmatist philosopher and psychologist, give a talk.

Meyer described himself as a 'mental hygienist' and assisted in the foundation of the (American) National Committee of Mental Hygiene (Wilcock 2001a). The mental hygiene movement held the following objectives:

- to work for the conservation of mental health
- to promote the study of mental disorders and mental effects in all their forms and relations
- to obtain and disseminate reliable data concerning them
- to help raise the standard of care and treatment (Henderson 1923).

These apparently philanthropic aims are, however, tainted by an aspect of Meyer's life that is less well known and has had little mention in occupational therapy literature. Meyer, like many others involved in the Mental Hygiene movement, was also a proponent of Eugenics. Eugenics is the proposed improvement of the human species by encouraging or permitting reproduction of only those individuals with genetic characteristics judged desirable. The Mental Hygiene movement was permeated with Eugenic thought, a philosophy most notoriously and extremely supported by the Nazis during the Second World War. From Meyer's perspective, Eugenics provided an opportunity to eradicate mental illness through the prevention of reproduction by people with mental illness. It has since been broadly discredited. Eugenic organizations do, however, continue to the present day and Meyer's membership and espousal of such a philosophy provides a different perspective of the man who is credited as providing the first conceptual model of occupational therapy (Meyer 1922, Reed & Sanderson 1999).

During his career, Meyer recognized the impact of instincts, habits and interests, as well as experiences on people's lives and because of this developed an interest in the impact of occupation with his patients (Wilcock 2001a). Indeed, such was his interest in the impact of occupation that he employed Eleanor Clarke Slagle, following her early occupational therapy training. During this period, Dr David Henderson, a young graduate from Scotland, came to work with Meyer. Henderson saw Slagle's work within the institution and was impressed by the impact she had on the patients with whom she worked (Wilcock 2001a). On his return to Scotland, it was Dr Henderson, inspired by the time he had spent with Meyer and Slagle, who opened the first occupational therapy department in the UK, at Gartnavel Royal Hospital, Glasgow, in 1919. In 1922, the first 'occupational therapist', Dorothea Robertson, was appointed within the same department.

British founders

Whilst Dr Henderson was the first individual to introduce occupational therapy to the UK and Dorothea Robertson the first appointed occupational therapist, two other key figures require presentation if we are to understand more fully the introduction of occupational therapy within the UK; they are Margaret Barr Fulton and Elizabeth Casson. Margaret Fulton was the first qualified occupational therapist in the UK. Born in Scotland and raised in England, Margaret Fulton trained to become an occupational therapist whilst in the USA. On her return she was put in contact with Dr Henderson; however, as he was unable to appoint, she was employed by the Aberdeen Royal Asylum. Whilst Margaret Fulton did not write or present a great deal on her philosophy of practice, her work stood out and gained her high office. In 1937, whilst working in Aberdeen, she met Alfred Adler, one-time colleague of Sigmund Freud and founder of Individual Psychology (Wilcock 2001a). He was later to comment, 'I was particularly struck with the Occupational Therapy department and with the high degree of interest which is shown in psychological problems' (Aberdeen Press and Journal 1937). Fulton's capabilities are also apparent in her election to the position of first president of the World Federation of Occupational Therapists (Wilcock 2001a).

Another key British founder of occupational therapy is Elizabeth Casson. Born in 1881, Elizabeth was brought up amongst a family of varied artistic talents, so it is not surprising that the young Elizabeth was noted to be good with her hands, demonstrating practical as well as academic talents (Wilcock 2001a). Following an initial period of secretarial work, Casson worked with Octavia Hill (1838–1912), a remarkable women who is credited with the foundation of several organizations and professions, including the Open Space Movement, the National Trust, housing management and social work (Wilcock 2001b). Hill is believed to have had a considerable effect on Casson during their period together at the Red Cross Hall, where Hill employed Casson as a secretary (Wilcock 2001a). Casson became very involved in the practical activities of the tenants, for whom she organized a variety of educational and recreational activities. Casson then surprised those closest to her by announcing to everyone that she intended to study medicine. Graduating in 1929 as the first female doctor from the University of Bristol, Casson herself states that her 'real introduction' to occupational therapy came through reading a description of Henderson's work in Glasgow. Casson's medical training and intrigue, coupled with her personal and family talents and social commitment, naturally fostered a profound interest in occupational therapy. This interest culminated in her establishment and development of the first British occupational therapy school at Dorset House, Bristol (Wilcock 2001a). Casson's importance to the development of occupational therapy in Britain today is honoured by the College of Occupational Therapists through the Casson Memorial

Lecture, an annual event at the college's annual conference.

This overview of some of the historical developments of occupational therapy is provided to demonstrate the very real connections between the external influences on the early development of the profession and the foundations of the profession as we know it today. The history of occupational therapy is a rich tapestry, upon which this text has only fleetingly touched. Interested readers are guided to two fascinating volumes on the subject, from a predominantly British perspective (Wilcock 2001a,b).

Paradigm shifts in occupational therapy

Having reviewed the philosophical basis and the influential individuals who were responsible for the foundation of the profession, it is important to examine the theoretical developments of occupational therapy. Such developments are perhaps best understood through the concept of paradigms and paradigm shifts. Kuhn (1970) understood that members of a profession were bound by a shared vision of what it meant to be. Paradigms represent the shared consensus regarding the most fundamental beliefs of a profession. Paradigm shifts, therefore, are the moments in which the shared vision and understanding of a field changes and a new consensus regarding the fundamental beliefs of the profession is adopted. Understandably, as paradigms represent the core of a profession, such shifts are both rare and traumatic to the field. The concept of paradigms has been developed by a variety of individuals, including Tornebohm (1986) and MacIntyre (1980). Tornebohm (1986) views a profession's paradigm as the defining feature of a profession and believes that within it can be found a profession's vision of practice. MacIntyre (1980) argues that paradigms provide professions with their values and concerns for practice.

Within occupational therapy, it is the work of Professor Gary Kielhofner (2009) that is most closely associated with the paradigmatic conceptualization of occupational therapy's professional development. Kielhofner (2009) develops the work of Kuhn (1970), Tornebohm (1986) and MacIntyre (1980) in his understanding of the paradigmatic content of occupational therapy, and suggests that the occupational therapy paradigm consists of three elements: core constructs, focal viewpoints and integrated values.

'Core constructs' of the profession tackles the issues regarding a profession's service provision. 'Core constructs' relate to the need for the profession, the problems it focuses on and the manner in which it addresses such problems. The 'focal viewpoint' of a paradigm is interested in the way in which a profession views, understands and interprets the world. The 'focal viewpoint' of a profession will also influence the knowledge that is deemed important within the profession. Finally, 'values' highlight the level of importance that a profession places on issues from its own perspective (Kielhofner 2004a).

Kielhofner (2009) outlines three different paradigms that have existed in occupational therapy since its inception (Table 3.1): the occupational paradigm, the mechanistic paradigm and the contemporary paradigm. The original paradigm (the occupational paradigm) arose from the work of the profession's founders and was based on their core construct, views and values. During the 1940s and 1950s, occupational therapy was placed under increasing pressure from the medical profession to become objective and create an empirical basis for its intervention (Kielhofner 2004a). In search of professional acceptance, occupational therapy increasingly focused on biomedical explanations for practice; thus the mechanistic paradigm period of occupational therapy was born. During the mechanistic period, occupational

Table 3.1 Paradigmatic shifts in occupational therapy

The nature of paradigms	Core constructs	Focal viewpoint	Integrated values
Paradigm of occupation (1900s–1940s)	Occupation is essential to life and influences people's health Occupation includes thinking, acting and existing, and requires each of these elements to be balanced in daily life Mind and body are intrinsically linked Occupation can be used to regain function	Focusing on both personal motivation and the effect of the environment on performance	Human dignity is realized through performance of occupation Occupation is important for health Holism
Crisis	Occupational therapy is placed under increasing pressure from medicine to become objective Occupational therapy seeks professional recognition through the adoption of biomedical explanations and approaches to dysfunction		
Mechanistic paradigm (1960s–1970s)	Performance is dependent on the functioning of inner systems: intra-psychic, nervous and musculoskeletal Damage to any of the above systems causes dysfunction Functional performance is regained through addressing or compensating for deficits in these systems	This period focused on the internal mechanisms described in the above core constructs	In-depth knowledge of inner systems Objectivity Use of occupation to address and measure disordered inner systems precisely
Crisis	The acceptance of reductionism and focus on inner systems were recognized as incomplete Prominent occupational therapy figures called for a return to occupation, with a focus on the importance of occupation to health		
Contemporary paradigm (1980s onwards)	Occupation has a central role in human life. It provides motive and meaning to life Lack of access (or restricted access) to occupations may have a negative effect on health and quality of life The use of occupation to address impacts on health or quality of life is the core of occupational therapy	This person focuses on a return to occupation and a focus on the whole, rather than its component parts	Respect for the value of human life The importance of individuals' empowerment and engagement in occupation The integration of individuals into life through meaningful occupation

therapists become increasingly competent at measuring and attempting to objectify their practice. However, such developments caused the profession to lose sight of its roots and the original impetus for the profession's birth. The initial call for the profession to return to its original vision came from Mary Reilly, a highly influential scholar in the history of modern occupational therapy (Kielhofner 2004a). Reilly's original call for the return of occupational therapy's focus on occupation came in her Eleanor Clarke Slagle Lecture in 1961. During this keynote speech to the annual conference of the American Occupational Therapy Association, she gave a poetic (but from our current perspective completely un-evidence-based) vision of the impact of occupation on health, stating that 'man through the use of his hands, as they are energized by his mind and will, can influence the state of his own health' (Reilly 1962, p.1). Through this clarion call to the profession, a new crisis emerged as practitioners sought to return once again to being occupationally focused, whilst retaining the developments in objectivity and professional status they had gained during the mechanistic period. The return to occupation heralded the contemporary paradigm, in which occupation is understood in a new and more complex manner and the importance of occupation in health has once again been established.

Professional paradigms are dynamic in nature. Whilst whole-scale paradigm shifts are relatively rare, occupational therapy is constantly evolving and developing. This process, whilst perhaps not quite as traumatic as a paradigm shift, can none the less be painful and challenging. Contemporary debates regarding approaches to theoretical development within occupational therapy constitute one such challenge. Whilst the contemporary paradigm is not being questioned, the manner in which knowledge is developed to support the paradigm undoubtedly is. Wilcock (1998) recognized at an early stage that the developing complexity of occupational therapy theory would lead to 'heated debate' between professionals (p.203). Despite acknowledging that 'heated debate about the profession's foundation is not part of occupational therapists' tradition' (p.203), she felt that such debate was important and would ultimately benefit the profession. This position is supported by Bannigan (2001), who also recognized occupational therapists' reluctance to argue but supports the requirement of professional argument in order to develop a robust knowledge base and pursue excellence in practice.

Theoretical developments within occupational therapy

Possibly the first elucidation of the theoretical (as opposed to the philosophical) basis of occupational therapy was in 1940, with the publication of a text entitled *Theory of Occupational Therapy for Students and Nurses* (Haworth & Macdonald 1940). Whilst theoretical developments have emerged throughout each of the profession's paradigms, it is during the period of the contemporary paradigm that occupational therapy research and theoretical developments have truly gathered pace. These developments are the natural evolution from the paradigm of occupation that has now emerged and established itself as the central focus of occupational therapists' concern (Kielhofner 2004a).

Theory is a term that is readily used in our everyday conversations (for example, 'In theory I could do this but . . .'); however, within occupational therapy, theoretical approaches are not always as easily articulated. Mitcham (2003) describes a scenario that will be recognized by many students and practitioners. Discussing the complexity of theory in practice, she states:

> we panic when a keen, bright eyed student asks us in the clinic one day, 'which theoretical approach guides your practice?' We stumble and mumble a response along the lines of, 'Oh, I haven't touched that theory stuff since I graduated', or 'I'm eclectic, I use a little of everything'. (p.65)

Such a scenario is commonly recounted by students undertaking fieldwork placements. Whilst the reasons for a practitioner's inability to justify their practice theoretically may be various, such a response in effect perpetuates the theory–practice divide and suggests to the practitioners of the future that theory is not important in practice. This is not the case and the aim of this text is to demonstrate the importance of theory to practice, to assist students and practitioners to make sense of theory in practice, and to develop understanding of how theory can be developed and implemented in practice.

So, what is theory? Reed (1997) defines it as 'an organized way of thinking about given phenomena . . . It attempts to:

- Define and explain the relationships between concepts or ideas related to phenomena of interest;

- Explain how these relationships can predict behaviour or events; and
- Suggest ways that phenomena can be changed or controlled' (p.521).

Kielhofner (2009) offers another definition, stating that theory is 'A network of explanations that provides concepts that label and describe phenomena and postulates that specify relationships between concepts' (p.8).

Creek (2002) defines theory as a 'conceptual system or framework used to organize knowledge. A theory consists of a description of a set of phenomena, an explanation of how and under what circumstances they occur, and a demonstration of how they relate to each other' (p.46).

Various definitions of theory have been offered and agreement is clear between authors cited.

Theory and practice

The relationship of theory to practice varies in different professions. Radiology, for example, draws heavily upon knowledge that has been developed in the fields of chemistry, physics, anatomy and physiology. Radiology places less emphasis on the social sciences than occupational therapy. Furthermore, unlike occupational therapy, radiology has not developed its own theoretical understandings to guide practice. Each of these issues can help us understand why some professions do not appear to have a theory–practice dilemma, whilst others, such as occupational therapy, do (Mitcham 2003).

The issue of the theory–practice gap and the manner in which theory is built, tested, understood and applied to practice form the basis for an important and current debate in occupational therapy. This debate is core, as it presents conceptually differing approaches to theory and knowledge development.

Basic science

Basic sciences emerged from the development of logical positivism previously discussed in Chapter 2 (p.11). The focus of basic research is the development of pure theory. No consideration is given to its potential application. Basic research can certainly be influential in applied settings. Esdaile and Roth (2003) provide two examples of how basic research has caused an impact in applied situations. Compact disks use a coding system (pure theory) that was

originally developed by Gaulois, an 18th century French mathematician. More recently, nuclear magnetic resonance (which was discovered in 1938) was integrated into this technology several decades later to assist in the early detection of diseases. Whilst the time taken to integrate these research findings into practice is considerable, it could be argued that the delay in application was a result of having to wait for technology to catch up, before such basic science could be applied. The study of the therapeutic effects of aspirin, however, highlights that, even when research can be easily applied, with life-saving effects, considerable delays occur in the transference of knowledge.

Aspirin's role in preventing heart attacks first emerged in 1948. Dr Lawrence Craven, a general practitioner in California, undertook a small study of 400 men whom he placed on an aspirin regimen. Over a period of 2 years, no participants suffered a heart attack. The initial study was expanded, and in 1956 it was reported that a study of 8000 men found that those who took one or two aspirin tablets daily did not suffer heart attacks. In 1988 Harvard University undertook a study of 22 000 male doctors and found that those who took one 325 milligram aspirin tablet every second day had 44 per cent fewer heart attacks than those who did not. The study had been scheduled to last 8 years but the researchers found the results so positive that ethically they did not feel they should withhold aspirin's benefits from the control placebo group (Steering Committee of the Physicians' Health Study Research Group 1988). Further studies have amended the dosage of aspirin required to prevent a heart attack and the population who would most benefit from such usage; however, aspirin continues to be underused for conditions in which its efficacy is well established (Reilly & Fitzgerald 2002). It would appear, therefore, that basic research can influence practice, but that there may be a time delay and the influence of such research on practice can be accidental or unplanned.

Occupational therapy's relationship with basic science

Mosey (1992) distinguishes theory that explains phenomena (basic science) from the integration of such research into practice (application). Mosey (1992) argues that occupational therapy's remit is solely within the application of theory to practice and suggests that such theory can be found in the scientific disciplines of biology, sociology, philosophy and so on. In doing so, Mosey (1992) supports the

Fig. 3.1 • The application of basic science to practice.

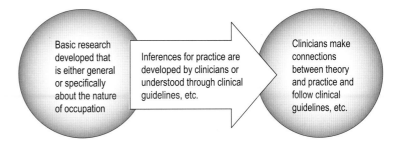

separation of theory from practice and the basic science approach to knowledge generation. Mosey (1992) supports the application of existing knowledge to support occupational therapy. Others have argued, however, that it is necessary to create a basic science of occupation. This approach, known as Occupational Science (Clark et al 1991), is discussed in greater depth in Chapter 18.

Basic science is based on the premise of technical rationality (Schon 1983). Technical rationality assumes that knowledge that is generated in basic research will naturally lead to applications of knowledge in practice (Fig. 3.1). Viewed from this perspective, knowledge is seen as hierarchical in nature, with the highest position given to the developers of knowledge, whilst lower positions are occupied by problem-solving and other applications (Schon 1983). The transference of such knowledge into practice, however, is not as linear as the technical rational perspective suggests. A major criticism of the basic science approach to integrating theory into practice is that it does not provide either evidence or applications that are directly applicable in practice (Taylor et al 2002). In recent years a whole field of research has emerged that focuses on improving the communication of knowledge between research and practice. Alternatively referred to as knowledge transfer and knowledge exchange, it is both a technical and a social process that emphasizes the mutual learning that can occur between practice and research (see Bannigan 2009 for further information).

In recognition of the difficulties of implementing basic research into practice, several mechanisms have been developed to assist practitioners in the process. One example of a mechanism designed to assist practitioners in integrating theoretical findings into practice is the 'learning through discussion process' (Rabow et al 1994). Fawcett Hill's process ensures that practitioners understand what they are reading, can clearly conceptualize what the author is trying to

convey, and evaluate the applicability of the material to the wider field and to an individual's practice. The process suggests an eight-step written process used to guide discussion and understanding (Table 3.2).

Journal clubs are another mechanism that is designed to assist individuals to appraise new knowledge critically and understand its implication in practice. Journal clubs have been used within medicine for several years (Taylor 2003) and their use is also promoted within occupational therapy and other allied health professions (Bannigan 2002).

Whilst these mechanisms, along with others such as checklists (Thompson 2003) and clinical guidelines (Duncan et al 2000), are of great value in increasing practitioners' critical appraisal skills and use of theory in practice, they are limited in the extent to which they can guide and influence practice.

It is increasingly recognized, within the allied health professions, that the development of clinically relevant knowledge is a truly collaborative process. Occupational therapists, amongst others, must strive to develop the highest quality of evidence-based theories, relevant to the individuals receiving the service and demonstrably effective in practice. Such high expectations cannot be developed in isolation. Collaborations between academics, practitioners and service users, as equal partners in the development and implementation of theory into practice, are essential.

Scholarship of practice

The scholarship of practice is a method of knowledge generation that has gained momentum within occupational therapy practice. Schon (1983) is widely credited with developing the concept of scholarship in practice. As with other areas of theory and knowledge development, the term 'scholarship of practice' is understood by differing theorists in different ways. Esdaile and Roth (2003) describe a scholarship of

Table 3.2 Learning through discussion

Step	Focus
1	**Definition of terms and concepts.** All words or terms that the reader is unfamiliar with should be listed and explored
2	**Statements of the author's message(s).** Participants should write down a summary of the main message
3	**Identification of major themes.** In this step, participants identify the main and sub-themes of the paper
4	**Allocation of time.** This section is for explicitly stating which areas you had difficulty understanding and on which you feel you should focus
5	**Discussion of major themes and sub-themes.** The purpose of this step is to provide background material so that the participants do not have to refer continually to the original source
6	**Integration of material with other knowledge.** Participants should list other material that backs up or challenges the paper under review
7	**Application of material.** This section focuses the participants on how the material can apply to one's own situation and the implications it has for practice
8	**Evaluation of author's presentation.** Participants should form an opinion on the work reviewed and clearly be able to highlight how it is or is not useful

practice 'in terms of an integrated model in which basic research from both the physical and social sciences informs practice, and practice generates further questions for research' (p.161). From Esdaile and Roth's (2003) perspective, the focus of scholarship of practice is on:

- discovery — not only of research, but also of practice observations, often achieved in collaboration between academics and clinicians
- integration — including information from other disciplines; crucially, integration is seen as the process through which academics and practitioners are linked
- application — using evidence-based techniques and models or frames of reference on practice
- teaching — continuous professional development and the sharing of knowledge with peers, students, clients and carers.

Scholarship of practice within the Model of Human Occupation

The term 'scholarship of practice' is used in a particular way to describe the process of knowledge development within the Model of Human Occupation. Within this model, the scholarship of practice is described as a dialectic (that is, a discussion or debate) between theory and practice (Hammel et al 2002,

Kielhofner 2004a, Kielhofner et al 2004). Furthermore, Forsyth et al (2005b) describe the scholarship of practice as a partnership between academia and practice, 'in which theoretical and empirical knowledge is brought to bear on the practical problems of therapeutic work and in which the latter raise questions to be addressed through scholarship' (p.260). This scholarship of practice approach focuses on:

- research that is carried out and contributes directly to *practice*
- partnerships that are developed outside academic institutions; such partnerships provide new research, **practice** and educational opportunities
- the creation of effective collaborations that advance both academia and *practice* (Forsyth, Summerfield-Mann & Kielhofner 2005b) [emphasis added]

In order to develop effectively as a 'practice scholar' (Forsyth, Summerfield-Mann & Kielhofner 2005b), who builds and implements knowledge directly relevant to practice, an alternative approach to research, other than the technical rational approach of basic research described above, must be considered. It is necessary to create equal partnerships, between clinicians, academics and the recipients of services, in knowledge development: partnerships that reflect a true collaboration and power sharing so that 'all participants may have a degree of responsibility, voice and decision-making about all aspects of knowledge generation' (Kielhofner 2005).

Scholarship of practice recognizes the strengths of all approaches that support the development of practice-related research. However, in order to engage in a scholarship of practice approach to knowledge development, Kielhofner (2009) advocates for the development of an 'engaged scholarship' (Boyer 1990) that examines alternative ways of addressing and resolving the everyday life difficulties of people and society. Whilst positivistic approaches can achieve this (Gitlin et al 2001), engaged scholarship requires a re-evaluation of how knowledge is best developed.

An alternative method for developing knowledge, used within this scholarship of practice approach, is 'participatory action research' (Waterman et al 2001). Participatory action research is incorporated within the scholarship of practice approach, as it provides an alternative method of knowledge generation that supports partnership working and leads to change within the practice setting (Forsyth, Summerfield-Mann & Kielhofner 2005a, Kielhofner 2004b).

Kurt Lewin (1890–1947) is credited with coining the phrase 'action research', an approach that he initially used to study inter-group relations and issues of minority groups in the USA (Meyer 2000). Action research is a cyclical process that intertwines action, reflection and research. Key elements of action research include the clear definition of phases of the study, a clear description of everyone involved, consideration of the local context throughout the study and the nature of the relationship between the researchers and participants (Waterman et al 2001). Action research has been recognized as a solution to the theory–practice gap (Meyer 2000).

Participatory action research has been advocated for use within an occupational science framework (Wilcock 1998). However, its use within this scholarship of practice approach is focused on research that is centred on practice. Moreover, the adoption of participatory action research within an engaged scholarship approach does not require a total dismissal of previous research approaches.

Kielhofner (2009) recognizes the importance of preserving the positive components of traditional methods of knowledge generation, whilst engaging with contemporary approaches (such as participatory action research) that are more suited to creating theories that both are global and have a concurrent practical utility. Therefore, scholarship of practice supports the development of a knowledge-creating system (Senge & Scharmer 2001). This system integrates research and theory development, capacity-building amongst professionals and practical utility, through the development of tools for practice, into a single process of combined strength. In this manner, the divide of knowledge development and application found in basic science is removed (Kielhofner 2004b) (Fig. 3.2).

Fig. 3.2 • A knowledge-creating system. Reprinted from Kielhofner G., 2005. Scholarship and practice: bridging the divide. American Journal of Occupational Therapy 59 (2), 231–239.

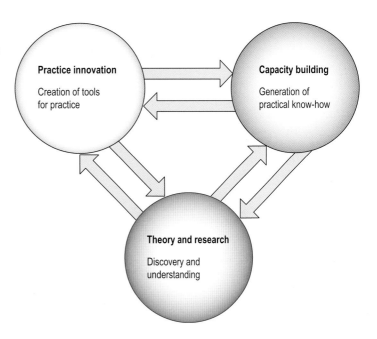

Kielhofner's approach to the scholarship of practice, whilst originating from the USA, is gathering pace throughout the international occupational therapy community. Forsyth et al (2005b) describe how a forensic occupational therapy service in Scotland has developed a scholarship of practice approach to research and practice. Other scholarship of practice collaborations are developing. The scholarship of practice approach has been used for several years in practice; it is only one type of knowledge exchange that occurs in occupational therapy. Other types of knowledge exchange activity have been presented by Bannigan (2009).

Knowledge development — an important debate

This section of the chapter has provided an introductory analysis of the conceptually diverse methods of theoretical knowledge development within occupational therapy. The importance of this debate regarding approaches to knowledge development within occupational therapy is reflected in a series of letters written to the editor of the *British Journal of Occupational Therapy* (BJOT) between August 2001 and June 2002. In total, 17 letters were exchanged on the subject of the appropriate approach to knowledge development in occupational therapy and related issues. This series of letters was initiated in response to the College of Occupational Therapists' publication of its research development strategic vision and action plan (Ilott & White 2001), in which occupational science was listed as a specific priority for research.

These letters have been variously described as 'a passionate intellectual debate' (Butler & Ilott 2001, p.41), 'invidious confrontation' (van Dam 2001, p.580), 'good examples of how worthy it is to pursue argument[s] of concern' (Summerfield-Mann 2001, p.620) and 'individual criticism' (Wilcock 2002, p.97). Whatever one's perspective, the sheer volume of correspondence is indicative of the relevance and importance of the manner in which knowledge is currently being developed within occupational therapy today.

Complexity

The word 'complexity' has lay and technical meanings. In practice' clinicians will often refer to the 'complexity' of practice; however, this is, more often than not, using the lay definition of the term. Just because something appears complex in a general sense does not necessarily mean (and mostly will not mean) that it is also complex in the technical sense of the word. The technical senses of 'complexity' are, well, complex (sic)!

Complexity theory is one technical explanation of complexity. It explores how complex systems (such as humans) sometimes behave in the real world and how complex systems can generate simple outcomes. Complexity theory views all living creatures as complex adaptive systems (Lewin 1993). Such complexity is easy to witness. Consider the sight of a flock of geese flying south in a 'V' formation in the autumn or a flock of swifts that twist and turn in harmony in the dusk of a city landscape. Such sights are truly wondrous. Complex adaptive systems are also observable in humans at a multitude of levels. Consider the complexity of getting out of bed in the morning and getting yourself to university or work. Such complexity is then magnified when we consider the systems in which such an activity occurs (e.g. the other people you meet on your way to university, the environment in which you live, and so on). Humans do not exist in isolation and complexity theory acknowledges the importance of understanding the interconnectedness of nature. Despite such complex interactions, complexity scientists have discovered that complex behaviour can emerge from the existence of a few simple rules. Geese fly in the manner that causes least resistance — their bodies are shaped to decrease wind resistance when they fly diagonally to each other. Swifts have a simple rule of staying an equal distance from their fellow birds and flying in roughly the same direction.

A further component of complexity theory is the recognition of small changes that potentially lead to larger effects. This is commonly known as the 'butterfly effect', as it has been shown that a butterfly flapping its wings in India can cause changes in air currents that lead to an eventual windstorm in Chicago. Within occupational therapy, it could be argued that Reilly's call for a return to occupation-focused activity (Reilly 1962) sparked a similar wave of effects that resulted in a professional paradigm shift and influenced the practice of occupational therapists internationally. Within occupational therapy practice, it is observable that a small positive action or interaction within an occupational therapy session can have significant effects on the whole of a person's functioning. Similarly, provision of a simple piece of adaptive kitchen equipment can lead to someone returning to previously valued occupations and life roles — small changes can have a big effect on the whole system.

It is not, therefore, surprising that complexity theory has gained attention within healthcare research.

Another related but separate issue is that of complex interventions. Complex interventions have many different components to them, and it can at times be hard to tell which of them is the crucial one or the 'active ingredient'. Just having an intervention with many components does not mean that the components interact with each other according to complexity theory. Indeed, there may be a very simple interaction between the elements (and thus it is a complex intervention); the only way truly to tell is by conducting research into the action of the intervention. The Medical Research Council (MRC) of the UK has recognized the importance of complexity interventions in healthcare. In 2000 it published its first guide to developing and evaluating complex interventions (Medical Research Council 2000). This was later substantially updated (Medical Research Council 2008). Creek (2003) used the original MRC framework to study occupational therapy as a complex intervention. Creek (2003) viewed occupational therapy as a complex intervention that meets the MRC definition of comprising 'a number of separate elements which seem essential to the proper functioning of the intervention although the "active ingredient" of the intervention that is effective is difficult to specify' (Medical Research Council 2000, p.1). Creek's (2003) work focuses on the establishment of the theoretical basis and 'modelling' which represents an attempt to separate occupational therapy's component parts and illustrate how they inter-relate to each other. This document was published by the College of Occupational Therapists (COT). More recently, an overview into the use of the document was conducted by Creek (2009). Interestingly, Creek's definition of occupational therapy as a complex intervention has not been used for its original purpose (research), but has instead been used and misused by academics and practitioners trying to explain or describe the occupational therapy process (Creek 2009). Considerable confusion has arisen surrounding whether occupational therapy is a complex intervention, whether some occupational therapy interventions are complex interventions, or whether in fact some occupational therapy interventions can be better understood by complexity theory. A robust discussion occurred in the literature on these very issues (Creek et al 2005, Duncan et al 2007, Lambert et al 2007); the interested reader is guided to these articles for further information and consideration of the issues.

Summary

This chapter has provided an overview of the internal influences on the theoretical foundations of occupational therapy. These influences were first placed within their historical context. Following this, an overview of the various contemporary influences on theory development within occupational therapy was given.

The challenges of the issues presented and multiple uses of similar terms are often disheartening for students and practitioners who are trying to grapple with the theoretical influences of the profession. There can be a temptation either to look for a single theoretical answer or to give up and conclude that theory is not important. Both are erroneous views. Theory and knowledge are vital to practice, and practice is the crucible in which new theories are evaluated. Without a theoretical basis, the profession would crumble. The multiplicity of views and debate within the profession serves only to progress our theoretical understanding of the effect of occupation on health. Debate fosters development and this would not occur if a single perspective were consistently taken. Furthermore, without knowledge and understanding of the theoretical basis for practice, a practitioner's intervention may be viewed as unethical. How can a professional work in an ethical way without knowing the theoretical basis for such intervention? It is important, therefore, to grapple with the literature and engage in the debate surrounding theory development and its application in practice.

This review of the internal influences on theory development is, by necessity, partial. Other themes are picked up on in subsequent chapters and debated more fully. Having read and reflected on the issues raised within this chapter, readers are encouraged to explore other internal influences discussed by other authors in this text and beyond and to explore the issues in greater depth.

Reflective learning

- History is made in the present. What are the current influences that will shape the future of occupational therapy?
- What are the key paradigm shifts in occupational therapy to date? Are we anywhere near another? If so, what could it be?
- In your own words, describe the difference between a lay meaning of complexity and the ideas of complexity theory and complex interventions.

References

Aberdeen Press and Journal, 1937. Welfare Work in Aberdeen. Professor Adler Pays Tribute. Aberdeen Press and Journal.

Bannigan, K., 2001. Use argument to deliver excellence. British Journal of Occupational Therapy 64 (3), 113.

Bannigan, K., 2002. How journal clubs can overcome barriers to research utilization. British Journal of Therapy and Rehabilitation 9 (8), 299–303.

Bannigan, K., 2009. Knowledge Exchange. In: Duncan, EAS (Ed.), Skills for Practice in Occupational Therapy. Elsevier/Churchill Livingstone, pp. 231–248.

Boyer, E., 1990. Scholarship Reconsidered: Priorities of the Professorate. Carnegie Foundation for the Advancement of Teaching, Princeton.

Butler, J., Ilott, I., 2001. R&D strategy: New Year's resolutions [letter]. British Journal of Occupational Therapy 65 (1), 41–42.

Clark, F.A., Parham, D., Carlson, M.E., et al, 1991. Occupational science: academic innovation in the service of occupational therapy's future. American Journal of Occupational Therapy 45 (4), 300–310.

Creek, J., 2002. The knowledge base of occupational therapy. In: Creek, J. (Ed.), Occupational Therapy and Mental Health. Churchill Livingstone, Edinburgh.

Creek, J., 2003. Occupational Therapy Defined as a Complex Intervention. College of Occupational Therapists, London.

Creek, J., Ilott, I., Cook, S., Munday, C., 2005. Valuing occupational therapy as a complex intervention. British Journal of Occupational Therapy 68 (6), 281–284.

Creek, J., 2009. Occupational Therapy defined as a complex intervention: a 5-year review. British Jounral of Occupational Therapy 72 (3), 105–115.

Duncan, E.A.S., Thomson, L.D.G., Short, A., 2000. Clinical guidelines within mental health services: an overview of the appraisal and implementation process. British Journal of Occupational Therapy 63 (11), 557–560.

Duncan, E.A.S., Paley, J., Eva, G., 2007. Complex interventions and complex systems in occupational therapy. British Journal of Occupational Therapy 70 (5), 199–206.

Esdaile, S.A., Roth, L.M., 2003. Creating scholarly practice: integrating and applying scholarship to practice. In: Brown, G., Esdaile, S.A., Ryan, S.E. (Eds.), Becoming an Advanced Healthcare Practitioner. Butterworth–Heinemann, London.

Forsyth, K., Duncan, E.A.S., Summerfield-Mann, L., 2005a. Scholarship of practice in the United Kingdom: an occupational therapy service case study. Occupational Therapy in Healthcare 19 (1–2), 17–29.

Forsyth, K., Summerfield-Mann, L., Kielhofner, G., 2005b. Scholarship of practice: making occupation focused, theory driven, evidence based practice a reality. British Journal of Occupational Therapy 68 (6), 260–268.

Gitlin, L.N., Corocoran, M., Winter, L., et al, 2001. A randomized control trial of a home environmental intervention. Effect on efficacy and uptake in caregivers and on daily function of persons with dementia. Gerontologist 41, 4–14.

Hammel, J., Finlayson, M., Kielhofner, G., et al, 2002. Educating scholars of practice: an approach to preparing tomorrow's researchers. Occupational Therapy in Healthcare 15 (1/2), 157–176.

Haworth, N.A., MacDonald, E.M., 1940. Theory of occupational therapy for students and nurses. Bailliere, Tindall and Cox, London.

Henderson, D.K., 1923. Mental hygiene. Glasgow Medical Journal, June.

Ilott, I., White, E., 2001. College of Occupational Therapists research and development strategic vision and action plan. British Journal of Occupational Therapy 64 (6), 270–277.

Kielhofner, G., 2005. Scholarship and practice: bridging the divide. American Journal of Occupational Therapy 59 (2), 231–239.

Kielhofner, G., 2009. Conceptual Foundations of Occupational Therapy, fourth ed. FA Davis, Philadelphia.

Kielhofner, G., Hammel, J., Helfrich, C., et al, 2004. Studying practice and its outcomes: a conceptual approach. American Journal of Occupational Therapy 58, 15–23.

Kuhn, T., 1970. The Structure of Scientific Revolutions. University of Chicago, Chicago.

Lambert, R., Harrison, D., Watson, M., 2007. Complexity, occupational therapy, unpredictability and the scientific method: a response to Creek et al (2005) and Duncan et al (2007). British Journal of Occupational Therapy 70 (12), 534–536.

Lewin, R., 1993. Complexity: Life on the Edge of Chaos. Phoenix, London.

Llobera, J., 1998. Historical and comparative research. In: Seale, C. (Ed.), Researching Society and Culture. Sage, London.

MacIntyre, A., 1980. Epistemological crisis, dramatic narrative, and the philosophy science. In: Gutting, G. (Ed.), Paradigms and Revolutions: Appraisals and Applications of Thomas Kuhn's Philosophy of Science. Notre Dame Press, Notre Dame.

Medical Research Council, 2000. A Framework for the Development and Evaluation of RCTs for Complex Interventions to Improve Health. Medical Research Council, London.

Medical Research Council, 2008. Complex Interventions Guidance. Medical Research Council, London.

Meyer, A., 1922. Philosophy of occupation therapy. Archives of Occupational Therapy 1 (1), 1–10.

Meyer, J., 2000. Using qualitative methods in health related action research. British Medical Journal 320, 178–181.

Mitcham, M.D., 2003. Integrating theory and practice: using theory creatively to enhance professional practice. In: Brown, G., Esdaile, S.A., Ryan, S.E. (Eds.), Becoming an Advanced Healthcare Practitioner. Butterworth–Heinemann, London.

Mosey, A.C., 1992. Applied Scientific Inquiry in Health Professions. American Occupational Association, Rockville.

Rabow, J., Charness, M.A., Kipperman, J., et al, 1994. William Fawcett Hill's Learning Through Discussion, third ed. Waveland, Long Grove, Il.

Reed, K.L., 1997. Theory and frame of reference. In: Neistadt, M.E., Crepeau, E.B. (Eds.), Willard and Spackman's Occupational Therapy. Lippincott Williams & Wilkins, Philadelphia.

Reed, K.L., Sanderson, S.N., 1999. Concepts of Occupational Therapy. Lippincott Williams & Wilkins, Philadelphia.

Reilly, M., 1962. Eleanor Clarke Slagle Lecture. Occupational therapy can be one of the great ideas of 20th century medicine. American Journal of Occupational Therapy 16, 1–9.

Reilly, M., Fitzgerald, G., 2002. Gathering intelligence on antiplatelet drugs: the view from 30000 feet. British Medical Journal 324, 59–60.

Schon, D., 1983. The Reflective Practitioner. Basic, New York.

Schwartz, C., 1994. Chambers Dictionary. Chambers, Edinburgh.

Senge, P., Scharmer, O., 2001. Community action research. In: Reason, P., Bradbury, H. (Eds.), Handbook of Action Research: Participatory Inquiry and Practice. Sage, London.

Steering Committee of the Physicians' Health Study Research Group, 1988. Findings from the aspirin of the ongoing Physicians Health Study. New England Journal of Medicine 318, 262–264.

Summerfield-Mann, L., 2001. The real issue at stake. British Journal of Occupational Therapy 64 (12), 620–621.

Taylor, M.C., 2003. Evidence-based practice: informing practice and critically evaluating related research. In: Brown, G., Esdaile, S.A., Ryan, S. (Eds.), Becoming an Advanced Healthcare Practitioner. Butterworth–Heinemann, London.

Taylor, R., Braveman, B., Forsyth, K., 2002. Occupational science and the scholarship of practice: implications for practitioners. New Zealand Journal of Occupational Therapy 49 (2), 37–40.

Thompson, C., 2003. Finding, appraising and using research evidence in practice. In: Pickersing, S., Thompson, J.

(Eds.), Clinical Governance and Best Value. Butterworth–Heinemann, Edinburgh.

Tornebohm, H., 1986. Caring, Knowing and Paradigms. University of Goteborg, Goteborg.

van Dam, J., 2001. The grand design. British Journal of Occupational Therapy 64 (11), 580.

Waterman, H., Tillen, D., Dickson, R., et al, 2001. Action research: a systematic review and guidance for assessment. Health Technology Assessment 5 (23).

Wilcock, A.A., 1998. An Occupational Perspective of Health. Slack, Thorofare, NJ.

Wilcock, A.A., 2001a. Occupation for Health: a Journey from Prescription to Self Health. British College of Occupational Therapists, London.

Wilcock, A.A., 2001b. Occupation for Health: a Journey from Self Health to Prescription. British College of Occupational Therapists, London.

Wilcock, A., 2002. Improving health and wellbeing through occupation. British Journal of Occupational Therapy 65 (2), 97–98.

Skills and processes in occupational therapy

4

Edward A.S. Duncan

OVERVIEW

This chapter focuses on theoretical foundations of what occupational therapists 'do'. As the preceding chapter concluded, humans and the systems and environments in which they exist are complex processes. Describing occupational therapy, which focuses on individuals within the context of their physical and social environments, is not, therefore, quite as simple as it may at first appear. This chapter commences with a brief summary of occupational therapy definitions. Over the years, there has been considerable interest within occupational therapy literature regarding the nature of practice and the skills of an occupational therapist. In order to address this, the chapter will examine the various skills (core, shared and specialist) of an occupational therapist. The chapter then concludes by examining the occupational therapy process.

Key points

This chapter:
- highlights the core skills and processes of occupational therapy
- separates skills into those that are core, shared or specialist for practice
- outlines the occupational therapy process and its cyclical nature
- examines issues arising in assessment, goal-setting and evaluation.

Defining occupational therapy

Definitions are important. To define something is to clarify a topic and provide a vision of its function. Definitions also set boundaries and limitations. Therefore, definitions should be a useful tool in the description of occupational therapy. However, as previously acknowledged, defining occupational therapy can be complex. Despite or perhaps because of this, a multiplicity of occupational therapy definitions exist. The College of Occupational Therapists (COT) provides the following brief description of occupational therapy,

> Occupational Therapy enables people to achieve health, well being and life satisfaction through participation in occupation. (College of Occupational Therapists 2004a)

The World Federation of Occupational Therapists (WFOT) describes occupational therapy as:

> a health discipline which is concerned with people who are physically and/or mentally impaired, disabled and/or handicapped, either temporarily or permanently. The professional qualified occupational therapist involves the patients in activities designed to promote the restoration and maximum use of function with the aim of helping such people meet the demands of their working, social, personal and domestic environment, and to participate in life in its fullest sense. (World Federation of Occupational Therapists 2003)

This definition is significant, as it considers the role of the occupational therapist in relation to the environment, an area of increasing relevance in contemporary practice.

The WFOT (2003) provides a further 37 definitions of occupational therapy that have been developed by its national member associations. Reviewing comparative definitions of occupational therapy, it is apparent that there is substantial consensus of opinion regarding the definition of occupational therapy. National differences appear more reflective of the differing layers of complexity considered rather than significant differences of opinion.

Defining the skills of an occupational therapist

The skills of an occupational therapist are many and varied, and are often presented in seemingly simple ways. This is both the profession's strength and greatest challenge. A key skill of an occupational therapist is their ability to bring an occupational perspective, in terms of both a person's ability and their identity, to the therapeutic context. Within this context, occupational therapists work with client's strengths and address areas of occupational dysfunction. To achieve this, occupational therapists use a range of skills: core, shared (sometimes referred to as 'generic') and specialist.

Core skills in occupational therapy

> The 'core' of an object is it most important part. From there everything else develops. (Schwartz 1994)

If an uninformed observer were to witness the work of occupational therapists from different specialties, their initial impression might be, at least on a superficial level, that they have little in common. Therapists working in social services, mental health and physical rehabiliation often appear, at first glance, to be doing different things. In all honesty, it must be admitted that at times they are — practice in some areas has lost its focus. This, however, is not how it should be.

Defining practice and developing a shared understanding of a profession's key competencies and processes are vital to its development. Mosey was perhaps the first theorist to tackle the concept of core skills in occupational therapy rigorously

(Mosey 1986). Within the UK, the 1990s witnessed considerable interest and effort invested in further identifying and describing occupational therapy's core skills (Thorner 1991, Renton 1992, Hollis 1993a,b, Hollis & Clark 1993, Phillips & Renton 1995). The reason that such discussion was stimulated is reflective of the complexity of occupational therapy and the multi-layered components of each skill.

The COT outlined seven core skills (College of Occupational Therapists 2004a):

- collaboration with the client
- assessment
- enablement
- problem-solving
- using activity as a therapeutic tool
- group work
- environmental adaptation (Creek 2003).

Hagedorn recognized the complexity of occupational therapy and the difficulties that are faced when attempting to define the core skills of the profession, stating that:

> Our core competencies and processes must somehow encompass the nebulous aspects of professional judgment and reasoning, problem solving and research as well as the 'hands on' forms of therapeutic knowledge and skill … This exercise will probably demonstrate that it is far from easy to untangle the things which are *only* done by occupational therapists from those which many other professions may do. (Hagedorn 2001, p.34)

Analysis and adaptation of occupations

The analysis of occupations and their use in therapy has also been recognized as a core skill of the occupational therapist (Hagedorn 2001). The analysis and prescription of occupations have two purposes:

- to deal with problems experienced by the client in all aspects of their everyday life — frequently classified as work, leisure and self-care
- the use of occupations as specific therapeutic interventions to address occupational perfomance difficulties and assist in the development of a positive occupational identity.

Activity analysis involves dissection of an occupational form into its component parts (tasks) and sequence, looking at its stable and situational components and evaluating its therapeutic potential. In doing so, it finds or adjusts an occupation for therapeutic benefit and enables a person to engage or re-engage in some form of occupation (Kielhofner & Forsyth 2009). Occupational therapists carry out activity analysis in order to consider:

- the kind(s) of performance needed to achieve the occupational form, e.g. cognitive, motor, physical, interpersonal (the headings used for detailed analysis will depend on the selected conceptual model or frame of reference)
- the degree of complexity of the activity
- the social or cultural associations
- defining the component tasks of which the occupational form is composed
- analysing the sequence of task performance and whether this is fixed or flexible
- defining the tools, furniture, materials and environment required for completion of the occupational form
- defining and taking account of safety precautions or risk factors.

Environmental analysis and adaptation

This is another skill used in a way that is core to occupational therapy practice. Occupational therapists recognize that the physical and social environments can have an important beneficial or detrimental effect on the individual. Environmental analysis may provide information on the causes of problems for the individual, explanations for behaviour or ideas or suggestions for therapeutic adaptation.

As conceptual models of practice have developed within occupational therapy, core skills have become increasingly linked to theory. Conceptual models can provide assessment(s) and taxonomies that assist in the detailed and structured analysis of occupations (see Kielhofner & Forsyth 2009 and Chapter 6 for an example of this). Frames of reference provide theoretical frameworks to support the therapeutic use of self (read Chapters 6–8 for further information).

Shared skills

It is acknowledged that, as well as their core skills, each occupational therapist has a variety of shared skills. Whilst shared, these skills are no less essential to practice. Occupational therapists draw on the wealth of assessments and interventions that have not been developed by occupational therapists but facilitate the development of occupational performance and assist in the creation of a greater occupational self-identity.

The use of interventions that are not occupational therapy-specific is a contentious topic, as the profession becomes ever more deeply occupation-focused. Do non-occupational therapy-specific interventions have a place in the profession today? Several of the chapters in this book address this issue, either directly or indirectly.

Occupational therapists have a range of shared skills. Some of the most central are described below.

Leadership and management

Often placed together, leadership and management are two important but distinct skills.

Management

Occupational therapists have to manage services, a case load, an academic department or research team resources, and, importantly, themselves. The therapist needs to set standards, monitor quality and audit performance. These findings need to be communicated within the profession and to others. The therapist must be critically aware of their performance, seeking regular supervision and evaluating and updating personal knowledge. Management is not, therefore, a skill that is the remit of the head of a service, but the responsibility of all staff, albeit in differing ways. Furthermore, as well as managing others, therapists must also be able to manage themselves. Self-management consists of the actions and strategies we use to direct our own activity and ensure that we remain fit for purpose at work and at home. Bannigan (2009) describes the importance of self-management and the development of professional resilience in the face of the many challenges that arise in the workplace.

Leadership

Leadership is different from management. Whilst management has been defined as the 'bottom line ... how can I best accomplish things', leadership has been defined as knowing 'what are the things I want to accomplish' (Covey 1989, p.101). Leaders in occupational therapy develop innovative approaches to intervention, work with clients in new ways, spot opportunities and develop services. The historical view of management and leadership as components of the same role is increasingly recognized as ineffectual. Indeed, the developing roles of consultant and clinical specialist occupational therapists (within the UK) appears to recognize that certain career pathways offer and require particular leadership qualities. Managing a service is an alternative professional pathway. Therefore, the leader of an occupational therapy team is not necessarily the manager, but may be a senior clinician with the vision and skills to move the service forward. Developing as a leader, however, is more than merely a professional skill; it is a personal and professional quality.

An awareness of one's need for continuous self-improvement and openness to others' perspectives of our own leadership qualities is essential. Whilst everyone will have their own leadership style, lots can be learned from other people. Often the best way to start devloping this quality is to observe leaders you admire (both within and outside the profession), taking a bird's-eye view of their practice/life. What do they do that makes you admire them? How do they deal with other people? How do they deal with themselves? What is their vision? How do they maintain their integrity in difficult situations? Conversely, the same exercise can be carried out with individuals whose practice you may not like to emulate! Reflect on these observations and consider any lessons that can be learnt. What would you wish to integrate into your practice/life?

As well as observation, a lot can be learnt from the wealth of literature that is available on this subject (e.g. Covey 1989, Goleman et al 2002). Christiansen (2009) writes on leadership with direct reference to leadership in occupational therapy. Ultimately, however, leadership qualities are lived, developed and refined over a lifetime.

Therapeutic use of self

The therapeutic use of self is arguably one of the most important skills a therapist has. Mosey (1986) describes an occupational therapist's use of self as a concsious therapeutic tool and suggests that there is a difference between a spontaneous interaction that is unplanned and a planned interaction that, whilst appearing spontaneous, is guided and informed. Yarwood and Johnstone (2002) suggest four issues that essentially relate to the therapeutic use of self and the development of a therapeutic relationship:

- 'Establish rapport;
- Respect the wishes of the client;
- Use honesty and strive to develop a collaborative approach; and
- Adapt to communicate effectively with all kinds of people' (p.327).

Occupational therapists have adopted various theoretical frameworks that assist in the development of the therapeutic use of self in differing ways. These include the client-centred, the cognitive behavioural and the psychodynamic frames of reference (see Chapters 11, 12 and 13 for further information).

Research

Research is a central component of occupational therapy practice (Ilott & White 2001) and the emphasis on research is arguably the single most significant development that has occurred in occupational therapy in the last 20 years (Duncan 2009). Every occupational therapist is required to use skills in research. This does not mean that every occupational therapist must carry out independent research, but at the very least everyone should be effective and critical consumers of research (Ilott & White 2001). The skills required to do this include:

- information and communication technology skills, to search and locate the literature
- critical appraisal skills, to evaluate research
- development of a personal evaluative perspective, to challenge custom and practice
- ability to integrate research into practice, in order to deliver consistently the highest quality of service available.

Specialist skills

Specialist skills are skills that cannot be expected of a competent clinician without further training, supervision and expertise (Duncan 1999). Occupational therapists can develop specialist skills that are either an extension of their core skills, such as specialist assessments (e.g. the Assessment of Motor and Process Skills (AMPS); Fisher 1997), or an extension of their shared skills, such as undertaking advanced splinting or psychotherapy training (Duncan 1999).

Defining the occupational therapy process

The occupational therapy process is the name given to the series of actions a therapist initiates in order to provide services to their client. This process is clearly not unique to occupational therapy. It is a form of problem analysis and solution that has been used by various healthcare professionals. There have been several representations of the process in occupational therapy, each differing a little from the others in accordance with each author's personal concept of the sequence. Generally, there is close agreement on the basic format. This involves gathering information concerning the client, their situation and challenges, carrying out assessments, identifying and formulating the problem or need, setting goals, setting consequent priorities for action, deciding on how to achieve these, implementing action and evaluating the outcome. Creek (2003) illustrates this process in a linear model (Fig. 4.1). Hagedorn (2001) uses similar points but illustrates the process's cyclical nature (Fig. 4.2). In practice, the occupational therapy process is often not linear (Creek 2003) or even cyclical. Frequently, these activities occur in synchrony and are repeated at various stages of therapy. The process is therefore circuitous, with overlapping and interwoven aspects of the process occurring throughout.

As shown in Figure 4.2, a referral is received by the therapist. This starts the intervention sequence. The therapist will then enter the cycle of information-gathering and problem analysis, decision-making, implementation of action and review of outcome, which is repeated until intervention is judged to be completed.

Throughout this process, the occupational therapist employs the unique combination of knowledge, skills and values that form the practice of occupational therapy. The way in which this happens is often informed and directed by conceptual models of practice and frames of reference, several of which are outlined in Chapters 6–14.

Assessment

Why assess?

Assessment is the gathering of relevant information that informs the prioritization and development of clinical goals for intervention. Assessments also assist in measuring change during interventions and evaluation of interventions at their conclusion. All assessment procedures require a basis of theoretical knowledge and practical experience and expertise. There are several basic skills required to carry out effective assessments:

- clinical judgement of what is to be assessed
- decision-making regarding the most appropriate assessment methods to use
- objectivity
- good observation skills

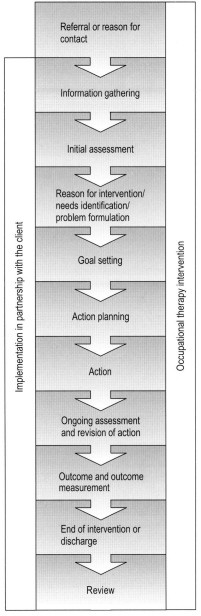

Fig. 4.1 • The occupational therapy process viewed linearly. Reproduced by permission of the College of Occupational Therapists from Creek 2003.

- production of consistent, accurate and, where possible, replicable results
- communicating results clearly to others
- client sensitivity.

Assessment should be recognized as a means to an end — identification of the problem; definition of a starting point for intervention; measurement of

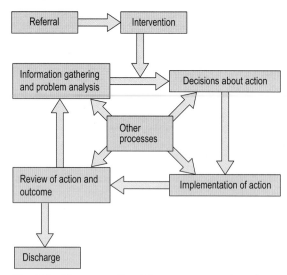

Fig. 4.2 • The occupational therapy process viewed cyclically.

- self-report or checklists — e.g. to provide a client perspective
- performance tests — e.g. of physical or cognitive ability
- measurement techniques — e.g. of physical performance.

In practice, a combination of these methods is often used; observation may be combined with interview, a structured assessment with an unstructured assessment. Therapists may interview a client, watch them carry out a task or occupational form, and ask them to complete a checklist or self-report instrument. Frequently, some of these assessments will be unstructured. Recently, a structured approach to multiple data-gathering has developed. The Model of Human Occupation (see Chapter 6) has developed some structured assessments that utilize a combined method of assessment. This is an innovative approach to structured assessment, as the use of mutiple methods causes statistical challenges in developing the reliability of the assessment. These assessments represent a useful addition to the repertoire of available assessments.

progress; evaluation of outcome. As well as assessing an individual's ability, it is also important to assess the context in which they are carrying out the task — the environment.

Environmental assessment

The way in which an environmental analysis is carried out depends on both the needs of the client and the conceptual model/frame of reference within which the therapist is working, as these will alter the significance of the components that are observed.

In general terms, the occupational therapist will observe and accurately record the physical environment (e.g. buildings, interiors, heat, light, sound) and the social environment (e.g. How many people are in the environment? What is the nature of the relationships? How supportive are they? and so on) that contribute to or detract from a client's performance and positive occupational identity.

How do you assess?

Assessments can be carried out in either a structured or an unstructured manner; depending on their aim, both can be valid (Kielhofner & Forsyth 2008). Using either structured or unstructured procedures, assessment information can be gathered through a variety of methods:

- observation — e.g. of a client performing an *occupational form*
- interview — e.g. with the client or relevant others

Unstructured assessment

Unstructured assessments are also referred to as informal, ad hoc or unstandardized. Many unstructured assessments are constructed by occupational therapists who may have developed them to meet local needs. Whilst unstructured assessments can never provide the reliability of structured assessments, several reasons exist that can justify their use:

- lack of an appropriate structured assessment
- lack of acceptability of structured assessments to a client
- use of unstructured assessments to add to information previously gained through structured assessment
- lack of time to complete a structured assessment
- structured assessments not available at an unforeseen opportunity to gather more information (Kielhofner & Forsyth 2008).

Structured assessment

Structured or standardized assessments have been rigorously developed over a period of time and are designed to be dependable. Two specific issues are of particular importance in the development and appraisal of a structured assessment: validity and reliability.

Validity

Validity concerns whether the assessment actually deals with matters that are appropriate to the situation and measures the right things. There are various different forms of validity (Oppenheim 1992):

- *Face validity*. Does the assessment look as if it does the things it is supposed to?
- *Concurrent validity*. Does the assessment gather relevant and associated information?
- *Predictive validity*. Can reliable conclusions be drawn from the assessment's findings?

Depending on the focus of the assessment, a structured assessment may require more than one form of validity to be evaluated in its development and appraisal. Furthermore, an assessment's validity grows with each study that develops its evidence base.

Reliability

Reliability means that you can be sure that, each time the test is used, the findings can be depended upon. Fundamentally, there are two forms of reliability:

- *Test–retest reliability*. The assessment is repeated and the same findings result.
- *Inter-rater reliability*. The assessment is repeated by different therapists, with the same result.

There are numerous structured assessments on the market. Several of them are discussed in this text. Whilst many structured assessments can be used by all qualified occupational therapists, there are some that require specific further training (e.g. AMPS; Fisher 1997).

Goal-setting

Having assessed the client and formed a professional perspective of a person's priorities and needs, it is important to set collaborative goals for intervention. 'Goals are targets that the client hopes to reach through involvement in occupational therapy' (Creek 2002, p.129). Developing goals is a vital component of the occupational therapy process. However, as Wade (2009) clearly states, 'setting goals with patients and monitoring their achievement is a core practice within much of rehabilitation, but the evidence base behind this practice is patchy' (Wade 2009, p.291). Despite such a lack of evidence, and in anticipation of greater clarity regarding its effectiveness as an intervention, goal-setting is likely to remain a central feature of practice. Park (2009) provides a good overview of the goal-setting process in occupational therapy. Without goals, neither client nor therapist can have any idea of when to finish their intervention or develop new goals. This, however, does not mean that goals cannot be amended during the therapeutic process. It may be that the initial goals were either too easy or too ambitious and a reappraisal is required.

Developing goals

Fundamentally, two types of goal exist:

- *Long-term goals*. These are the major goals, the final destination where both client and therapist view therapy as having been successful. Long-term goals are also referred to within the literature as 'aims' (Foster 2002).
- *Short-term goals*. These are the more immediate goals of therapy, the stepping stones to achieving the longer-term goal or aim. Short-term goals often form the component parts of a longer-term goal (e.g. making a cup of tea may be a short-term goal leading to independent meal preparation). In order to maintain motivation and build upon skill development, short-term goals are often developed in a hierarchical structure (Creek 2002).

Creek (2002) also refers to the development of intermediate goals, defined as 'clusters of skills to be developed or barriers to be overcome on the way to achieving the main goals of therapy' (p.122). Creek's (2002) rationale for intermediate goals is that the long-term goal may appear too distant or challenging, and the setting of intermediate goals provides a more realistic or achievable option.

Agreeing goals

Involvement of clients in the decision-making process surrounding setting goals is crucial. Neistadt (1995) found that clients who participated in the development of their goals made statistically and clinically significant gains in their performance ability.

Whilst structured methods for developing goals exist (Ottenbacher & Cusick 1990), the majority of therapists develop their own goals without using such procedures. It has, however, been suggested that such decision support aids are a useful component of therapy (Barclay 2002). The advantages of decision support aids in the development of short- and long-term goals constitute an area that deserves further research and evaluation.

Regardless of whether a structured method of setting goals is used or not, goals should be measurable and clear to all parties. An example of an unclear goal would be 'eat more healthily', whilst a clearer and more measurable goal might read 'be able to prepare and cook four separate meals using at least five different vegetables and including either chicken or fish'.

Interventions

Therapy, treatment and intervention are largely synonymous terms; however, each suggests certain philosophical beliefs about the position and role of the client in relation to the therapist. For example, the term 'treatment' suggests a largely passive experience where a person is done to instead of done with. The term 'intervention' is preferred in this text, as it recognizes the intrusion (however welcome) in a person's life and indicates a broadly based form of service provision. In one of the UK's earliest theoretical texts on occupational therapy, it was suggested that the range of occupational forms that could be used for therapeutic intentions was infinite. Of greater importance was the aim of their use and whether this was suitable and achievable (MacDonald 1960). This perspective remains as true today as it did then.

Application of occupational forms as therapy

The selection of an occupational form as a therapeutic intervention requires that a balance be achieved between the needs and interests of the client, the personal repertoire of skills possessed by the therapist, and the requirements of the conceptual model or frame of reference within which the therapist chooses to work. Occupational forms should be specifically selected for the individual client in respect of the developed goals.

Occupational forms may be used casually for recreation or as pastimes; such use is perfectly valid in the right context; however, their use in this way is diversional occupation, not occupational therapy.

Adapting occupational forms

The occupational form may be presented in an unadapted manner or may be adapted to meet the specified goals. Types of adaptation that may be required to assist the client to achieve their goals include:

- *environmental*, e.g. location, setting, milieu
- *equipment*, e.g. quantity of tools/materials, adaptation to tools
- *social*, e.g. number of people, degree of interaction
- *physical*, e.g. position, strength, range of movement
- *cognitive*, e.g. complexity, sequence, need for instructions
- *emotional*, e.g. interest, meaning, self-expression
- *temporal*, e.g. duration, repetition
- *structural*, e.g. order of tasks, omission of non-essential tasks.

The amended factors of an occupational form can then be graded over time to increase the client's occupational performance and development of a positive occupational identity.

Environmental context of interventions

Interventions can occur in a client's natural environment (such as their home or community), in proximate environments (such as a group home/hostel or a local community near their current residency) or in artificial environments (such as hospitals or prisons). Within these settings, interventions may take place in various forms of group setting (whether naturally occuring groups such as a football team, or artificial groups such as an on-ward cooking group) or individually.

Environmental adaptation

The therapist may suggest adapting, removing or adding to elements of the physical environment — e.g. physical features of buildings, access, sound, colour, lighting level, temperature, decor, furniture, information content — in order to remove obstacles to performance or to enhance the opportunities for performance, learning or development. Occupational therapists should also consider adapting the social environment (i.e. the groups of people that a person is involved with in their environment), as these can also postively or negatively affect the client in achieving their goals.

Specific interventions are shaped and influenced by the frames of reference and conceptual models of practice that guide them. Interventions from each of these theoretical constructs are described in detail in the following chapters.

Evaluation

Evaluating the effectiveness of occupational therapy is an ethical and professional imperative.

Individual evaluation

Evaluation is the method by which the client, therapist and other relevant individuals (such as carers) or bodies (such as the multidisciplinary team) know if the agreed goals have been met. Whilst evaluation is an ongoing process throughout therapy, it is the final evaluation that is often most significant. Measuring 'success' is often achieved using the same assessment measures employed at the initial and on-going assessment and looking for significant changes in the desired direction. Evaluation can also be measured by examining whether the specified goals have been met and by discussing the client's perspective of the situation.

Service evaluation

As well as evaluating individual client's interventions, occupational therapists can and should periodically evaluate their service as a whole. Several mechanisms can be used to assist in this process.

Reviewing existing service strategy

The service strategy (or a document with a similar title and aim) outlines an occupational therapy service's aims, guiding philosophy and objectives. This is an important document, which can be appropriately adapted to communicate the workings of an occupational therapy service to clients, carers, new members of staff, other members of staff not engaged in occupational therapy, students and the public. Service strategies should include:

- an executive summary
- historical background to the service
- current strategic drivers (e.g. relevant national, professional and local policies)
- the vision for the service (aim, philosophy of care, clinical perspective/conceptual model of practice used etc.)
- specific objectives against which the service can be measured.

Audit service against existing standards

These may be clinical standards set by national organizations (e.g. the National Institute for Health and Clinical Excellence (NICE) or Quality Improvement Scotland (QIS)) or standards set by professional bodies such as COT (College of Occupational Therapists 2004b) or AOTA (American Occupational Therapy Association 2005).

Gaining feedback from clients who have used the service

This could be achieved through either questionnaire or interview procedures.

Gaining feedback from colleagues

This can also be achieved through either questionnaire or interview procedures.

Summary

This chapter has explored the theoretical foundations of what occupational therapists 'do'. Differing definitions of occupational therapy were presented and referred to. It is recognized that each definition holds a commonly shared vision of the profession.

Occupational therapy's apparent simplicity is both its strength and its greatest challenge. This chapter's brief review of an occupational therapist's skills and the component parts of the occupational therapy process illustrates that, whilst occupational therapy interventions are not always complex in the technical sense of the word (Duncan et al 2007), they can certainly be multi-factorial and challenging to describe. Perhaps it is for this reason that the challenging nature of delivering sophisticated occupational therapy interventions is not always immediately apparent to those who observe them but do not appreciate the process at work.

Reflective learning

- What do you consider to be the key skills you use in practice? How aware of them are you when you use them?
- How do you choose which method of assessment to use with each client?
- Have you seen or do you use goal-setting in practice? What are its strengths and limitations?
- How do you evaluate your practice?

References

American Occupational Therapy Association, 2005. Standards of Practice for Occupational Therapy. http://www.aota.org/general/otsp.asp (accessed 25.01.05).

Bannigan, K., 2009. Management of self. In: Duncan, E.A.S. (Ed.), Skills for Practice in Occupational Therapy. Churchill Livingstone, Edinburgh, pp. 231–248.

Barclay, L., 2002. Exploring the factors that influence the goal setting process for occupational therapy intervention with an individual with spinal cord injury. Australian Journal of Occupational Therapy 49, 3–13.

Christiansen, C., 2009. Leadership skills. In: Duncan, E.A.S. (Ed.), Skills for Practice in Occupational Therapy. Churchill Livingstone, Edinburgh, pp. 313–322.

College of Occupational Therapists, 2004a. Definitions and Core Skills for Occupational Therapy. College of Occupational Therapists, London.

College of Occupational Therapists, 2004b. Professional Standards for Occupational Therapy Practice. College of Occupational Therapists, London.

Covey, S., 1989. The 7 Habits of Highly Effective People. Simon & Schuster, London.

Creek, J., 2002. Treatment planning and implementation. In: Creek, J. (Ed.), Occupational Therapy in Mental Health, third ed. Churchill Livingstone, Edinburgh, pp. 119–138.

Creek, J., 2003. Occupational Therapy Defined as a Complex Intervention. College of Occupational Therapists, London.

Duncan, E.A.S., 1999. Occupational therapy in mental health: it is time to recognise that it has come of age. British Journal of Occupational Therapy 62 (11), 521–522.

Duncan, E.A.S., 2009. Developing research in practice. In: Duncan, E.A.S. (Ed.), Skills for Practice in Occupational Therapy. Churchill Livingstone, Edinburgh, pp. 279–292.

Duncan, E.A.S., Paley, J., Eva, G., 2007. Complex interventions and complex systems in occupational therapy.

British Journal of Occupational Therapy 70 (5), 199–206.

Fisher, A., 1997. Assessment of Motor and Process Skills. Three Star, Fort Collins.

Foster, M., 2002. Skills for practice. In: Turner, A., Foster, M., Johnson, E.S. (Eds.), Occupational Therapy and Physical Dysfunction: Principles, Skills and Practice. Churchill Livingstone, Edinburgh, pp. 85–105.

Goleman, D., Boyatzis, R.E., McKee, A., 2002. Primal Leadership: Realizing the Power of Emotional Intelligence. Harvard Business School, Harvard.

Hagedorn, R., 2001. Foundations for Practice in Occupational Therapy. Churchill Livingstone, Edinburgh.

Hollis, V., 1993a. Core skills and competencies: what is experience? Part 1. British Journal of Occupational Therapy 56 (2), 48–50.

Hollis, V., 1993b. Core skills and competencies: application and expectation. British Journal of Occupational Therapy 56 (5), 181–184.

Hollis, V., Clark, C.R., 1993. Core skills and competencies: the competency conundrum. Part 2. British Journal of Occupational Therapy 56 (3), 102–106.

Ilott, I., White, E., 2001. College of Occupational Therapists research and development strategic vision and action plan. British Journal of Occupational Therapy 64 (6), 270–277.

Kielhofner, G., Forsyth, K., 2008. Assessment: choosing and using structured and unstructured means of gathering information. In: Kielhofner, G. (Ed.), Model of Human Occupation: Theory and Application, fourth ed. Lippincott Williams & Wilkins, Baltimore, pp. 155–170.

Kielhofner, G., Forsyth, K., 2009. Activity analysis. In: Duncan, E.A.S. (Ed.), Skills for Practice in Occupational Therapy. Churchill Livingstone, Edinburgh, pp. 91–104.

MacDonald, E.M., 1960. Occupational Therapy in Rehabilitation. Baillière, Tindall & Cox, London.

Mosey, A.C., 1986. Psychosocial Components of Occupational Therapy. Raven, New York.

Neistadt, M.E., 1995. Methods of assessing clients' priorities: a survey of adult physical dysfunction settings. American Journal of Occupational Therapy 49, 428–436.

Oppenheim, A.N., 1992. Questionnaire Design. Interviewing and Attitude Measurement. Continuum, London.

Ottenbacher, K.J., Cusick, A., 1990. Goal attainment scaling as a method of service evaluation. American Journal of Occupational Therapy 44. 519–525.

Park, S., 2009. Goal Setting in Occupational Therapy: a client centred perspective. In: Duncan, E. (Ed.), Skills for Practice in Occupational Therapy 105–122.

Phillips, N., Renton, L., 1995. Is assessment of function the core of occupational therapy? British Journal of Occupational Therapy 58 (2), 72–74.

Renton, L.B.M., 1992. Occupational therapy core skills in mental handicap: a review of the literature. British Journal of Occupational Therapy 55 (11), 424–428.

Schwartz, C., 1994. Chambers Dictionary. Chambers, Edinburgh.

Thorner, S., 1991. The essential skills of an occupational therapist. British Journal of Occupational Therapy 54 (6), 222–223.

Wade, D., 2009. Goal setting in rehabilitation: an overview of what, why and how. Clinical Rehabilitation 23, 291–295.

World Federation of Occupational Therapists, 2003. Definitions of Occupational Therapy. http://www.wfot.org.au/Document_Centre/default.cfm (accessed 25.01.05).

Yarwood, L., Johnstone, V., 2002. Acute psychiatry. In: Creek, J. (Ed.), Occupational Therapy and Mental Health, third ed. Churchill Livingstone, Edinburgh, pp. 317–333.

An introduction to conceptual models of practice and frames of reference

5

Edward A.S. Duncan

OVERVIEW

This chapter provides an introduction to frames of reference and conceptual models of practice within occupational therapy. It commences by exploring the rationale for having theoretical constructs in practice. It continues by examining the challenges that theoretical terminology has posed occupational therapists, before defining key terms used in this text. The proliferation of frames of reference and conceptual models of practice is then discussed and a guide for future theoretical development and evaluation presented. Following this, the relationship between conceptual models of practice and frames of reference in this text is explained.

Key points

This chapter:
- introduces conceptual models of practice and frames of reference
- emphasizes the importance of language and understanding theoretical terminology
- discusses the development of theory in occupational therapy
- examines the stages of theoretical development of conceptual models of practice.

Why have frames of reference or conceptual models of practice?

Imagine the following scenario. After a few weeks of feeling unwell, you consult your doctor, who decides that you should go to see a consultant surgeon. Your consultation goes as follows:

You: Doctor, I haven't felt well for several weeks. My stomach's upset. I've lost my appetite and some weight, and I don't feel that I have the same energy and get up and go that I normally have.

Consultant surgeon: I see. Well, I tell you what . . . why don't I do some tests?

You: What are you testing for?

Consultant surgeon: Not sure, really. I have a few personal favourite tests that I've used a lot. Did I tell you I've been qualified for over 20 years? So I think I'll use those and see what they show up. I reckon I know what I'm going to do anyway.

How would you feel leaving this consultation? It probably wouldn't engender much confidence that your health was being considered in a structured, evidence-based manner.

It is difficult to come up with 'answers' in healthcare, and all the more so in professions such as occupational therapy that have inherently broad aims. However, it is known that professionals' individual perspectives are highly vulnerable to a range of biases and heuristics when making clinical judgements (Gilovich et al 2002), regardless of their clinical 'expertise'. It is also true that experience and 'time served' as a practitioner are fairly consistently shown to have no effect on improving clinical judgements (Grove & Meehl 1996, Grove et al 2000). Knowledge of such inherent limitations of individual perspectives supports the acceptance and development of evidence-based decision-making approaches to therapeutic interventions. Frames of reference and conceptual models of practice are an ideal way in which clinicians can use theory, in a structured manner, to conceptualize clients' difficulties, shape intervention and evaluate success. Using a well-developed frame of reference and/or conceptual model of practice encourages therapists to consider a whole range of options that they would perhaps be less likely to do if left to their own devices.

In her review of the history of occupational therapy in the UK, Wilcock (2001) attributes the first use of the terms 'frame of reference' and 'model' to Miss McLean, an American occupational therapist working as a lecturer in England (McClean 1974). McClean's rationale for the development of a structured theory to underpin occupational therapy practice was financial. Hospital management, McClean (1974) argued, was no longer willing to tolerate therapeutic interventions for reasons of enjoyment alone. The requirement to demonstrate the value of practice had dawned and the development of theories, McClean suggested, would enable the evaluation of practice and research to be undertaken (McClean 1974). In today's world of clinical governance and evidence-based practice, finance remains a dominant driver in the development of theory. It is certainly true, now more than ever, that the demonstration of effectiveness is of vital importance — not only for the good of the patients who receive the service, but also for the good of the profession as it faces increasingly probing questions about its worth in a financially challenging climate.

Structured theories develop out of a desire to explain the function and mechanisms of impact of occupational therapy, and help explain why a person is experiencing a particular problem, what a potential solution could be and why a particular intervention works. Structured theories provide explanations and describe the relationship between different aspects of a person (Kielhofner 2009). Theories also identify occupational therapy's unique contribution to health and assist in defining professional boundaries (Feaver & Creek 1993b).

Supporting the use of structured theory in practice does not negate the requirements for occupational therapists to use their judgement. Occupational therapists have to decide which conceptual model provides the best evidence base and supporting structure for the setting in which they work. Sometimes this will be self-evident; it is highly unlikely that a psychodynamic frame of reference would be a useful *primary* frame of reference in an orthopaedic ward; the occupational therapist is more likely to use a biomechanical frame of reference and an associated conceptual model of practice. At other times, however, the case may not be so clear and a careful appraisal of the available evidence is required to inform theoretical decisions and the directions of practice.

Defining and understanding theoretical terminology

Having articulated the rationale for having a structured theoretical basis for practice, we must now examine the importance of developing a clear understanding of the key terms that are used to articulate them. This is not straightforward as 'different writers use them [theoretical terms] in different ways and their meaning is modified by the context in which they are used' (Feaver & Creek 1993a, p.4).

The description of occupational therapy theory rapidly evolved from the mid-1980s on. Contemporaneously, the language that described theory developed and terms such as *paradigm*, *model*, *frame of reference* and *approach* were often used interchangeably and with different meanings by various authors (e.g. Reed 1984, Mosey 1986, Creek 1992, Kielhofner 1992, Young & Quinn 1992, Hopkins & Smith 1993). Such variation adds considerably to the confusion of clinicians, students and academics who try to understand and evaluate contrasting conceptual foundations of practice. Hagedorn (2001) likened the struggle to understand the various uses of terminology in occupational therapy to the following discourse between Alice in Wonderland and Humpty Dumpty (Lewis Carroll, *Alice Through the Looking Glass*):

> 'There's glory for you!'
>
> 'I don't know what you mean by "glory",' Alice said.
>
> 'I meant, "there's a nice knock-down argument for you!"'
>
> 'But "glory" doesn't mean "a nice knock-down argument",' Alice objected.
>
> 'When *I* use a word,' Humpty Dumpty said in a rather scornful tone, 'it means just what I choose it to mean — neither more nor less.'

Whilst the debate about the 'correct' use of terminology appears to have abated, it is important to remain mindful that specific terms are still being used by different people in different ways. One solution to this is the development of internationally recognized standard definitions of theoretical terms and concepts. However, whilst this is a tempting proposal, it is questionable whether it could be meaningfully achieved. Differences in definitions of terminology are not simply semantic; they frequently expose an author's conceptual bias. By way of example, two contemporary definitions of 'models', developed by theoretical leaders in the field, are provided here. Creek (2003, p. 55) defines a model as a *'simplified representation* of the structure and content of a phenomenon or system that describes or explains certain data or relationships and integrates elements of theory and practice', whilst Forsyth and Kielhofner (2005, p. 91) highlight how 'the strength and application of MOHO [a well-known conceptual model of practice] is *neither simple nor formulaic*. Instead it aims to understand important multiple dimensions of each client's unique experience and bring a sophisticated understanding to bear on the life issues facing each client in practice' (author's emphasis added).

These contrasting contemporary definitions of models of practice illustrate:

- the reason why a universally defined shared terminology is unlikely to work
- the continuing importance of truly understanding the perspective of an author(s) when reading and appraising literature relating to occupational therapy theory and practice.

Whilst theory should never be presented as unnecessarily complicated, neither should its inherent complexity be watered down towards an unachievable simplicity. Theoretical terminology is important; it defines key terms and enables the succinct communication of complex ideas. However, terminology can require effort to understand. It is easy to become disheartened when faced with a massive amount of new theoretical 'language' to grapple with. As a result, some students and clinicians may venture no further with such texts. This elective loss of knowledge is not simply a personal issue; one's professional capacity is also diminished through a lack of engagement with the profession's rich knowledge base. Students, clinicians and academics are therefore encouraged to grapple with their frustration (if they have any) and engage with theoretical terminology where it exists, in both this text and others. The investment of time and reflective thought, as well as discussions with peers and colleagues, will all assist in further understanding the concepts that are being communicated. If you sustain your engagement with such literature, you will encounter a wealth of knowledge that you would otherwise have left undiscovered.

Theoretical definitions used in this book

In order to give meaning to the structure of this book and to assist the reader in following the arguments and propositions contained within, it is necessary to define some key theoretical terms. Where possible, these definitions have been adhered to throughout the text. In defining theoretical terms, consideration has been given to lessening confusion by providing clear and (hopefully) uncontroversial taxonomy. Some terminology has already been introduced in the preceding chapter; however, it is repeated here for clarity.

- *Paradigm.* The shared consensus regarding the most fundamental beliefs of the profession.
- *Frame of reference.* Theoretical or conceptual ideas that have been developed outside the profession but which, with judicious use, are applicable within occupational therapy practice.
- *Conceptual model of practice.* Occupation-focused theoretical constructs and propositions that have been developed specifically to explain the process and practice of occupational therapy.

Occupational therapy's theoretical proliferation

The development of formalized theory came relatively late in the genesis of occupational therapy. Whilst its development is welcomed, the manner in which it has occurred has, perhaps, not always been helpful. One example of this is the variance in theoretical depth of some of the profession's 'models' of practice.

Hagedorn (2001, p.131) outlined 11 person–environment–occupational performance models (termed conceptual models of practice in this current edition). Some of these were based on ongoing research; others represented the perspectives of an individual or a small group of occupational therapists at a particular moment in time. Whilst the publication of scholarly debate on occupational therapy's theory base is invaluable, the proliferation of personal perspectives shaped as nascent conceptual models of practice does not meaningfully support the development of occupational therapy's knowledge base and can increase confusion amongst clinicians and students in an already complex field.

Conversely, occupational therapy should not necessarily be limited to the few conceptual models or frames of reference that have an established evidence base. The profession's theoretical development would be poorer if the above call for rationalization of personal conceptual models was understood as an attempt to stifle novel ideas and innovations. New conceptual models of practice/frames of reference, which recognize or perceive limitations in existing theories or practice and aim to address these, should be welcomed. They will enhance the knowledge base and encourage greater debate and understanding within the profession. However, these developments should contain sound theoretical arguments and vision of future development.

Kielhofner (2009) suggests that sustained development of a conceptual model of practice is required to ensure that its theoretical constructs are valid and useful. Furthermore, as well as providing a theoretical structure, a conceptual model of practice should also develop appropriate assessments and technology (e.g. intervention protocols) for use in practice (Kielhofner 2009). As such developments require to be gradually developed and tested, it is perhaps useful to consider what the developmental stages of a conceptual model of practice should be.

Proposed stages of theoretical development

The following stages are based on a review of conceptual models to date and outline a proposed developmental sequence that illustrates the required developmental stages of contemporary conceptual models of practice. Frames of reference, as applied knowledge, are likely to have undergone a similar process within their original knowledge base. The process of integrating frames of reference is therefore different and is referred to throughout this text (see Chapters 6–10).

Whilst the developmental stages of conceptual models of practice suggest a general progression, it is acknowledged that some of these stages may occur simultaneously.

Develop initial conceptual ideas

- Why is a new theoretical construct necessary?
- Form a basis for a new theoretical perspective.
- What are the factors that differentiate this construct from existing conceptual models?

Refine conceptual ideas

- Present the conceptual model to the occupational therapy community.
- Work with others (academics, clinicians and clients) to refine ideas and understandings.
- Continue to present refinements for critical appraisal and debate.

Test theory in practice

- This can be achieved through the use of a variety of research methods to examine the validity of the developing theories' claims in practice situations.

Develop tools for practice (technology for application) (Kielhofner 2009)

- Develop self-report assessments, interview schedules, observation measures etc.
- Develop protocols that support the clinician to enable them to use the information they gain using the model and associated tools to assist the client.

Increase the evidence base for the conceptual model

- Refine the theoretical arguments and understanding on the basis of research carried out in clinical settings.
- Build the evidence base for the validity, reliability and utility of the conceptual model and its associated tools for practice.

Verify the conceptual modal and associated tools for practice externally

- Theoretical constructs are rigorously tested by people with no personal bias as regards their success or failure.
- The tools for practice are evaluated by people with no personal bias as to their success or failure.
- Publications from independent research support the conceptual model's theoretical basis and utility in practice settings.

The relationship between conceptual models of practice and frame of reference

Developed and evidence-based conceptual models of practice provide a rigorous organizational structure that avoids personal biases and heuristics. In doing so, such models also ensure that interventions remain occupation-focused. Frames of reference are useful supports to conceptual models of practice and bring with them additional knowledge, tools and priorities. Frequently, occupational therapists will use one or more frames of reference in conjunction with their selected conceptual model of practice. The frames of reference should be selected before the assessment and goal-setting commence, as they may shape and influence the information that is gathered and the interventions that are employed to meet a client's goals (Fig. 5.1).

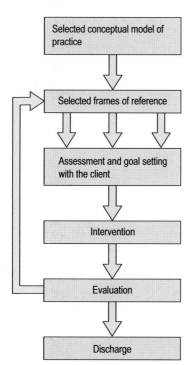

Fig. 5.1 • The relationship between conceptual models of practice and frames of reference.

Selection of frames of reference and conceptual models of practice in this book

Amongst other theoretical developments, this book provides a detailed introduction to five frames of reference and five conceptual models of practice. The selection of each theoretical approach was not an arbitrary one, but was based on their prominence within the literature, developing evidence base or commonality of use in practice. Not all the models and frames of reference presented in this text have equal evidence to support their practice. Indeed, at least one of them (the *Kawa* (River) Model) challenges the nature of evidence-based practice (Iwama 2006). Inclusion in this book should not therefore be seen as a form of endorsement. The reader is presented with a range of conceptual models and frames of reference to inform their thinking, and asked to critique each to decide what influence these will go on to have on their practice.

Summary

This chapter has introduced the importance, use and relationships of frames of reference and conceptual models of practice in occupational therapy. Their importance in assisting structured clinical decision-making has been highlighted. The chapter explains the relationship between conceptual models and frames of reference, underlines the importance of their continued development, and introduces the rationale for the selection of the frames of reference and conceptual models of practice introduced in this text.

Reflective learning

- In your own words, describe what a conceptual model of practice and a frame of reference are.
- Imagine you are explaining the importance of conceptual models of frames of reference to someone in your family. What would you say?
- What basis would you use when considering which conceptual model and/or frame of reference to use in practice?

References

Creek, J., 1992. Occupational Therapy and Mental Health. Churchill Livingstone, Edinburgh.

Creek, J., 2003. Occupational Therapy Defined as a Complex Intervention. College of Occupational Therapists, London.

Feaver, S., Creek, J., 1993a. Models for practice in occupational therapy: Part 1. Defining terms. British Journal of Occupational Therapy 56 (1), 4–6.

Feaver, S., Creek, J., 1993b. Models for practice in occupational therapy: Part 2. What use are they? British Journal of Occupational Therapy 56 (2), 59–69.

Forsyth, K., Kielhofner, G., 2005. The Model of Human Occupation: embracing the complexity of occupation by integrating theory into practice and practice into theory. In: Duncan, E.A.S. (Ed.), Hagedorn's Foundations for Practice, fourth ed. Churchill Livingstone, Edinburgh.

Gilovich, T., Griffen, D., Kahneman, D., 2002. Heuristics and Biases: The Psychology of Intuitive Judgement.

Cambridge University Press, Cambridge.

Grove, W.M., Meehl, P.E., 1996. Comparative efficiency of informal (subjective, impressionistic) and formal (mechanical, algorithmic) prediction procedures: the clinical/statistical controversy. Psychology, Public Policy, and Law 2, 1–31.

Grove, W.M., Zald, D.H., Lebow, B.S., et al, 2000. Clinical vs mechanical prediction: a meta analysis. Psychological Assessment 12, 19–30.

Hagedorn, R., 2001. Foundations for Practice in Occupational Therapy. Churchill Livingstone, Edinburgh.

Hopkins, H., Smith, H., 1993. Willard and Spackman's Occupational Therapy, eighth ed. Lippincott, Philadelphia.

Iwama, M., 2006. The Kawa Model. Culturally Relevant Occupational Therapy. Elsevier, Edinburgh.

Kielhofner, G., 1992. Conceptual Foundations of Occupational Therapy. FA Davis, Philadelphia.

Kielhofner, G., 2009. Introduction to the model of human occupation. In: Kielhofner, G. (Ed.), Model of Human Occupation: Theory and Application, fourth ed. Lippincott Williams & Wilkins, Philadelphia, pp. 1–7.

McClean, H., 1974. Towards developing a frame of reference and defining a treatment model in occupational therapy as applied to psychiatry. British Journal of Occupational Therapy 37 (11), 196–198.

Mosey, A.C., 1986. Psychosocial components of occupational therapy. Raven, New York.

Reed, K.L., 1984. Models of Practice in Occupational Therapy. Williams & Wilkins, Baltimore.

Wilcock, A.A., 2001. Occupation for Health: A Journey from Prescription to Self Health. College of Occupational Therapists, London.

Young, M., Quinn, E., 1992. Theories and Practice of Occupational Therapy. Churchill Livingstone, Edinburgh.

Section 2

Conceptual models of practice

The Model of Human Occupation

6

Embracing the complexity of occupation by integrating theory into practice and practice into theory

Kirsty Forsyth   Gary Kielhofner

OVERVIEW

Every day, occupational therapists must answer questions such as:

- What are the occupational needs of this client?
- How do I best support the client to engage in this activity?
- What goals does this client want and need to achieve?
- How can I assist in the achievement of these goals?

To answer these and other practice questions, occupational therapists need comprehensive ways of understanding the client situation.

Evidence suggests that, worldwide, occupational therapists use the Model of Human Occupation (MOHO) more than any other framework to address these types of practice question (Law & McColl 1989, Haglund et al 2000, National Board for Certification in Occupational Therapy 2004, Lee et al 2009, Taylor et al, 2009). Widespread use of this model reflects the fact that MOHO has the concepts, evidence and practical resources to enable occupational therapists to plan and implement high-quality, evidence-based, client-centred and occupation-focused practice.

This chapter will first take an overview of how and why MOHO was developed. It will then introduce its major concepts and note their relevance to understanding clients and to therapy. Following this, the chapter discusses some of the available resources for using MOHO in practice. Finally, the use of MOHO will be illustrated through a case example.

Key points

- MOHO is a client centred, occupation focused, evidence based conceptual model of practice
- MOHO provides a way of embracing the complexity of client's occupational needs
- MOHO provides specific occupationally focused outcomes measures to measure occupational participation
- MOHO provides a range of therapeutic intervention options
- MOHO has been applied successfully across cultures and used extensively internationally

Why and how MOHO was developed

From the 1960s onward, there was a recognition that occupational therapy had become too concerned with remediating impairment and needed to recapture its original focus on occupation (Reilly 1962, Shannon 1970, Kielhofner & Burke 1977). The Model of Human Occupation (MOHO) was the first occupation-focused model to be introduced in the profession (Kielhofner 1980a,b, Kielhofner & Burke 1980, Kielhofner et al 1980). It was developed by three occupational therapy practitioners who wanted to organize concepts that could guide their *delivery of occupation-focused practice*. In the three decades since MOHO was first formulated, numerous practitioners and researchers throughout the world have contributed to its development. Today, a literature of approximately 500 published works undergirds this model, making it the most evidence-based, occupational-focused model in the field.

The developers of this model have always sought to ensure that its concepts and tools are relevant and useful in practice. MOHO has been developed through an approach called 'the scholarship of practice'. This approach emphasizes the importance of an ongoing dialogue between theory/research and practice (Taylor et al 2002). Consequently, the scholarship of practice represents a commitment to scholarship, which supports occupational therapy practice, as well as a commitment to partner clinicians who are involved in the application of MOHO (Fig. 6.1). Moreover, the collaboration ensures that the needs and circumstances of practice shape theory development and research. All participants (for example, clients, therapists, managers, educationalists, students, researchers) take on the role of 'practice scholars', sharing responsibility for developing and applying MOHO. MOHO is, therefore, driven by practice concerns, and practice shapes how its theory is articulated and applied. This approach has not only assured MOHO's usefulness in practice, but has also enhanced the profile of occupational therapists, resulting in greater client understanding and satisfaction, and more respect for the occupational therapy contribution made by managers, policy-makers and interdisciplinary colleagues.

In 1985 the book *A Model of Human Occupation: Theory and Application* introduced an expanded theory and a wide range of clinical applications (Kielhofner 1985). Revisions of the model were

completed in 1995 and 2002, and the fourth edition (Kielhofner 2008) presents the authoritative and most current understanding of this theory and its application; it should be considered the primary reference on the model. For therapists who wish to apply MOHO, this text is a necessary resource.

Other published literature provides additional sources of theoretical discourse, discussions of programmatic applications, cases examples and research findings. The literature on this model is published worldwide. A current bibliography of literature, an evidence-based search engine and hundreds of evidence briefs, along with a wide range of assessment tools and intervention protocols on the model, can be found on a website: http://www.moho.uic. edu/. The website also provides an opportunity to join a list serve where students and practitioners can post practice questions and receive expert advice.

MOHO theory

A conceptual model of practice proposes theory to address certain phenomena with which the model is concerned (Kielhofner 2008). MOHO provides theory to explain occupation and occupational problems that arise in association with illness and disability. Its concepts address:

- the motivation for occupation
- the routine patterning of occupational performance
- the nature of skilled performance
- the influence of environment on occupation.

The following section will address the main conceptual ideas in MOHO (Fig. 6.2), namely:

1. embracing the complexity of human occupation
2. components of the person
3. environment
4. occupational performance.

Embracing the complexity of human occupation in practice

MOHO recognizes that occupation (i.e. what a person does in work, play and self-care) is influenced by many factors inside and outside the person. MOHO further emphasizes that each person's inner characteristics and external environment are linked

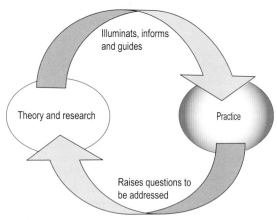

Fig 6.1 • Scholarship of practice. Reproduced with the permission of Professor G. Kielhofner from Challenges of the New Millennium: Keynote Address, WFOT Conference, Stockholm 2003.

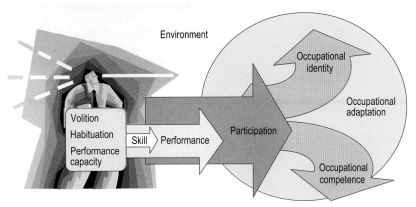

Fig 6.2 • MOHO concepts. Reproduced from Kielhofner, G., 2008. A Model of Human Occupation: Theory and Application, 4th edn, published by Lippincott Williams & Wilkins, Baltimore

together into a dynamic whole. In order to embrace this complexity, MOHO theory includes a range of concepts. These concepts seek not only to offer explanations of the factors that influence occupation, but also to provide a framework for gathering data about a client's circumstances, generating an understanding of the client's occupational strengths and limitations, and selecting and implementing a course of occupational therapy.

Further, MOHO theory views therapy as a process in which people are helped to do things in order to shape their occupational abilities and occupational identities. MOHO provides a framework for successfully and meaningfully engaging people in occupations, which helps to maintain, restore, or reorganize their occupational lives.

Components of the person

To explain how occupational participation is chosen, patterned and performed, MOHO conceptualizes people as composed of three interconnected ideas:

- volition
- habituation
- performance capacity.

Volition refers to the process by which persons are motivated toward and choose what they do. Habituation refers to a process whereby doing is organized into patterns and routines. Performance capacity refers to both the underlying mental and physical abilities and the lived experience that shapes performance. Each of these three components of the person is discussed in more detail below.

Volition

Volition refers to the process by which people are motivated toward and choose what they do. The concept of volition asserts that all humans have a desire to engage in occupations, and that this desire is shaped by ongoing experiences as we do things. Volition consists of thoughts and feelings that occur in a cycle of anticipating possibilities for doing, choosing what to do, experiencing what one does, and subsequent interpretation of the experience. These thoughts and feelings are concerned with three issues:

1. how effective one is in acting on the world (personal causation)
2. what one holds as important (values)
3. what one finds enjoyable and satisfying (interests).

Personal causation

Personal causation is reflected in our awareness of present and potential abilities (Harter 1983, Harter & Connel 1984) and our sense of how able we are to do what we want to do (Rotter 1960, Lefcourt 1981). Our own culture and social environment tell us what capacities we should have and why they matter. For example, a performer on stage, a taxi driver in a large city, a secondary school teacher, and a farmer in the countryside will each be concerned about very different kinds of ability. Also, developmental level will affect the experience of personal causation. A young child typically will be concerned with developing such skills as walking and playing with toys. An older child may be mostly concerned with school performance and ability to get along with peers and perform in sports. Adolescents usually begin to think about capacity for further education and entry into a line of work. Adults will focus on such things as the capacity for work performance and management of other adult responsibilities such as parenting. Older adults will often be concerned with loss of capacity associated with ageing and how to maintain abilities for personally important things.

Consequently, personal causation is never static, but rather a dynamic unfolding set of thoughts and feelings about our capacities and our efficacy in doing what we want to do. Our unique personal causation influences how we anticipate, choose, experience and interpret what we do. Consequently, the thoughts and feelings that make up personal causation are powerful motivational influences and they also guide how we experience what we do and how we look forward to the future.

Values

Choices of occupations are also influenced by our values. Values are beliefs and commitments that define what we see as good, right and important; they shape our sense of what is worth doing, how we ought to act, and what is the right way of doing things (Lee 1971). The child who plays nicely with other children because he has learned that playing in this way is important is expressing values. The worker who feels she needs to excel, the father who believes it is important to spend time with his children, and the old person who feels compelled to volunteer his services to his church are all examples of people whose values shape what they do. When we cannot live up to our values, we may feel guilty or inadequate and we experience a lack of meaning (Bruner 1990). The worker who has a stroke and subsequently loses his job, the mother whose mental illness interferes with parenting her child, the child whose learning disability makes it difficult to do as well in school as he thinks he should, and the elderly person whose fear of falling interferes with being able to engage in meaningful occupations are all examples of persons who are unable to enact their values.

Interests

Being interested in an occupation means that one feels an attraction based on anticipation of a positive experience in doing that occupation. The experience of pleasure and/or satisfaction in doing something may come from positive feelings associated with either the exercise of capacity, intellectual or physical challenge, fellowship with others, aesthetic stimulation, or other factors. We are more likely to enjoy what we can perform with some level of proficiency when skill is involved in the performance. Csikszentmihalyi (1990) describes flow, a form of ultimate enjoyment

in occupations that occurs when a person's capacities are optimally challenged. Often, this preference is manifested as a pattern of related interests such as athletic interest or cultural interests, including theatre and art. Preferring certain occupations over others influences what we are motivated to choose to do.

Illness or impairment can interfere with doing what one is interested in. For instance, a person might lose the capacity to do something he previously enjoyed, or an individual may find that engaging in an interest is no longer pleasurable because it evokes too much pain or fatigue. Persons with depression may find that they no longer enjoy doing what was previously pleasurable. Being able to engage in occupations that interest us and provide us with enjoyment and satisfaction is essential to well-being, and when illness or impairment interferes with this engagement, quality of life is reduced.

Summary

Our interests, values and personal causation affect what everyday activity we are motivated to do, what activities we choose to engage in and how we experience doing them. Illness and disability can interfere with volition in many ways. When this is the case, occupational therapists need to be able to assess and address volitional problems.

Additionally, volition is critical to the occupational therapy process. In order to provide therapy, occupational therapists must enable clients to engage in meaningful activity. Choosing a therapeutic activity and experiencing it as meaningful is a function of volition. Therapy cannot be meaningful unless occupational therapists attend to their client's volition.

The outcomes of therapy also depend on volition. It is not enough to improve a client's capacity. If the client leaves therapy and has no volitional motivation to use that capacity by engaging in activities of value and interest, then the client will not use what he or she has gained in therapy. Thus, therapy should always support the client's volition. Good therapy outcomes require that clients will *choose* to use their capacity, to develop new capacities, or make adjustments for their limitations because they can see these efforts as providing a life with value and satisfaction over which they can exercise reasonable control.

Habituation

Occupation is more than simply doing things. Every person has some kind of life pattern that is made up of everyday routines and roles. Habituation refers to the process by which people organize their occupational performance into the recurrent patterns of behaviour. These patterns integrate us into our physical and temporal world (when and where we do things) and our social and cultural world (doing things that reflect what we are expected to do by virtue of our position in society). Moreover, they allow us to carry out our daily lives efficiently and automatically. Habituated patterns of action are governed by:

- habits
- roles.

Habits

Habits involve learned ways of doing occupations that unfold automatically. The way we bathe and dress ourselves each morning, and how we drive, take a bus or ride a bike to work or school are examples of habits. We learn these habits through repeated experience. When we learn a habit, we acquire a way of appreciating and behaving in our familiar environments. So, for instance, we recognize the ring of the alarm clock as an indication that it is time to rise and bathe and dress; we know where to find the toothbrush and reach for it without thinking. We know how to turn on the shower and do it unreflectively. Because we do not have think about these things as we go about our morning routine, our routines take less effort and concentration. Our habits always involve cooperation with our environment (Dewey 1922). When our environment changes, our habits may no longer work automatically. For instance, when we find ourselves in an unfamiliar environment such as a hotel room, we may suddenly find that we have consciously to think about and figure out how to do a routine task such as turning on the shower. As the example illustrates, when habits cannot guide our behaviour automatically, it takes more concentration and effort to complete our routines. Consequently, habits give us our bearings throughout daily life and allow us to do routine things with relative ease.

Habits also organize our underlying capacities. When we reach for the toothbrush or turn on the shower, we are using our vision, our cognition and our motor capacity. If we were to experience a loss of any of these capacities, our habits would disintegrate. For example, if the power is out and one has to feel one's way about the bathroom at night without the benefit of sight, habits go out of the window. If one has a broken arm and one's dominant hand is in a cast, simple things like turning on the shower, brushing one's teeth or putting on clothes take a lot more thinking and effort or may be impossible. When clients develop impairments, their habits become disrupted

and their everyday routines take additional effort and thought or cannot be done without help. When one suddenly must use a wheelchair, the environment is changed and familiar habits no longer work. Getting into the shower and reaching to the medicine cabinet for the toothbrush are suddenly no longer habitual or possible. All the familiarity and ease of everyday life is disrupted. An important function of occupational therapy is to help clients develop new habits of everyday life in order to restore some of the ease and familiarity of daily life.

Roles

People see themselves as students, workers and parents, and recognize that they should behave in certain ways to enact these roles. Much of what we do is done *as* a spouse, parent, worker, student and so on (Mancuso & Sarbin 1983). The presence of these and other roles helps assure that what we do is regular (e.g. we go to school or work according to a schedule). Roles also give us a sense of identity and belatedly a sense of what we are obligated to do. When we tell someone we are a parent, a student, a worker or a member of some group, we are telling them who we are. Moreover, we know what is expected of us in those roles. Parents take care of children. Students attend lectures, study and take exams. Members of a bicycling club plan and go on bicycle trips together.

The roles that we have internalized serve as a kind of framework for looking out on the world and for engaging in occupation. When one is engaging in an occupation within a given role, it may be reflected in how one dresses, one's demeanour, the content of one's actions and so on. For instance, one would dress differently for work from when engaging in a leisure role. We do quite different things when we are in the role of student from when we are in the role of a friend.

Having an impairment can compromise one's ability to engage in meaningful life roles. If the impairment is severe, it can prevent or alter the way a person engages in all of their life roles. People with chronic disabilities often inhabit many fewer roles than those who do not have impairments. As a consequence, they have fewer opportunities to develop a sense of identity and to fill their lives with meaningful activities. In order to understand fully how a disability has influenced a client, the occupational therapist must understand its impact on their roles. Moreover, the aim of occupational therapy should be to support clients to enable them to engage in those roles that are most important or necessary for them.

Summary

Habituation regulates the patterned, familiar and routine features of what we do. Habits and roles give regularity, character and order to what we do and how we do it. They make our everyday lives familiar and they give us a sense of who we are. Disability can invalidate established habits and roles. Having a disability may require one to develop new habits for managing everyday routines and it may interfere with being able to engage in a role or alter how one can do that role. Understanding how a disability affects any person requires that the occupational therapist pays careful attention to the client's habituation.

Moreover, it is not sufficient that a client develops skills for doing everyday routines; it is also critical that the client develops the habits to integrate these skills into effective ways of doing everyday life tasks. Similarly, having abilities does little good, if clients are not able to access and identify with roles that call upon them to use those abilities. Therapy that focuses only on augmenting capacity without considering how the client will go about organizing everyday life is incomplete. Moreover, knowing what roles and habits are part of a client's life will also provide important information to enable us to prioritize the kinds of skill development on which to focus. Clients do not simply do things; they do them in order to enact daily routines and discharge their roles.

Performance capacity

The capacity for performance is affected by the status of one's musculoskeletal, neurological, cardiopulmonary and other bodily systems. A number of occupational therapy frameworks provide detailed concepts for understanding performance capacity. For example, the biomechanical framework seeks to explain human movement as the function of a complex organization of muscles, connective tissue and bones (Trombly 1989), while the sensory integration framework (Ayres 1972, 1979, 1986) explains how the brain organizes sensory information for executing skilled movement. Because these frameworks already address performance capacity, MOHO does not address this aspect of performance capacity. Consequently, occupational therapists using MOHO routinely use other frameworks for understanding and addressing performance capacity.

MOHO (Kielhofner et al 2008) concepts offer a different but complementary way of thinking about performance capacity. This view of performance capacity builds upon phenomenological concepts from philosophy (Husserl 1962, Merleau-Ponty 1962) and focuses on the subjective experience of performing. It asks occupational therapists to pay more attention to how it feels to perform with a disability. By having a better understanding of a client's pain, fatigue, confusion or other subjective aspects of performance, therapists can be more client-centred and more helpful in assisting clients to learn or relearn skills.

Interweaving of volition, habituation and performance capacity

The things we do reflect a *complex* interplay of our motives, habits and roles, and performance capacity. Volition, habituation and the subjective experience of performance always operate in concert with each other. We cannot fully understand a client's occupation without considering all these contributing factors. For example, a person with low personal causation will tend to feel anxious when attempting to perform. This anxiety in turn can negatively affect performance. Another example is that if a person does not have interests and values that lead him to use his capacities, those capacities will diminish through disuse. For this reason, it is important that occupational therapists gather information about all the aspects of a client (performance capacity, values, interests, personal causation, roles and habits) in order truly to understand that client and provide the best services.

The environment

Just as volition, habituation and performance capacity are inter-related and interdependent, people and their environments are also inseparable (Kielhofner 2008). Our environments offer us opportunities, resources, demands and constraints. Whether and how these environmental potentials affect us depends on our values, interests, personal causation, roles, habits and performance capacities. Because each individual is unique, any environment will have somewhat different effects on each individual within it.

The physical environment consists of natural and human-made spaces and the objects within them. Spaces can be the result of nature (e.g. a forest or a lake) or the result of human fabrication (e.g. a house, classroom or theatre). Similarly, objects may be those that occur naturally (e.g. trees and rocks) or those that have been made (e.g. books, cars and computers). The social environment consists of groups of persons, and the occupational forms or tasks that persons belonging to those groups perform. Groups allow and prescribe the kinds of thing their members can do. Occupational forms or tasks refer to the things that are available to do in any social context (for example, in a classroom the kinds of thing that are typically done include writing notes, giving a lecture, answering questions, taking exams and so forth). Every context has certain occupational forms or tasks associated with it.

Any setting within which we perform is made up of spaces, objects, occupational forms/tasks and/or social groups. Typical settings in which we engage in occupational forms are the home, neighbourhood, school or workplace.

The environment can be both a barrier and an enabler for disabled persons. For example, snow dampens the sound used by blind persons to help navigate without sight and may make the pavement inaccessible to the wheelchair user. Much of the built environment limits opportunities and poses constraints on those with disabilities because it often has been designed for persons without impairments. On the other hand, careful design of spaces can facilitate daily functioning of disabled persons. Similarly, while most fabricated objects in the environment are created for use by able-bodied, sighted, hearing and cognitively intact individuals, there are also a large number of objects designed to compensate for impairments. Occupational therapists are experts in providing and training clients in the use of these specialized objects.

People with a physical and mental impairment often contradict cultural values, making others uncomfortable and evoking a range of reactions. These attitudes can limit the person with disability. Moreover, disability may remove people from or alter the positions they can assume in social groups. The occupational forms available to the person with a disability may be limited or altered. Performance limitations can make doing some occupational forms impossible. Persons with disabilities often must give up or relinquish to others occupational forms that have become impossible to do.

In short, the physical and social environment can have a multitude of positive or negative impacts on the disabled person, which can make all the difference in that person's life. The environment is not only a pervasive factor influencing disability. It is a critical tool for supporting positive change in the disabled person's life. A therapist may purposefully alter the physical setting to remove constraints or to facilitate function. An example of this is a ramp that replaces inaccessible steps. Therapists can remove objects that are barriers or provide objects such as assistive technology that facilitate functioning. The therapist may provide, monitor or seek to change social groups such as families or work colleagues. Finally, the therapist may provide or help a client select occupational forms to undertake, or to modify how an occupational form is done.

Understanding occupational performance

Personal causation, values and interests motivate what we choose to do. Habits and roles shape our routine patterns of doing. Performance capacities and subjective experience provide the capacity for what we do. The environment provides opportunities, resources, demands and constraints for our doing. We can also examine the doing itself and what consequence it has over time. Doing can be examined at different levels:

- skills
- occupational performance
- occupational participation
- occupational identity/occupational competence
- occupational adaptation.

Skills

Within occupational performance we carry out discrete purposeful actions called skills. For example, making a cup of tea has a culturally recognizable occupational form in the UK. To do so, one engages in such purposeful actions as *gathering* together tea, kettle and a cup, *handling* these materials and objects, and *sequencing* the steps necessary to brew and pour the tea. These actions that make up occupational performance are referred to as skills (Fisher & Kielhofner 1995, Fisher 1999a, Forsyth et al 1998). In *contrast* to performance capacity (which refers to underlying ability, e.g. range of motion, strength, cognition), skill refers to the discrete actions seen *within* an occupation performance. There are three types of skill: motor skills, process skills, and communication and interaction skills.

If a person has difficulty 'reaching', an occupational therapist may conclude that the client has a limited range of motion in the shoulder joint. However, using Figure 6.2 to support theoretical clinical reasoning, we could hypothesize other reasons for the client not 'reaching'. For example, the client may not think he has the capacity to reach (personal causation); he may not see the activity as important and therefore fail to reach (values); he may not find the activity satisfying or enjoyable and therefore fail to reach (interest); it may not be part of his role responsibilities and therefore he fails to reach as he knows someone else will do this for him (roles); the environment may not be supporting the reach; the occupational form may not be within the person's culture and so they do not know they need an object to complete the occupational form and so fail to reach; and so on. Skills can therefore be influenced by a range of personal and environmental factors. Having a theoretical framework supports clinical reasoning to understand why a client is having difficulty exhibiting skill to complete the occupational form.

Occupational performance

When we complete an occupational form or task, we perform. Occupational forms for a lecturer may include lecturing, writing, administering and marking exams, creating courses and counselling students. Taking care of ourselves may involve performing the occupational forms of showering, dressing and grooming. Other examples of occupational performance are when persons do such tasks as walking the dog, baking a chicken, vacuuming a rug or mowing the lawn. These people are performing those occupational forms.

Occupational participation

Participation refers to engagement in work, play, or activities of daily living that are part of one's socio-cultural context and are desired and/or necessary to one's well-being. Examples of occupational participation include working in a full- or part-time job, engaging routinely in a hobby, maintaining one's home, attending school and participating in a club or other organization. This definition is consistent with the World Health Organization's view that participation is 'taking part in society along with their experiences within their life context' (World Health Organization 1999, p.19). Each area of occupational participation involves a cluster of related things that one does. For example, maintaining one's living space may include paying the rent, doing repairs, and cleaning.

Occupational identity and occupational competence

Our participation helps to create our identities. Occupational identity is defined as a composite sense of who one is and who one wishes to become as an occupational being, generated from one's history of occupational participation. Occupational identity includes one's sense of capacity and effectiveness for doing; what things one finds interesting and satisfying to do; who one is, as defined by one's roles and relationships; what one feels obligated to do and holds as important; a sense of the familiar routines of life; perceptions of one's environment and what it supports and expects. These are garnered *over time* and become part of one's identity. Occupational identity reflects accumulative life experiences that are organized into an understanding of who one has been and a sense of desired and possible directions for one's future.

Occupational competence is the degree to which one sustains a pattern of occupational participation that reflects identity. Competence has to do with putting your identity into action. It includes *fulfilling* the expectations of one's roles and one's own values and standards of performance; *maintaining* a routine that allows one to discharge responsibilities; *participating* in a range of occupations that provide a sense of ability, control, satisfaction and fulfilment; and *pursuing* one's values and taking action to achieve desired life outcomes.

Occupational adaptation

Occupational adaptation is the construction of a positive occupational identity and achieving occupational competence over time in the context of the environment.

Resources for practice

MOHO was initiated with the specific goal of *developing resources to guide and enhance occupation-focused practice*. Practitioners have collaborated in the development of a wide range of tools for partnerships. Academic/practice partnerships were built around how the tools developed. This ensured that the tools were theoretically driven and had robust research to support them while simultaneously being flexible and useful within busy clinical workplaces.

MOHO tools are specifically built to support occupation-focused practice. Examples are:

- a range of assessments that operationalize concepts from the model (Box 6.1 and Fig. 6.3)

- published case examples, as well as videotapes, illustrating application of the model in assessment, treatment planning and intervention (Box 6.2)
- published papers and manuals describing the implementation of programmes

 ## Box 6.1

MOHO assessment tools

Overview assessments

Occupational Performance History Interview (OPHI-II)

As a historical semi-structured interview, the OPHI-II seeks to gather information about a patient or client's past and present occupational performance. The OPHI-II is a three-part assessment, which includes:

- a semi-structured interview that explores a client's occupational life history
- rating scales that provide a measure of the client's occupational identity, occupational competence and the impact of the client's occupational behaviour settings
- a life history narrative designed to capture salient qualitative features of the occupational life history.

Occupational Circumstances Interview and Rating Scale (OCAIRS)

The OCAIRS is a semi-structured interview focused on the present and seeks to understand clients' occupational abilities on the full range of MOHO issues. It is an outcome measure. It is appropriate for clients who are conversational and is used when time is limited, as it is shorter than the OPHI-II interview.

Assessment of Occupational Functioning (AOF)

The AOF is a semi-structured interview, designed to identify strengths and limitations in areas of occupational functioning derived from MOHO (personal causation, values, roles, habits and skills). The AOF includes two parts:

- an interview schedule
- a rating scale.

Occupational Self-Assessment (OSA) and the Child Occupational Self-Assessment (COSA)

The OSA is an update of the Self-Assessment of Occupational Functioning (SAOF) and is designed to capture clients' perceptions of their own occupational competence and of the impact of their environment on their occupational adaptation. As such, the OSA is designed to be a client-centred assessment, which gives voice to the client's view. Once clients have had an opportunity to assess their occupational behaviour and their environments, they review the items in order to establish priorities for change, which can be translated into therapy goals.

Model of Human Occupational Screening Tool (MOHOST) and Short Child Occupational Profile (SCOPE)

These are relatively new assessments based on MOHO. Similar in format and administration, they were developed with clinicians in response to their request for a comprehensive assessment that is quick and simple to complete. MOHOST and SCOPE may be scored by the therapist using any combination of observation, interview, information from others who know the client, and chart audit. Because of their flexibility, the two tools can be used in a wide range of settings and with a wide range of clients. Moreover, the tools can be administered in a way that is client-centred.

Observational assessments

Assessment of Communication and Interaction Skills (ACIS)

The ACIS is a formal observational tool designed to measure an individual's performance in an occupational form and/or within a social group of which the person is a part. The instrument aims to assist occupational therapists in determining a client's ability in discourse and social exchange in the course of daily occupations.

Assessment of Motor and Process Skills (AMPS)

The AMPS (Fisher 1999b) represents a fundamental and substantive reconceptualization in the development of occupational therapy functional assessments. The AMPS is a structured, observational evaluation. It is used to evaluate the quality or effectiveness of the actions of performance (motor and process skills) as they unfold over time when a person performs daily life tasks.

Volitional Questionnaire (VQ) and the Paediatric Volitional Questionnaire (PVQ)

Traditionally, it has been difficult to assess volition in clients who have communication and cognitive limitations, due to the complex language requirements of most assessments of volition. The Volitional Questionnaire is an attempt to recognize that, while such clients have difficulty formulating goals or expressing their interests and values verbally, they are often able to communicate them through actions. The client is observed in a number of occupational behaviour settings so that a picture of the person's volition and the environmental supports required to support the expression can be identified.

(Continued)

Box 6.1

MOHO assessment tools—cont'd

Self-reports

Interest Checklist and the Paediatric Interests Profiles (PIP)

Although a number of versions of the Interest Checklist exist, the revised version appears to be the one most commonly used by occupational therapists utilizing the Model of Human Occupation and will be the one referred to in this discussion. This version consists of 68 activities or areas of interest. A revision within the UK is currently under way. There is a paediatric version available.

National Institutes of Health Activity Record (ACTRE)

The NIH ACTRE was developed as an outcome measure for a study of patients with rheumatoid arthritis. This instrument provides a 24-hour log of a patient's activities and is an adaptation of the Occupational Questionnaire (described below). The ACTRE aims to provide details of the impact of symptoms on task performance, individual perceptions of interest, significance of daily activities, and daily habit patterns.

Occupational Questionnaire (OQ)

The OQ is a pen-and-paper, self-report instrument that asks the individual to provide a description of typical use of time and utilizes Likert-type ratings of competence, importance, and enjoyment during activities. The client completes a list of the activities they perform each half-hour on a typical weekday. After listing the activities, the client is asked to answer four questions for each activity.

Role Checklist

The Role Checklist is a self-report checklist that can be used to obtain information about the types of role people engage in and which organize their daily lives. This checklist provides data on an individual's perception of their roles over the course of their life and also the degree of value, i.e. the significance and importance that they place on those roles. The Role Checklist can be used with adolescents, adults or geriatric populations.

Vocational assessments

Worker Role Interview (WRI)

The WRI is a semi-structured interview designed to be used as the psychosocial/environmental component of the initial rehabilitation assessment process for the injured worker. The interview is designed to have the client discuss various aspects of their life and job setting that have been associated with past work experiences. The WRI combines information from an interview with observations made during the physical and behavioural assessment procedure of a physical and/or work capacity assessment. The intent is to identify the psychosocial and environmental variables that may influence the ability of the injured worker to return to work.

Work Environment Impact Scale (WEIS)

The WEIS is a semi-structured interview designed to gather information about how individuals with disabilities experience and perceive their work settings. The focus of the interview is the impact of the work setting on a person's performance, satisfaction and well-being. An important concept underlying this scale is that workers are most productive and satisfied when there is a 'fit' or 'match' between the worker's environment and their needs and skills. Hence, the same work environment may have a different impact on different workers. It is important to remember that the WEIS does not assess the environment. Rather, it assesses how the work environment affects a given worker.

School assessments

Occupational Therapy Psychosocial Assessment of Learning (OT PAL)

The OT PAL is an observational and descriptive assessment tool. It assesses a student's volition (ability to make choices), habituation (roles and routines), and environmental fit within the classroom setting. The observational portion consists of 21 items that address the major areas of making choices, habits/routines and roles. In addition to the observation portion, there is a pre-observation form and interview guidelines. The pre-observation form is designed to gather environmental information, as well as assist in determining an appropriate time to complete the observation. The semi-structured interviews of the teacher, the student and the parent(s) are designed to have the teacher, student and parent describe various psychosocial aspects of learning related to school.

The School Setting Interview (SSI)

The SSI is a semi-structured interview designed to assess student–environment fit and identify the need for accommodations for students with disabilities in the school setting. The SSI is a client-centred interview intended to assist the occupational therapist in the planning of intervention by examining the student's interaction with the physical and social environments at school. The SSI provides the occupational therapist with a picture of the child's functioning in 14 content areas. This assessment is designed to be used collaboratively with the student and is therefore intended for students who are able to communicate adequately enough to discuss their feelings.

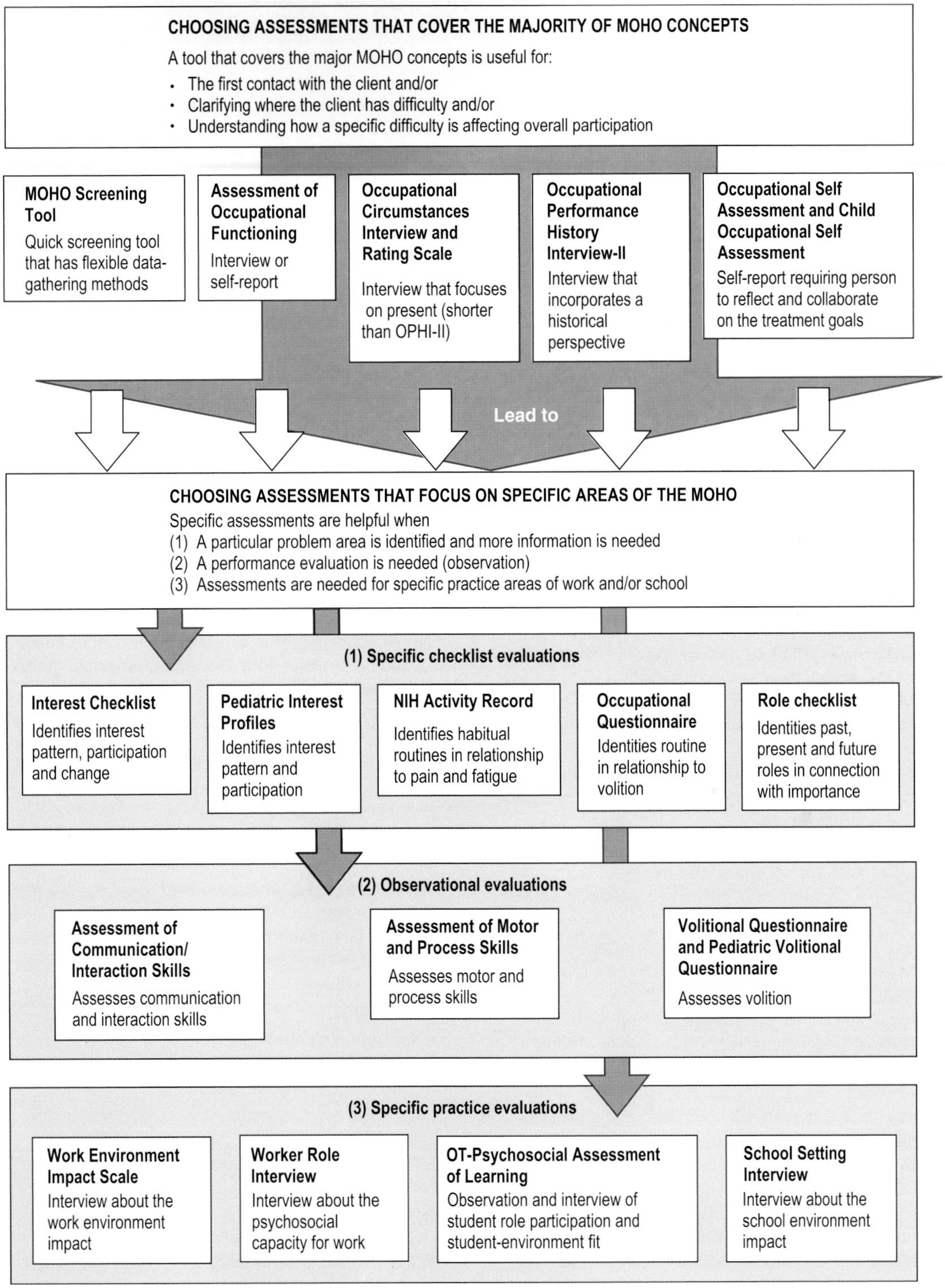

CHOOSING ASSESSMENTS THAT COVER THE MAJORITY OF MOHO CONCEPTS

A tool that covers the major MOHO concepts is useful for:
- The first contact with the client and/or
- Clarifying where the client has difficulty and/or
- Understanding how a specific difficulty is affecting overall participation

MOHO Screening Tool	**Assessment of Occupational Functioning**	**Occupational Circumstances Interview and Rating Scale**	**Occupational Performance History Interview-II**	**Occupational Self Assessment and Child Occupational Self Assessment**
Quick screening tool that has flexible data-gathering methods	Interview or self-report	Interview that focuses on present (shorter than OPHI-II)	Interview that incorporates a historical perspective	Self-report requiring person to reflect and collaborate on the treatment goals

Lead to

CHOOSING ASSESSMENTS THAT FOCUS ON SPECIFIC AREAS OF THE MOHO

Specific assessments are helpful when
(1) A particular problem area is identified and more information is needed
(2) A performance evaluation is needed (observation)
(3) Assessments are needed for specific practice areas of work and/or school

(1) Specific checklist evaluations

Interest Checklist	**Pediatric Interest Profiles**	**NIH Activity Record**	**Occupational Questionnaire**	**Role checklist**
Identifies interest pattern, participation and change	Identifies interest pattern and participation	Identifies habitual routines in relationship to pain and fatigue	Identities routine in relationship to volition	Identities past, present and future roles in connection with importance

(2) Observational evaluations

Assessment of Communication/ Interaction Skills	**Assessment of Motor and Process Skills**	**Volitional Questionnaire and Pediatric Volitional Questionnaire**
Assesses communication and interaction skills	Assesses motor and process skills	Assesses volition

(3) Specific practice evaluations

Work Environment Impact Scale	**Worker Role Interview**	**OT-Psychosocial Assessment of Learning**	**School Setting Interview**
Interview about the work environment impact	Interview about the psychosocial capacity for work	Observation and interview of student role participation and student-environment fit	Interview about the school environment impact

Fig 6.3 • Choosing a MOHO assessment. (NIH = National Institutes of Health). Reproduced from Kielhofner, G., 2008, A Model of Human Occupation: Theory and Application, 4th edn, published by Lippincott Williams & Wilkins, Baltimore

Box 6.2

Published articles and videotapes

There are a large number of published case examples, as well as videotapes, illustrating application of the model in assessment, treatment planning and intervention. A selection are referenced below:

Case illustrations through articles

Affleck A, Bianchi E, Cleckley M et al 1984 Stress management as a component of occupational therapy in acute care settings. Occupational Therapy in Health Care 1(3):17–41

Baron KB, Littleton MJ 1999 The model of human occupation: a return to work case study. Work: A Journal of Prevention, Assessment & Rehabilitation 12(1):37–46

Barrett L, Beer D, Kielhofner G 1999 The importance of volitional narrative in treatment: an ethnographic case study in a work program. Work: A Journal of Prevention, Assessment & Rehabilitation 12(1): 79–92

Curtin C 1991 Psychosocial intervention with an adolescent with diabetes using the model of human occupation. Occupational Therapy in Mental Health 11(2/3):23–36

DePoy E, Burke JP 1992 Viewing cognition through the lens of the model of human occupation. In Katz N (ed.), Cognitive Rehabilitation: Models for Intervention in Occupational Therapy. Butterworth-Heinemann, Stoneham, MA, pp.240–257

Froehlich J 1992 Occupational therapy interventions with survivors of sexual abuse. Occupational Therapy in Health Care 8(2/3):1–25

Gusich R 1984 Occupational therapy for chronic pain: a clinical application of the model of human occupation. Occupational Therapy in Mental Health 4(3):59–73

Helfrich C, Kielhofner G 1994 Volitional narratives and the meaning of occupational therapy. American Journal of Occupational Therapy 48:319–326

Helfrich C, Kielhofner G, Mattingly C 1994 Volition as narrative: an understanding of motivation in chronic illness. American Journal of Occupational Therapy 42:311–317

Kavanaugh J, Fares J 1995 Using the model of human occupation with homeless mentally ill patients. British Journal of Occupational Therapy 58(10): 419–422

Mentrup C, Niehaus A, Kielhofner G 1999 Applying the model of human occupation in work-focused rehabilitation: a case illustration. Work: A Journal of Prevention, Assessment & Rehabilitation 12(1):61–70

Neville A 1985 The model of human occupation and depression. Mental Health Special Interest Section Newsletter 8:1–4

Oakley F 1987 Clinical application of the model of human occupation in dementia of the Alzheimer's type. Occupational Therapy in Mental Health 7(4): 37–50

Pizzi MA 1990 The model of human occupation and adults with HIV infection and AIDS. American Journal of Occupational Therapy 44:257–264

Pizzi MA 1990 Occupational therapy: creating possibilities for adults with human immunodeficiency virus infection, AIDS related complex, and acquired immunodeficiency syndrome. Occupational Therapy in Health Care 7(2/3/4):125–137

Series C 1992 The long-term needs of people with head injury: a role for the community occupational therapist? British Journal of Occupational Therapy 55(3):94–98

Woodrum SC 1993 A treatment approach for attention deficit hyperactivity disorder using the model of human occupation. Developmental Disabilities Special Interest Section Newsletter 16(1):1–2

Case illustrations through videotapes

Facilitating Empowerment and Promoting Self-Advocacy: ADA
  Population: Disabled workers
  Author: Renee Moore-Corner

OPHI-II
  Population: Adults who can reflect upon and talk about their life history
  Authors: Gary Kielhofner, Trudy Mallinson, Carrie Crawford, Meika Nowak, Matt Rigby, Alexis Henry, Deborah Walens

Understanding the Work-hardening Client
  Population: Injured workers
  Authors: Clare Curtin, Trudy Mallinson

Work Environment Impact Scales
  Population: Adult workers with recent/current work experience
  Authors: Renee Moore-Corner, Linda Olson, Gary Kielhofner

Worker Role Interview
  Population: Injured workers
  Authors: Craig Velozo, Gary Kielhofner, Gail Fisher

Box 6.3

Example manuals for MOHO-based programmes

The Banfield Assessment
Population: Disabled long-term residential clients
Authors: Hazel Broadley, Guylaine Desharnais
Remotivation Manual
Population: People with poor volitional status
Author: Carmen Gloria de la Heras
Wellness and Lifestyle Renewal: A Manual for Personal Change
Population: 'Worried well' adults
Author: Mark S. Rosenfeld
Work Readiness: Day Treatment for Persons with Chronic Disabilities
Population: Unemployed adults with chronic disabilities
Author: Linda Olson
Work Rehabilitation in Mental Health Programs
Population: Adults with mental illness
Authors: Trudy Mallinson, Dorianne LaPlante, Jan Holmann-Smith

---

based on the model (Box 6.3). There is an evidence-based search engine and downloadable evidence briefs on the MOHO website to make it easier for practitioners to focus on the evidence for their areas of practice.

Questions and answers

Since its inception and over the past four decades, the development of this model has been accompanied by a history of questions and critiques. Central questions have been:

- Can MOHO be used with other models of practice?
- Is MOHO client-centred?
- Is MOHO flexible enough to embrace a range of social, geographic and cultural environments?
- Why is there specific language?
- Can MOHO embrace the complexity of human occupation?
- Is MOHO applicable to lower functioning clients?
- Is MOHO an evidence-based choice?
- Can MOHO be used when selecting adaptive equipment?

We will attempt to address these issues through a series of questions and answers.

Can MOHO be used with other models of practice?

Yes. A common question is, 'Is it MOHO or nothing?' This question involves the extent to which MOHO can be used in an integrative way with other models of practice. As mentioned above, MOHO does not provide theoretical arguments to understand the capacity for performance that is supported by one's musculoskeletal, neurological, cardiopulmonary, mental or cognitive abilities such as memory, and planning and other bodily systems. A number of occupational therapy conceptual models of practice seek to explain performance capacities that make possible occupational performance. These models provide detailed concepts for understanding some aspect of performance capacity. Consequently, occupational therapists using MOHO will also need to use other frameworks in order to understand and address performance capacity. A combination of frameworks can, therefore, be used to support a full understanding of the client's occupational engagement. Figure 6.4 identifies how this can be achieved. Overarching values and beliefs of occupation therapy (e.g. occupation is important for health, it is important to consider both the mind and the body, it is important to be client-centred, and so on) inform occupation-focused conceptual models of practice (e.g. MOHO). MOHO has very specific detail on how to carry out occupation-focused practice. Both the values and beliefs of occupational therapy and MOHO provide support for the concept of an 'occupation filter' (Mallinson & Forsyth 2000). The occupation filter is a way of viewing knowledge from outside occupational therapy and bringing it into our practice in an occupation-focused way (Fig. 6.5). This allows the integration of a range of theories, yet avoids the 'cutting and pasting' of bodies of knowledge from outside occupational therapy into our practice and calling it occupational therapy when it in fact closely resembles other professionals' practice. For example, 'cutting and pasting' cognitive behavioural therapy into occupational therapy without using an 'occupation-focused filter' will result in practice that looks like that of a psychologist and perpetuate role confusion within occupational therapy.

Is MOHO client-centred?

MOHO is recognized as a model consistent with client-centred practice (Law 1998; Sumsion 1999). MOHO concepts require therapists to have

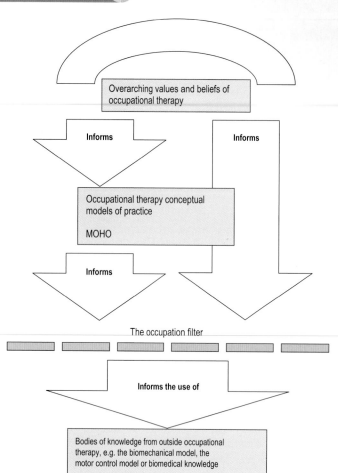

Fig 6.4 • MOHO integration. Reproduced with permission from Forsyth & McMillan, personal communication, 2001.

knowledge of their client's values, sense of capacity and efficacy, value, roles, habits, performance experience and personal environment. MOHO-based assessments are designed to gather information on and provide clients with opportunities to provide their perspectives on these factors. The client's unique characteristics, in combination with the theory, guide the development of an understanding of the client's unique situation. The understanding of the client, in turn, provides the rationale for therapy. Moreover, since MOHO conceptualizes the client's own doing, thinking and feeling as the central dynamic in achieving change, therapy must support the client's choice, action and experience.

MOHO is, therefore, inherently a client-centred model in two important ways. Firstly, it views each client as a unique individual whose characteristics fundamentally influence the rationale for and nature of the therapy goals and strategies. MOHO theory both focuses the therapist on the unique characteristics of the client and provides concepts that allow the therapist to appreciate the client's perspective and situation more deeply. Secondly, MOHO views what the client does, thinks and feels as the central mechanism of change (Kielhofner 2002). MOHO concepts also propose that the client's occupational engagement (i.e. what the client does, thinks and feels) is the central dynamic of therapy (Kielhofner 2002). MOHO-based intervention supports the client's doing, thinking and feeling in order to achieve change. MOHO-based practice, therefore, requires a client–therapist relationship in which the therapist must understand, respect and support their client's values, sense of capacity and efficacy, value, roles, habits, performance experience and personal environment.

Fig 6.5 • Components of the occupational filter. Reproduced with the permission of T Mallinson & K Forsyth, personal communication, 2000

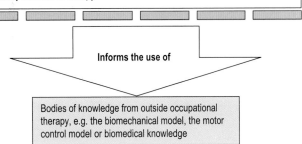

(a) Persons occupational performance
The primary concern is the understanding of how the phenomena from bodies of knowledge from outside occupational therapy (e.g. strength, memory, coordination) influence a person's performance of occupational forms or life roles

(b) Assess through occupation
Evaluate/assess the phenomena from bodies of knowledge from outside occupational therapy (e.g. strength, memory, coordination) within the context of the person's performance of occupational forms or life roles

(c) Occupation restores/maintains
Emphasises the person's performance of occupational forms and life roles in the restoration and/or maintenance and/or compensation of the phenomena from bodies of knowledge from outside occupational therapy (e.g. strength, memory, coordination)

(d) Outcome of OT is satisfying/meaningful performance in occupations
Views the satisfying, meaningful performance of occupational forms or life roles as the primary outcome of therapy

Informs the use of

Bodies of knowledge from outside occupational therapy, e.g. the biomechanical model, the motor control model or biomedical knowledge

Is MOHO flexible enough to embrace a range of social, geographic and cultural environments?

Some have questioned whether MOHO is flexible and pragmatic enough to be used in a wide range of social, geographic and cultural environments.

With respect to the social environment, the third edition of MOHO has been influenced by the disabilities studies literature (Miller & Oertel 1983, Hull 1990, Gill 1997). This literature argues that many of the problems faced by persons with disabilities can more properly be located in the environment —in everything from physical barriers to stigmatizing attitudes and outright discrimination. A growing theme is that disability occurs because of a lack of fit between person and environment. This implies, of course, that change must include altering the environment. Accordingly, MOHO calls attention to the environment as both an enabler of and a barrier to occupation (Kielhofner 2002). Throughout, an effort has been made to call attention to circumstances both within the person

and within the environment that contribute to a person's motivation, patterns of behaviour and occupational performance. The assessment tools that have been developed routinely contain an environmental component and examine the fit between the person and their environment. A MOHO-based assessment that is entirely focused on the environment has been developed (Moore-Corner et al 1998), and others incorporate the environment as an aspect of the assessment.

There have been questions raised about the portability of MOHO to different geographic and cultural environments. The scholarship of practice approach to MOHO development has encouraged an international community of occupational therapists to use and contribute to the development of MOHO. MOHO has, therefore, become an international conceptual practice model. MOHO has received significant attention, including criticism, elaboration, application and empirical testing by occupational therapists throughout the world in such diverse countries as Australia, New Zealand, the Netherlands, Sweden, Denmark, Japan, Korea, Spain, Italy, Portugal, Chile and Colombia.

The theory itself incorporates a respect for each client's individuality and cultural narrative into its concepts, and many of the assessments are specifically designed to capture a client's unique cultural perspective. For example, the OPHI-II (Kielhofner et al 1997) elicits and considers culturally influenced values, interests and roles through the use of narrative ethnography as a predominant interviewing method. For this reason, the OPHI-II and similar assessments are particularly useful when therapists desire to gather information about the client's culturally influenced thoughts, feelings and actions. Concepts of occupational form can also be helpful in identifying how different cultures define how everyday occupations are completed. Each culture includes a wide range of occupational forms that constitute the opportunities and demands that culture will put on its members for doing everyday things. Knowing how occupational forms are culturally defined for each client (for example, the occupational form of dressing has different social expectations based on cultural norms from culture to culture) helps occupational therapists to be sensitive to cultural differences in the ways of doing everyday activity.

Assuring that assessments are relevant and valid with persons from diverse cultural backgrounds requires ongoing development and research. Such work is being undertaken across the MOHO-based assessments. Assessments have been developed in collaboration with therapists and clients representing multiple cultures and languages. Many of the MOHO standardized assessments are now translated into different language versions. Research indicates that many of the MOHO-based assessments do not reflect cultural biases. For example, studies of the WRI (Haglund et al 1997), the WEI (Kielhofner et al 1999), the OPHI-II (Kielhofner et al 2001), the ACIS (Forsyth, Salamy, Simon et al 1997 and the OS (Kielhofner & Forsyth 2001) indicate that these assessments are valid cross-culturally. The UK is very influential in the development of MOHO theory and application. An active group of both researchers and practitioners are working together to contribute to the development of MOHO.

Why is there specific language?

The words that are selected to describe therapy are very important. Complex conditions or procedures can be conveyed and immediately understood when such professional terminology is used. Occupational therapists acquire the professional languages of several disciplines. In college we learn medical language to support our communication with medical colleagues. For example, we can say 'Alzheimer's disease' and immediately the multidisciplinary team have a sense of the issues faced by the person under discussion and then can enter into specifics of how the condition has affected this particular person. The medical definition of Alzheimer's disease is very long and having language to name and frame the issue supports effective communication with others who are familiar with the terms. Therefore, one strength of having a unique language is that MOHO terminology can be used in consultation with others who are familiar with the model to convey complex concepts accurately and succinctly. For example, the term 'volition' conveys a complex set of ideas about how people are motivated toward their occupations. When someone refers to a client having a volitional challenge, those who know the terminology can anticipate that the challenge involves the client's values, personal causation and interests, and how this manifests in the way clients anticipate, choose, experience and interpret what they do every day. In this way, MOHO terminology can succinctly convey information.

Deciding whether and how to use MOHO terminology in communication and documentation requires consideration of several factors. MOHO terms, like those of any other professional language, offer benefits and pose challenges. The major disadvantage of *all* professional language is that everyone needs to have a common understanding of the terms. It is, therefore, ineffective to use MOHO terms (or, indeed, medical terms) with colleagues, clients and others who will not understand what the words mean. Therefore, therapists should carefully decide when and how they use MOHO terms in communicating to clients, lay persons and other professionals. Because practitioners, clients and settings differ greatly in terms of their knowledge and understanding of languages associated with particular theoretical models, it is ultimately the clinicians' responsibility and judgement that count in terms of translating the MOHO terms into verbal and written language that accurately conveys the intended knowledge. There follow two examples where MOHO was used to understand the client's situation. Example 1 involves a situation where the occupational therapist decided not to use MOHO terminology and example 2 describes a situation where the occupational therapist found it helpful to use the terminology.

EXAMPLE 1: OCCUPATIONAL THERAPIST DECIDES NOT TO USE MOHO TERMINOLOGY

The following is an example of an entry into a multidisciplinary record. It frames Sophie's occupational life using MOHO; however, specific MOHO terminology was not used because the multidisciplinary team was not familiar with MOHO language. MOHO constructs have been placed in brackets for illustration only.

> 'Sophie states she was previously a very active person (occupational identity). She worked behind the bar of a local pub (role) for 20 years before her retirement (role change) 5 years ago. She was very social and felt that a lot of the "regulars" at the pub were like friends (social environment). She enjoyed (interests) the social aspect of her job. Since retirement (role change) she has felt isolated (social environment). She is extremely house-proud (values), always had high standards (values) of cleaning and ran the household very efficiently (homemaker role). It was important (values) for Sophie always to present herself well. She took great care of her appearance (self-care role), liked to be "well turned out" (values) and had her hair set once a week (habit). She enjoyed spending time with her daughter and family (interest/social environment). She was particularly close to her granddaughter (role) and they had previously spent time together every Saturday out in the community (habit). She also enjoyed board games and knitting (interest). She previously volunteered at a local sheltered housing complex (role), where she made soup and meals. She was involved in church events (role) and ran charity events for the women's guild (role).'

EXAMPLE 2: OCCUPATIONAL THERAPIST DECIDES TO USE MOHO TERMINOLOGY

The following is an example of using MOHO language to help understand a client called Jane. An occupational therapist may routinely document in their notes the following statement:

Statement A
'Jane lacks confidence and is overly dependent.'

Using MOHO framework and language makes the definition of the challenge Jane faces more specific:

Statement B
'Jane's personal causation is characterized by lacking a clear sense of her own capacity. As a result, she anticipates performance situations with anxiety and frequently chooses to avoid doing things for

which she has adequate skills. She also habitually seeks advice and help from others, which leads to her being unnecessarily dependent on others.'

In this situation the therapist decided to use statement B because using the terminology of MOHO resulted in documentation that was more precise and detailed. Moreover, while statement A describes Jane's behaviour, it does not explain it. The MOHO framework and language in statement B offered an *explanation* that also provides a rationale for the following interventions:

- Advise Jane on a course of occupational therapy that will support a graded engagement in occupations to challenge her sense of capacity increasingly.
- Provide Jane with feedback around her occupational performance to enable a more accurate sense of her own capacities to engage in occupations.
- Encourage Jane to sustain occupational performance in the face of anxiety.
- Structure the environment to provide the opportunity for Jane to practise engaging in occupations with more autonomy.

Precision in language, including the use of theoretical terms, can clarify what we understand clients' occupational challenges to be and how we plan to address them.

Can MOHO embrace the complexity of human occupation?

Human occupation is complex (Creek 2003). Most people come into occupational therapy with significant impairments and major disruptions to their lives. Others struggle with declining function or recurring exacerbations of their diseases. A large proportion of clients face the task of rebuilding all or part of their lives. In short, their occupational problems tend to be complex and challenging. The strength and application of MOHO is neither simple nor formulaic. Instead, it aims to understand important multiple dimensions of each client's unique experience and bring a sophisticated understanding to bear on the life issues facing each client in practice.

In occupational therapy, a number of frameworks address aspects of occupational performance and the capacities that underlie it, but these theories tend to exist in isolation from one another. For example, occupational therapy theories that concentrate on physical performance have generally attended to the bodily components (brain and musculoskeletal system) involved in physical doing, while motives have been seen as part of a separate domain. By contrast, MOHO offers an approach to thinking about the capacity for occupational performance that complements existing theory. There is growing recognition of the importance of considering body and mind together in explaining phenomena (Kielhofner 1995, Trombly 1995). After all, motivation for a task can influence the extent of physical effort directed to that task (Yoder, Nelson, Smith 1989, Riccio et al 1990), while physical impairments can weigh down the desire to do things (Murphy 1987, Toombs 1992). Conceptually, MOHO seeks to avoid dividing humans into separate physical and mental components, and instead embraces the complexity of human occupation. MOHO seeks to explain how occupation is motivated, patterned and performed, and implicates both body and mind in each of these major concepts. By offering explanations of such diverse phenomena, MOHO offers a broad and integrative view of human occupation. Consequently, it can be used to explain and guide practice involving a wide range of phenomena and corresponding concepts. Moreover, as stated above, therapists often use MOHO in combination with other conceptual models of practice or with theories borrowed from other disciplines or professions.

Is MOHO applicable to lower-functioning clients?

Some have questioned the relevance of MOHO in addressing issues of motivation in children and in lower-functioning clients. This perception is perplexing, since those clients who are least able to self-describe and self-advocate most deserve careful assessment of their volition. This can be achieved through careful observation of the client's volitionally relevant actions. The VQ (de las Heras et al 2001), the PVQ (Geist et al 2001) and the MOHOST (Parkinson et al 2001) work well with such clients. A therapist can, therefore, readily gain insight into the volition of children or lower-functioning clients. Additionally, therapists can make good use of unstructured means of assessment for such clients (Kielhofner 2002) that allow for complete flexibility within the assessment process.

Is MOHO an evidence-based choice?

Yes. Since MOHO was first published in the early 1980s it has built up an evidence base (see http://www.moho.uic.edu/). The majority of these studies were completed in the last decade, indicating an accelerating growth in research on MOHO, and it is now the most internationally researched, occupation-focused, conceptual model of practice. MOHO provides theoretical evidence for its practice theory and it provides research evidence for its tools for practice.

Theoretical evidence for practice

Such research examines whether the concepts of MOHO theory are supported by evidence. It also involves asking whether the theory can account for and predict the kinds of client change it seeks to explain. Therefore, theoretical evidence on MOHO has included the following kinds of study:

* construct validity studies that seek to verify MOHO concepts
* correlative studies that examine the accuracy of relationships between constructs proposed in MOHO theory
* studies comparing groups on concepts from MOHO theory to test whether they explain group differences
* prospective studies that examine the potential of MOHO concepts and propositions to predict future behaviour or states
* qualitative studies that explore MOHO concepts and propositions in depth.

This kind of theoretical evidence for practice yields findings that may lead one to have confidence in the theory and/or to eliminate, change or expand a concept and/or proposition.

Evidence for technology for practice application

In addition to offering a practice-based theory to embrace the complexity of therapy, conceptual models of practice like MOHO additionally generated a technology for application (e.g. assessments and intervention strategies) for use in practice. Examples of this kind of research are:

* psychometric studies leading to the development of outcome measures
* studies of how MOHO concepts influence therapeutic reasoning and practice
* studies that examine what happens in therapy
* outcomes studies that identify the effectiveness of occupational therapy services

- predictive studies that identify whether certain occupational outcomes can be predicted by the occupational therapist.

This kind of research provides practical tools for therapists to use within their practice and evidence to argue for additional occupational therapy resources.

While we can distinguish theoretical and application research within the MOHO research base, it is important to recognize that many MOHO-based studies incorporate both theoretical and application research aims to be addressed simultaneously. This is reflective of a 'scholarship of practice' approach to building evidence for the field, whereby research for theory and application are simultaneously achieved. For example, some studies that primarily sought to examine the dependability of an assessment tool have identified new concepts that were later incorporated into the theory (Mallinson et al 1998).

Can MOHO be used when selecting adaptive equipment?

Yes. Social service colleagues have asked the question, 'How would I apply MOHO to a client who is having difficulty bathing?' A biomechanical way of framing this challenge may be to state that the person is having difficulty 'physically getting in and out of the bath'. A MOHO way of framing the challenge is to state that the person is having 'difficulty engaging in the bathing activity'. MOHO, therefore, supports therapists in embracing the complexity of bathing rather than reducing it to only an issue of moving the client's body into/out of the bath. MOHO would support the therapist in asking the following questions:

- Does the person feel confident doing this activity?
- Have they had difficult past experiences doing this activity? (personal causation)
- Do they find this activity enjoyable/satisfying? (interest)
- How important is this activity for them?
- How important is it that they complete the activity alone?
- What meaning will adaptive equipment have for the person? (values)
- Can they physically do the activity? (motor skills)
- Do they have enough concentration — sequencing and so on — to complete the activity? (process skills)

- Do they have the full responsibility for doing the activity? (role)
- Does someone help them? (social environment)
- Where do they bathe?
- Where do they undress?
- Do they have any equipment to help them?
- Can they describe the environment when the bath is full — slippy, with lots of steam and on on? (physical environment)
- Do they have a routine when doing this activity?
- What time of day do they bathe? (habits)
- Are they satisfied with their morning/evening routine and when bathing happens?
- How does the time of day affect their abilities to bathe? (habits)

MOHO can, therefore, provide a framework for understanding the life within which occupational therapy is entering and whether adaptive equipment is appropriate. It also provides an understanding of the meaning attached to the equipment and how it might be adapted into the routine of the client. A lack of attention to these details may mean that the equipment is hidden away due to the client not wanting to be seen as 'disabled', or the equipment being removed because it was not adopted into the client's habitual routine.

Can you use MOHO as an activity analysis structure?

Yes. The analysis of occupations and their use within therapy are among the unique skills of the occupational therapist (Hagedorn 2000). There are many structures that provide a framework for analysing activity (Fidler & Fidler 1963, Mosey 1986, Lamport et al 2001, Creek 2002, Foster & Pratt 2002). Recently, however, there has been some discussion that advocates using theories as a framework for activity analysis (Crepeau 2003, Toglia 2003).

> Practitioners analyse activities from the perspective of practice theories to understand problems in performance and intervention strategies.
>
> (Crepeau 2003, p.191)

MOHO provides an evidence-based practice theory that supports a therapist in *analysing* a person's occupational life. Practice-based theories have the added advantage of providing an understanding of how different elements of analysis relate to each other and provide an insight into the change process (Creek 2009). MOHO has an established evidence base to support how different theoretical constructs relate to each other (e.g. Lederer et al 1985, Barris et al 1986, Ebb et al 1989, Davies Hallet et al 1994, Peterson et al 1999, American Occupational Therapy Association, 2002) and has a theory of how therapeutically supported change happens (Kielhofner 2002). It could, therefore, be argued that using evidence-based theory (e.g. MOHO) to analyse activities has several advantages over traditional activity analysis frameworks. MOHO-driven activity analysis simultaneously:

- provides an analysis of the person's occupational life
- examines how the different aspects of this analysis relate to each other

- looks at how this analysis relates to the changes that potentially can be made to support the client's re-engagement in everyday life.

This view has been supported by the inclusion of motor and process skills (Fisher & Kielhofner 1995, Kielhofner 2002), along with communication and interactions skills (Forsyth et al 1998, Kielhofner 2000) in the occupational therapy practice framework (Butts, Nelson 2007). As described in a previous section, MOHO would need to be used with other frameworks (e.g. biomechanical, motor control, sensory integration and so on) to support a complete activity analysis that included analysing performance capacities.

CASE STUDY

The case below illustrates the use of the MOHO framework to understand the occupational participation of a client called Sophie Bronson. The occupational therapy report shown below was developed from observations of Sophie within her home environment, and from face-to-face discussion with Sophie and Sophie's husband, in addition to telephone contact with Sophie's daughter. The therapist decided not to use MOHO terminology in the report due to the multidisciplinary audience.

SOPHIE: OCCUPATIONAL THERAPY REPORT[1]

Name: Sophie Bronson
Address: 12 Church Street, Edinburgh
Date of Birth: 12.03.30
GP: Dr Watson
Consultant: Dr Wallace
Data sources:
14 March 2005 Home visit with Sophie and her husband present
     15 March 2005 Telephone contact with Sophie's daughter
Date of report: 16 March 2008

REFERRAL AND REASON FOR ASSESSMENT

The referral was received from Sophie's GP, Dr Watson, on 24 February 2005. The referral stated that Sophie was now reporting 'difficulties with coping and mobility'. It also stated that Sophie has been diagnosed as having early dementia and has a previous medical history of osteoarthritis and congestive heart failure. The reason for the assessment, therefore, was to look at Sophie's engagement with

everyday activity and make recommendations to support Sophie in feeling as if she can 'cope and manage her mobility' issues and with other potential unidentified difficulties engaging in activity.

Sources of information for report

This report is a compilation of information gathered on a home visit (Sophie, her husband and her occupational therapist present) and a telephone contact with Sophie's daughter.

HISTORY OF ACTIVITY

Information from Sophie

She was previously a very active person. She worked behind the bar of a local pub for 20 years before her retirement. She was very social and felt that a lot of the 'regulars' at the pub were like friends. She enjoyed the social aspect of her job. Since retirement she has felt isolated. She is extremely house-proud, always had high standards of cleaning and ran the household very efficiently. It was important for Sophie always to present herself smartly. She took great care of her appearance, liked to be 'well turned out' and had her hair set once a week. She enjoyed spending time with her daughter and family. She was particularly close to her granddaughter and they had previously spent time together every Saturday out in the community. She also enjoyed board games and knitting. She previously volunteered at a local sheltered housing complex, where she made soup and meals. She was involved in church events and ran charity events for the women's guild.

Information from Sophie's husband and daughter

They both confirmed the above information from Sophie and so it could be concluded that Sophie is an accurate historian. They stated that Sophie's activity levels reduced when she retired 5 years ago. There has been a gradual deterioration in activity levels over a 12-month period. She has

---

[1] The Model of Human Occupation Screening Tool (MOHOST) assessment was used to complete this assessment. Parkinson, S., Forsyth, K., Kielhofner, G., 2002. 'A User's Manual for the Model of Human Occupation Screening Tool (MOHOST), Version 1.0, Research Version, MOHO Clearinghouse, University of Illinois at Chicago.

been sitting in her chair all day doing very little since her recent hospital admission 6 months ago.

CURRENT MENTAL/PHYSICAL HEALTH

A. Current mental health

On the visit Sophie was observed to be responsive and cooperative; she reported that her mood has been low for 6 months and that she no longer took any interest in activities that were once meaningful. Sophie identified the source of her low mood as including

- her inability to mobilize out of doors
- her recent hospital admission (6 months ago)
- a flood incident in the flat above.

She states that she is not coping with any activities that were previously meaningful to her and she is frustrated by this.

Sophie's daughter feels that her mother's current low mood is due to social isolation since retiring and to having reduced mobility ascending/descending stairs because of her painful and swollen feet. Sophie's social isolation has worsened recently because she is not taking as much care of her physical appearance and now would not want anyone to see her in an unkempt state.

B. Current physical health

Sophie needs a Zimmer frame to mobilize around her environment. She was observed to mobilize in her flat independently and safely using this frame. She has not gone outside for the past 12 months due to her inability to ascend/descend stairs. She was observed to have swollen feet, with hyper-extended big toes. The podiatrist and physiotherapist are involved, which has improved the situation; however, Sophie still reports pain.
She wears glasses, although states she is able to read without them. She reports deteriorated eyesight since a cataract operation. She states that she has hearing aids, which she was not wearing during the visit. She was observed to be answering questions appropriately and followed the conversations; therefore, she could hear people talking.

CURRENT ENGAGEMENT IN ACTIVITY

A. Physical environment

Sophie was observed to live in a two-bedroom, first-floor flat. External access is by two steps (no rails) into the building, a 100-yard paved corridor, then 16 steps broken halfway with a landing (with rail right side ascending). The physical condition of the flat was well maintained; it is centrally heated and connected by a telephone.

B. Social environment

Sophie states that she has had a home carer for the last 3 months who attends three times per day, 7 days a week. Sophie says she has not been enjoying the company of her granddaughter recently and feels guilty about this.

Sophie lives with her husband and he states that he is in good health. He says he is frustrated by his wife's lack of engagement in activities and her perception that he is not completing tasks to her standards.

Sophie's daughter states that she and her husband live close by. They both work full-time but Sophie's daughter visits every evening to support her parents. She has two teenage children, a son and a daughter, who now only visit sporadically.

Sophie has asked friends not to visit any longer. She states that she does not want them to see her unkempt.

C. Daily routine

Sophie's husband states that she rises at 9am when the home care assistant attends. She goes through her morning routine then has breakfast at 9.30am. She sits in her lounge chair watching TV all day and evening. The homecare assistant attends at 1pm to carry out domestic tasks. She then attends at 10pm to support Sophie with her night routine. Sophie states that she is not happy with this routine but cannot 'be bothered to do anything'.

D. Roles

i. Self-care: Sophie's self-care routine takes place entirely within her bedroom. Sophie does not:

- strip-wash at the bathroom sink
- use the shower
- use the perch stool

due to lack of confidence in her balance. Sophie states that to wash herself she has an established routine and sits on the bedside commode. The care assistant arranges needed objects to support this lack of mobility and provides verbal encouragement (to support Sophie's lack of confidence). Sophie and her daughter both state that she then has the skills to dress herself independently on the commode. Grooming herself is very important to Sophie; she says that she is currently unable to set her hair and can no longer get out of her flat to access the hairdresser.

Sophie was observed on the visit to:

- independently transfer on/off a 40 cm high commode using a Zimmer frame with a safe technique
- independently transfer on/off a 40 cm high toilet, using a 5 cm raised toilet seat and right wall grab rail, with a safe technique.

Bed transfer was not observed. Sophie did not want to attempt shower transfer, as she is not currently using the shower and is comfortable with her current arrangement of strip-washing at the bedside.

ii. Productivity

- *Cooking.* The kitchen was observed to have a gas cooker with overhead grill, microwave, electric kettle, continuous surfaces, and a table and chairs. Although Sophie stated that she previously enjoyed cooking for the sheltered housing volunteer position, her husband now does all the cooking and hot drinks at home. She states that she has 'no interest' in cooking now, although does occasionally help prepare meals with her husband. She feels she cannot do the cooking now and feels she will not be able to do this independently. They have a diet of toast in the morning, banana and bread for lunch and a cooked meal in the evening. Sophie states that she does not eat the vegetables because her husband does not prepare them well enough. Sophie's husband feels that Sophie still has the skill, supportive environment and previous habits to cook but she is not motivated to do so. He is frustrated by his wife's lack of engagement with cooking.

- *Task on visit: making a hot drink.* Sophie stated that she would not be able to manage to complete the activity. She did, however, manage to make the hot drink independently with the following skill level:
  - ○ *Motor skills.* She was unsteady at times and slow, but managed physically without intervention. She demonstrated some stiffness and reduction in strength. She appeared to lack energy and sat at regular intervals during the activity.
  - ○ *Process skills.* Sophie managed to use knowledge, plan and organize the activity. She did, however, have challenges problem-solving.
- Sophie did not view this as an achievement because it was not completed to her standard.
- *Laundry/cleaning and shopping.* These activities are completed by the home carer and Sophie's husband. They are happy to continue to support; however, Sophie feels these activities are not completed to 'her standards'.
- *Volunteer job.* Sophie has not been involved with her volunteer job for 3 years. She states she misses the social contact and the feeling of 'being useful'.

iii. Leisure: Sophie could identify interests that she engaged in the past. She specifically identified the social aspect of these interests as being enjoyable and satisfying.

Sophie now appears to have reduced leisure opportunities. She could identify specific TV programmes that she enjoys watching. She now receives a weekly visit at home from the church. She could not identify anything else that she does that brings her enjoyment.

Sophie's daughter is particularly concerned that Sophie is not engaging with previous leisure activities. Her daughter states she feels that this is the key for supporting her mother to 're-engage in life'.

E. Goals

Sophie was unable to identify any goals for the future. Sophie feels very pessimistic about her ability to return

to a meaningful life. She states she feels 'hopeless' about the future.

F. Readiness for change

Sophie's current situation is not supportive of her mental or physical health. The combination of high performance standards and less skill means that Sophie lacks motivation to engage in doing activities that were meaningful to her in the past and she cannot identify any goals, develop plans and follow them through. Although socially isolated by not being able to ascend/descend external stairs, Sophie stated that she is not prepared to consider moving to alternative accommodation on the ground floor. The couple have been buying their council flat and moving would be 'too large an upheaval'. Sophie now has carer support and has developed strong habits and dependence on this support. Although Sophie is unhappy with her circumstances, she is not ready to change independently and, therefore, requires further extended occupational therapy input.

Occupational therapy perspective (Fig. 6.6)

Sophie gives the impression of a person who has given up on life. She has previously been an active woman but has had a reduction in activity in the past 5 years since retiring; this has further reduced in the past 12 months and was accelerated within the last 6 months following a hospital admission. This situation was brought about primarily by a difficult transition from working to retirement, physical limitations and pain when mobilizing. This has been compounded by the identification of the start of a dementia process.

Motivation for activity: Currently Sophie lacks motivation to engage in previously held meaningful activity. Specifically, she has difficulty appraising her own abilities, leading to her being dependent on others. She does not expect success in the future, which leads to fear of failing and not meeting her high standards. She cannot identify any activities that bring her enjoyment and is unable to set goals for the future. These characteristics create a situation where Sophie does not make choices to do activity, apart from basic self-care.

Pattern of activity: Sophie has had substantial role loss over the last 5 years, which has led to an empty routine, a poor sense of belonging and avoidance of previously held responsibility. She demonstrates an unwillingness to agree to changes in her current routines and ways of doing activities, even though these habits do not support her preferred lifestyle.

Skill for activity: Sophie has adequate communication and interaction skills but is now having challenges maintaining relationships. She has physical difficulties with balance, stiffness, strength and energy. She has adequate processing skills but has difficulty with problem-solving.

Environment: Sophie's physical environment is problematic, as her flat is accessed by stairs and she cannot ascend/descend them. This will not be easily resolved. Her social environment is very supportive; however, carers are not supporting the development of Sophie's ability to engage in daily activities.

Overall recommendation

Sophie's current situation is not supportive of her mental or physical health. Although Sophie wants to change her circumstances, she is not ready to change independently and therefore requires further extended occupational therapy input.

NAME: Kirsty Forsyth
GRADE: Senior I
LOCATION: Edinburgh Community Rehabilitation Team
cc: GP, PT

Client: Sophie Bronson				**Assessor:** K. Forsyth
Age: 70	**Date of birth:** 01/02/34			**Designation:** Senior IOT
Sex:	Male:	Female:		**Signature:**
Status:	Impatient:	Outpatient:		**Date of assessment:** 16/03/05
Ethnicity:	White:	Black:	Asian:	**Treatment setting:** Home
Disabling condition:	Dementia			

4	Strength	Supports occupational participation
3	Difficulty	Minor interference with or risk to occupational participation
2	Weakness	Major interference with occupational participation
1	Problems	Prevents occupational participation

ANALYSIS OF STRENGTHS AND LIMITATIONS

Sophie is currently having difficulty engaging in meaningful daily activity and appears to have given up on life. This situation is not supportive of her physical or mental health. Although Sophie is dissatisfied with her present circumstances she is not ready to independently change, and therefore requires further extended occupational therapy. See ratings below.

Fig 6.6 • The Model of Human Occupation Screening Tool (MOHOST). Copyright © Patkinson, S., Forsyth, K., Kielhofner, G., 2005. The Model of Human Occupation Tool (MOHOST), version 2.0. Reproduced with the permission of Parkinson, Forsyth & Kielhofner.

SUMMARY OF RATINGS

Motivation of occupation				Pattern of occupation				Communication and interaction skills				Process skills				Motor skills				Environment			
Appraisal of abilities	Expectation of success	Interest	Commitment	Routine	Adaptability	Responsibility	Roles	Non-verbal skills	Conversation	Vocal expression	Relationships	Knowledge	Planning	Organization	Problem-solving	Posture and mobility	Coordination	Strength and effort	Energy	Physical space	Physical resources	Social groups	Occupational demands
4	4	4	4	4	4	4	4	(4)	(4)	(4)	4	(4)	(4)	(4)	4	4	4	4	4	4	4	(4)	4
3	3	3	3	3	3	3	3	3	3	3	3	3	3	3	3	3	(3)	(3)	3	3	3	3	(3)
(2)	2	(2)	2	2	2	(2)	2	2	2	2	(2)	2	2	2	(2)	(2)	2	2	(2)	2	2	2	2
1	(1)	1	(1)	(1)	(1)	1	(1)	1	1	1	1	1	1	1	1	1	1	1	1	(1)	(1)	1	1

MOTIVATION FOR OCCUPATION		
Appraisal of ability Understanding of strengths and limitations Self-awareness and realism Belief in skill	4	Realistic, recognizes strengths, aware of limitations, shows pride in assets
	3	Reasonable tendency to over/underestimate own abilities, recognizes some limitations
	(2)	Over/underestimates own abilities leading to inappropriate occupations
	1	Does not reflect on skills, fails to realistically estimate or lacks pride in own abilities
		Comments: ....
Expectation of success Optimism Self-efficacy Sense of control Hope	4	Anticipates success and seeks challenges, confident about overcoming obstacles
	3	Has some hope for success, adequate self-belief but has some doubts, may need encouraging
	2	Requires support to sustain confidence about overcoming obstacles or overly confident
	(1)	Pessimistic, feels hopeless or highly overconfident, gives up in the face of obstacles
		Comments: ....
Interest Expressed enjoyment Satisfaction Curiosity Participation	4	Keen, curious, lively, tries new occupations, expresses pleasure, perseveres, appears content
	3	Has adequate interests that guide choices, has some opportunities to pursue interests
	(2)	Difficulty identifying interests, interest is short-lived, ambivalent about choice of occupations
	1	Easily bored, unable to identify interests, apathetic, lacks curiosity even with support
		Comments: ....
Commitment Values and standards Goals and projects Choices and preferences Sense of purpose	4	Clear preferences and sense of what is important, motivated to work towards occupational goals
	3	Mostly able to make choices, may need encouragement to set and work towards goals
	2	Difficulties identifying what is important or setting and working towards goals, inconsistent
	(1)	Cannot set goals, impulsive, chaotic, goals are unattainable or based on antisocial values
		Comments: ....

Fig 6.6—cont'd

PATTERN OF OCCUPATION

Routine	4	Able to arrange a balanced routine that supports responsibilities and goals (steady)
Balance	3	Generally able to maintain an organized and productive daily schedule
Structure	2	Difficulty organizing routines to meet occupational responsibilities without support
Productivity	(1)	Chaotic or empty routine, unable to support responsibilities and goals (erratic/imbalanced)
Activity		Comments: ....
Adaptability	4	Anticipates change, alters actions or routine to meet demand (flexible/accommodating)
Anticipation	3	Generally able to modify behaviour, may need time to adjust, hesitant
Flexibility	2	Difficulty adapting to change, reluctant, passive or habitually overreacts
Response to change	(1)	Rigid, unable to adapt routines or tolerate change
Frustration tolerance		Comments: ....
Responsibility	4	Willingly takes on responsibilities and meets expectations (reliable/dependable)
Awareness	3	Accepts responsibility for most personal actions, can generally utilize constructive feedback
Handling expectation		
Fulfilling obligations	(2)	Difficulty recognizing responsibilities, avoids extra responsibilities or feels over-responsible
Acceptance	1	Unable to recognize responsibilities, denies responsibilities or responds inappropriately
		Comments: ....
Roles	4	Has a sense of identity that comes from roles, is committed to their roles and fits in well
Involvement	3	Generally meets obligations of several roles or maintains one major productive role
Belonging	2	Limited involvement in roles or has difficulty meeting role demands due to overload/conflict
Response to demand	(1)	Poor sense of belonging, has negligible role demands, does not identify with any role
Role variety		Comments: ....

COMMUNICATION AND INTERACTION SKILLS

Non-verbal skills	(4)	Appropriate (possibly spontaneous) body language, given culture and circumstances
Physicality	3	Demonstrates questionable ability to display or control appropriate body language
Eye contact	2	Difficulty controlling/displaying appropriate body language (delayed/limited/disinhibited)
Gestures		
Orientation	1	Unable to display appropriate body language (absent/incongruent/unsafe/violent)
		Comments: ....
Conversation	(4)	Appropriately initiates, discloses and sustains conversation (clear/direct/open)
Disclosing	3	Demonstrates questionable ability to effectively exchange information
Initiating and sustaining	2	Difficulty initiating, disclosing or sustaining conversation (hesitant/abrupt/limited/irrelevant)
Speech content		
Language	1	Uncommunicative, disjointed, bizarre or inappropriate disclosure of information
		Comments: ....
Vocal expression	(4)	Assertive, articulate, uses appropriate tone, volume and pace
Intonation	3	Demonstrates questionable ability in vocal expression
Articulation	2	Difficulty with expressing self (unclear/pressured speech/monotone)
Volume	1	Unable to express self (incomprehensible/too quiet or loud/too fast)
Pace		Comments: ....

Fig 6.6—cont'd

(Continued)

Relationships	4	Sociable, supportive, aware of others, sustains engagement, friendly, relates well to others
Cooperation	3	Demonstrates questionable social skills
Collaboration	(2)	Difficulty with cooperation or makes few positive relationships
Rapport	1	Unable to cooperate with others or make positive relationships
Respect		*Comments:* ....

PROCESS SKILLS

Knowledge	(4)	Seeks and retains relevant information, selects tools appropriately, shows understanding
Seeking and retaining information	3	Demonstrates questionable ability to seek and retain information and use tools
	2	Difficulty selecting and using tools, difficulty in asking for help (forgetful/unaware/confused)
Use of knowledge, including use of objects	1	Unable to complete occupation, disoriented or lacking knowledge or ability to use tools
Understanding, orientation		*Comments:* ....

Planning	(4)	Plans ahead, sustains concentration, starts and completes occupation at appropriate times
Thinking through from beginning to end	3	Demonstrates questionable ability to plan for and during occupations
Timing	2	Difficulty planning, fluctuating concentration or distractible, difficulty initiating and completing
Concentration	1	Unable to plan ahead, unable to concentrate, unable to initiate or complete occupations
		Comments: ....

Organization	(4)	Efficiently searches for, gathers and restores tools/objects needed in occupation (neat)
Arranging space and objects	3	Demonstrates questionable ability to search, gather and restore needed tools/objects
Neatness	2	Difficulty searching for, gathering and restoring tools/objects, appears disorganized/untidy
Preparation	1	Unable to search for, gather and restore tools and objects (chaotic)
		Comments: ....

Problem-solving	4	Shows good judgement, anticipates difficulties and generates workable solutions (rational)
Judgement	3	Demonstrates questionable ability to make decisions based on difficulties that arise
Adaptation	(2)	Difficulty anticipating and adapting to difficulties that arise, seeks reassurance
Decision-making	1	Unable to anticipate and adapt to difficulties that arise and makes inappropriate decisions
Responsiveness		*Comments:* ....

MOTOR SKILLS

Posture and mobility	4	Stable, upright, independent, flexible, good range of movement (possibly agile)
Stability walking	3	Demonstrates questionable ability to maintain posture and mobility in occupation
Alignment reaching	(2)	Unsteady at times, slow or manages with difficulty
Positioning bending	1	Extremely unstable, unable to reach and bend or unable to walk
Balance transfers		*Comments:* ....

Coordination	4	Coordinates body parts with each other, uses smooth fluid movements (possibly dextrous)
Manipulation	(3)	Some awkwardness or stiffness
Ease of movement	2	Difficulty coordinating movements (clumsy/tremulous/awkward/stiff)
Fluidity	1	Unable to coordinate, manipulate and use fluid movements
Fine motor skills		*Comments:* ....

Fig 6.6—cont'd

Strength and effort	4	Grasps, moves and transports objects securely with adequate force/speed (possibly strong)
Grip lifting	③	Demonstrates questionable ability in strength and effort
Handling, transporting	2	Has difficulty with grasping, moving, transporting objects with adequate force and speed
Moving, calibrating	1	Unable to grasp, move, transport objects with appropriate force and speed (weak/frail)
		Comments: ....
Energy	4	Maintains appropriate energy levels, able to maintain tempo throughout occupation
Endurance	3	Demonstrates questionable energy (whether low or high)
Pace	②	Difficulty maintaining energy (tires easily/evidence of fatigue/distractible/restless)
Attention	1	Unable to maintain energy, lacks focus, lethargic, inactive or highly overactive
Stamina		*Comments:* ....

ENVIRONMENT		
Physical space	4	Affords a range of opportunities, supports and stimulates valued occupations
Home and neighbourhood	3	OT questions whether the physical space adequately supports valued occupations
Work and/or leisure facilities	2	Affords a limited range of opportunities and curtails performance of valued occupations
Privacy and accessibility	①	Restricts opportunities and prevents performance of valued occupations
Stimulation and comfort		*Comments:* ....
Physical resources	4	Allow occupational goals to be achieved safely, easily and independently
Finance	3	Have questionable impact on ability to achieve occupational goals
Equipment and tools	2	Restrict ability to achieve occupational goals safely, easily and independently
Possessions and transport	①	Have major impact on ability to achieve occupational goals, lead to high risks
Safety and independence		*Comments:* ....
Social groups	④	Offer practical support, values and attitudes support optimal functioning
Family dynamics	3	OT questions the support of social groups due to under- or over-involvement
Friends and social support	2	Offer reduced support, or detracts from functioning, supported in some groups but not others
Work climate	1	Do not support functioning due to lack of interest or inappropriate involvement
Expectations and involvement		*Comments:* ....
Occupational demands	4	Match well with abilities, interests, energy and time available
Social and leisure activities	③	OT questions whether the demands are consistent with abilities, interest, energy or time
Daily living tasks	2	Some inconsistencies with abilities and interest, or energy and time available
Work and/or domestic responsibilities	1	Inconsistent with abilities and motivation, under or overdemanding
		Comments: ....

Fig 6.6—cont'd

Summary

MOHO provides a way for occupational therapists to embrace the complexity of human occupation within their practice. It provides an understanding of the choice, order and performance of occupation within people's lives. It also provides assessment and intervention techniques to support the integration of MOHO theory into practice. MOHO is built for and with an international community of occupational therapists, with the ultimate goal of fully embracing the unique occupational characteristics of our clients and supporting them in their re-engagement with meaningful self-care, productivity and leisure.

Reflective learning

Think of a recent OT client you have been involved with (either as a student on placement or as a qualified OT) and ask yourself the following questions:

- What is the person's occupational identity? (Prompt: what roles do they identify with? Father, brother, sibling, worker)
- What is the person's occupational competence? (Prompt: what skills does the person feel they have to meet role responsibilities? Is this accurate appraisal?)
- What are the positive occupational issues for the person? (Prompt: Think about engagement in self-care, work and/or leisure & personal causation, values,

interests, habits, role, performance capacity, skills or environment? or a combination of these)

- Why is the person unable or having challenges engaging in occupations? (Prompt: Think about challenges engagement in self-care, work and/or leisure & personal causation, values, interests, habits, role, performance capacity, skills or environment? or a combination of these)
- Write a summary statement using the answers to the above questions in order to capture the main occupational issues for the client

References

American Occupational Therapy Association, 2002. Occupational therapy practice framework: Domain and process. American Journal of Occupational Therapy 56, 609–639.

Ayres, A.J., 1972. Sensory Integration and Learning Disorders. Western Psychological Services, Los Angeles.

Ayres, A.J., 1979. Sensory Integration and the Child. Western Psychological Services, Los Angeles.

Ayres, A.J., 1986. Developmental Dyspraxia and Adult Onset Apraxia. Sensory Integration International, Torrance, CA.

Butts, D.S., Nelson, D.L., 2007. Agreement between Occupational Therapy Practice Framework classifications and occupational therapists' classifications. American Journal of Occupational Therapy. Sep-Oct; 61 (5), 603–604.

Barris, R., Kielhofner, G., Burch, R.M., et al., 1986. Occupational function and dysfunction in three groups of adolescents. Occupational Therapy Journal of Research 6, 301–307.

Bruner, J., 1990. Acts of Meaning. Harvard University Press, Cambridge, MA.

Creek, J., 2002. The knowledge base of occupational therapy. In: Creek, J. (Ed.), Occupational Therapy and Mental Health. Churchill Livingstone, Edinburgh.

Creek, J., 2003. Occupational Therapy Defined as a Complex Intervention. College of Occupational Therapists, London.

Creek, J., 2009. Occupational therapy defined as a complex intervention: a 5-year review. British Journal of Occupational Therapy 72 (3), 105–115. Retrieved from CINAHL with Full Text database.

Crepeau, E., 2003. Activity analysis: a way of thinking about occupational performance. In: Crepeau, E.B., Schell, B., Cohn, E. (Eds.), Willard and Spackman's Occupational Therapy. Lippincott Williams & Wilkins, Philadelphia.

Csikszentmihalyi, M., 1990. Flow: The Psychology of Optimal Experience. Harper & Row, New York.

Davies Hallet, J., Zasler, N., Maurer, P., et al., 1994. Role change after traumatic brain injury in adults. American Journal of Occupational Therapy 48, 241–246.

de las Heras, C.G., Geist, R., Kielhofner, G., et al., 2001. The Volitional Questionnaire (VQ) (Version 4.1). Model of Human Occupation Clearinghouse. Department of Occupational Therapy, College of Applied Health Sciences, University of Illinois at Chicago, Chicago.

Dewey, J., 1922. Human Nature and Conduct. Henry Holt, New York.

Ebb, E.W., Coster, W., Duncombe, L., 1989. Comparison of normal and psychosocially dysfunctional male adolescents. Occupational Therapy in Mental Health 9, 53–74.

Fidler, G., Fidler, J., 1963. Occupational Therapy: a Communication Process in Psychiatry. Macmillan, New York.

Fisher, A., Kielhofner, G., 1995. Skill in occupational performance. In: Kielhofner, G. (Ed.), A Model of Human Occupation: Theory and Application. second ed. Williams & Wilkins, Baltimore.

Fisher, A.G., 1999a. Uniting practice and theory in an occupational framework. American Journal of Occupational Therapy 532 (7), 509–520.

Fisher, A.G., 1999b. Assessment of Motor and Process Skills (3rd ed.). Three Star Press, Ft. Collins, CO.

Forsyth, K., Salamy, M., Simon, S., et al., 1997. Assessment of Communication and Interaction Skills. University of Illinois, Model of Human Occupation Clearinghouse, Chicago.

Forsyth, K., Salamy, M., Simon, S., et al., 1998. A user's guide to the Assessment of Communication and Interaction Skills (ACIS) Chicago: Model of Human Occupation Clearinghouse. Department of Occupational Therapy, College of Applied Health Sciences, University of Illinois at Chicago, Chicago.

Foster, M., Pratt, J., 2002. Activity analysis. In: Turner, A., Foster, M., Johnston, S.E. (Eds.), Occupational Therapy and Physical Dysfunction: Principles, Skills and Practice. Churchill Livingstone, Edinburgh.

Geist, R., Kielhofner, G., Basu, S., et al., 2001. The Pediatric Volitional Questionnaire (PVQ) (Version 1.1). Model of Human Occupation Clearinghouse, Department of Occupational Therapy, College of Applied Health Sciences, University of Illinois at Chicago, Chicago.

Gill, C.J., 1997. Four types of integration in disability identity development. Journal of Vocational Rehabilitation 9, 39–46.

Hagedorn, R., 2000. Tools for Practice in Occupational Therapy. Churchill Livingstone, Edinburgh.

Haglund, L., Karlsson, G., Kielhofner, G., et al., 1997. Validity of the Swedish version of the Worker Role Interview. Scandinavian Journal of Occupational Therapy 4 (1–4), 23–29.

Haglund, L., Ekbladh, E., Thorell, L., et al., 2000. Practice models in Swedish psychiatric occupational therapy. Scandinavian Journal of Occupational Therapy 7 (3), 107–113.

Harter, S., 1983. The development of the self-system. In: Hetherington, M. (Ed.), Handbook of Child Psychology: Social and Personality Development, vol. 4. John Wiley, New York.

Harter, S., Connel, J.P., 1984. A model of relationships among children's academic achievement and self perceptions of competence, control, and motivation. In: Nicholls, J. (Ed.), The Development of Achievement Motivation. JAI, Greenwich, CT.

Hull, J.M., 1990. Touching the Rock: An Experience of Blindness. Vintage, New York.

Husserl, E., 1962. Ideas: General introduction to Pure Phenomenology. Collier, London (W.R.B. Gibson, Trans.).

Kielhofner, G., 1980a. A Model of Human Occupation, part three. Benign and vicious cycles. American Journal of Occupational Therapy 34, 731–737.

Kielhofner, G., 1980b. A Model of Human Occupation, part two. Ontogenesis from the perspective of temporal adaptation. American Journal of Occupational Therapy 34, 657–663.

Kielhofner, G., 1985. A Model of Human Occupation: Theory and Application. Williams & Wilkins, Baltimore.

Kielhofner, G., 1995. A Model of Human Occupation: Theory and Application, second ed. Williams & Wilkins, Baltimore.

Kielhofner, G., 1997. Conceptual Foundations of Occupational Therapy. FA Davis, Philadelphia.

Kielhofner, G., 2002. A Model of Human Occupation: Theory and Application, third ed. Williams & Wilkins, Baltimore.

Kielhofner, G., 2008. A Model of Human Occupation: Theory and Application, fourth ed. Lippincott Williams & Wilkins, Baltimore.

Kielhofner, G., Burke, J.P., 1977. Occupational therapy after 60 years: an account of changing identity and knowledge. American Journal of Occupational Therapy 31, 675–689.

Kielhofner, G., Burke, J., 1980. A Model of Human Occupation, part one. Conceptual framework and content. American Journal of Occupational Therapy 34, 572–581.

Kielhofner, G., Forsyth, K., 2001. Development of a client self-report for treatment planning and documenting therapy outcomes. Scandinavian Journal of Occupational Therapy 8 (3), 131–139.

Kielhofner, G., Burke, J., Heard, I.C., 1980. A Model of Human Occupation, part four. Assessment and intervention. American Journal of Occupational Therapy 34, 777–788.

Kielhofner, G., Mallinson, T., Crawford, C., et al., 1997. A user's guide to the occupational performance history interview-II (OPHI-II) (version 2.0). Model of Human Occupation Clearinghouse, Department of Occupational Therapy, College of Applied Health Sciences, University of Illinois at Chicago, Chicago.

Kielhofner, G., Lai, J.S., Olson, L., et al., 1999. Psychometric properties of the work environment impact scale: a cross-cultural study. Work: a Journal of Prevention. Assessment & Rehabilitation 12 (1), 71–77.

Kielhofner, G., Mallinson, T., Forsyth, K., et al., 2001. Psychometric properties of the second version of the Occupational Performance History Interview (OPHI-II). American Journal of Occupational Therapy 55, 260–267.

Lamport, N., Coffey, M., Hersch, G., 2001. Activity Analysis and Application Building Blocks of Treatment. Slack, Thorofare, NJ.

Law, M., 1998. Client-centred Occupational Therapy. Slack, Thorofare, NJ.

Law, M., McColl, M.A., 1989. Knowledge and use of theory among occupational therapists: a Canadian survey. Canadian Journal of Occupational Therapy 56 (4), 198–204.

Lederer, J., Kielhofner, G., Watts, J., 1985. Values, personal causation and skills of delinquents and non delinquents. Occupational Therapy in Mental Health 5, 59–77.

Lee, D., 1971. Culture and the experience of value. In: Maslow, A.H. (Ed.), Neural Knowledge in Human Values. Henry Regnery, Chicago.

Lee, S., Kielhofner, G., Taylor, R., 2009. Choice, knowledge, and utilization of a practice theory: a national study of occupational therapists who use the Model of Human Occupation. Occupational Therapy in Health Care 23 (1), 60–71.

Lefcourt, H.M., 1981. Research with the Locus of Control Construct, vol. 1: Assessment and Methods. Academic Press, New York.

Mallinson, T., Mahaffey, L., Kielhofner, G., 1998. The Occupational Performance History Interview: evidence for three underlying constructs of occupational adaptation. Canadian Journal of Occupational Therapy 65 (4), 219–228.

Mancuso, J., Sarbin, T., 1983. The self-narrative in the enactment of roles. In: Sarbin, T.R., Scheibe, K.E. (Eds.), Studies in Social Identity. Praeger, New York.

Merleau-Ponty, M., 1962. Phenomenology of perception. Translated by C. Smith from the French original version, Phénoménologie de la perception, Routledge & Kegan Paul, London.

Miller, J.F., Oertel, C.B., 1983. Powerlessness in the elderly: preventing hopelessness. In: Miller, J.F. (Eds.), Coping with Chronic Illness: Overcoming Powerlessness. FA Davis, Philadelphia.

Moore-Corner, R., Kielhofner, G., Olsen, L., 1998. Work Environment Impact Scale (WEIS) (Version 2). Model of Human Occupational Clearinghouse, Department of Occupational Therapy, College of applied Health Sciences, University of Illinois at Chicago, Chicago.

Mosey, A., 1986. Psychosocial Components of Occupational Therapy. Raven, New York.

Murphy, R., 1987. The Body Silent. Henry Holt, New York.

National Board for Certification in Occupational Therapy. (2004). A practice analysis study of entry-level occupational therapist registered and certified occupational therapy assistant practice. OTJR, Occupation, Participation and Health. Spring, Volume 24, Supplement 1,S3–31.

Parkinson, S., Forsyth, K., Kielhofner, G., 2001. The Model of Human Occupation Screening tool (MOHOST), version 1.0. Model of Human Occupation Clearinghouse, Department of Occupational Therapy, College of Applied Health Sciences, University of Illinois at Chicago, Chicago.

Peterson, E., Howland, J., Kielhofner, G., et al., 1999. Falls self-efficacy and occupational adaptation among elders. Physical & Occupational Therapy in Geriatrics 16, 1–16.

Reilly, M., 1962. Occupational therapy can be one of the great ideas of 20th century medicine. American Journal of Occupational Therapy 16, 1–9.

Riccio, C.M., Nelson, D.L., Bush, M.A., 1990. Adding purpose to the repetitive exercises of elderly women. American Journal of Occupational Therapy 44, 714–719.

Rotter, J.B., 1960. Generalized expectancies for internal versus external control of reinforcement. Psychological Monographs: General Applications 80, 1–28.

Shannon, P., 1970. The work-play model: A basis for occupational therapy programming. American Journal of Occupational Therapy 24, 215–218.

Sumsion, T., 1999. Client-centred Practice in Occupational Therapy: A Guide to Implementation. Churchill Livingstone, Edinburgh.

Taylor, R., Braveman, B., Forsyth, K., 2002. Occupational science and the scholarship of practice: implications for practitioners. New Zealand Journal of Occupational Therapy 49, 37–40.

Taylor, R.R., Lee, S.W., Kielhofner, G., Ketkar, M., 2009. Therapeutic use of self: A nationwide survey of practitioners' attitudes and experiences. American Journal of Occupational Therapy 63, 198–207.

Toglia, J.P., 2003. The multicontext treatment approach. In: Crepeau, E.B., Schell, B., Cohn, E. (Eds.), Willard and Spackman's Occupational Therapy. Lippincott Williams & Wilkins, Philadelphia.

Toombs, K., 1992. The Meaning of Illness: A Phenomenological Account of the Different Perspectives of Physician and Patient. Kluwer Academic, Boston.

Trombly, C.A., 1989. Occupational Therapy for Physical Dysfunction. Williams & Wilkins, Baltimore.

Trombly, C., 1995. Occupation: purposefulness and meaningfulness as therapeutic mechanisms. American Journal of Occupational Therapy 49, 960–972.

World Health Organization, 1999. ICIDH-2: International Classification of Functioning and Disability. Beta-2 draft, full version. WHO, Geneva.

Yoder, R., Nelson, D., Smith, D., 1989. Added-purpose versus rote exercise in female nursing home residents. The American Journal of Occupational Therapy: Official Publication of The American Occupational Therapy Association 43 (9), 581–586.

Applying the Canadian Model of Occupational Performance

7

Thelma Sumsion   Lesley Tischler-Draper   Sheila Heinicke

OVERVIEW

Client-centred practice now forms the foundation for interactions with people in many countries. Canadian occupational therapists created a model in the early 1980s to support the use of this approach and have continued to develop both the model and its application in a variety of clinical settings (see Chapter 11). Colleagues in many other countries are also developing expertise in the application of both the model and the outcome measure that arose from it. This chapter aims to ensure that students, therapists and educators understand the origins of this approach and how to apply the outcome measure. To accomplish this goal, a historical overview of the Canadian Model of Occupational Performance (CMOP) and the emergence of the Canadian Model of Occupational Performance and Engagement (CMOP-E), with a discussion of key components, has been provided. An overview of the Canadian Occupational Performance Measure (COPM) that arose from the model is also presented, together with detailed information about its application with two clients. In order to give a practical illustration of the model and outcome measure, particular reference is made to its application in a mental health setting.

Key points

This chapter examines:
- the development of the Canadian Model of Occupational Performance (CMOP)
- the emergence of the Canadian Model of Occupational Performance and Engagement (CMOP-E)
- the links between the CMOP and the Canadian Occupational Performance Measure (COPM)

Key points—cont'd

and provides:
- a description of the COPM
- two case examples showing the application of the COPM.

Introduction

This chapter aims to present the story of the development of the CMOP from a historical perspective, including the many revisions that have been made to the model and its consistent components, as well as its current format. The chapter then proceeds to apply the components of the model, and the outcome measure that arose from it, to two case studies.

Model of Occupational Performance

Historical perspective

The Model of Occupational Performance forms the basis of client-centred practice in occupational therapy in Canada and increasingly in other countries. A Canadian taskforce, jointly funded by the Canadian Association of Occupational Therapists (CAOT) and the Department of National Health and Welfare, developed the original Model of Occupational Performance that was based on the work of Reed and Sanderson (Law et al 1990).

In 1983 Reed and Sanderson proposed a Human Occupation Model that contained four concentric circles. The individual was in the centre of the model and therefore, by implication, was at the centre of the intervention. The second circle contained the five performance components or skills, which are 'areas a person develops to facilitate carrying out occupations' (p.11). These components are

- motor — composed of the neuromuscular/skeletal system
- sensory — the primary means of gaining information from the outside world
- cognitive — attending to tasks, problem-solving and memory
- intrapersonal — coping with reality and distinguishing it from non-reality
- interpersonal — relating to others in dyads or groups (pp.13–14).

Human occupation was shown in the third circle and was broken down into:

- self-maintenance — activities done to maintain the person's health and well-being in the environment
- productivity — activities or tasks done to enable the person to provide support to self and others
- leisure — activities or tasks done for enjoyment or renewal (p.10).

These occupations are the focus of occupational therapy. The outer circle was labelled 'adaptation to and with the environment' (p.6). People interact with the environment by using their occupational skills. In summary, this model outlined that the goal of occupational therapy was to promote or maintain health through performance of occupational skills throughout the lifespan, and in all stages of health and illness.

The early Canadian model (the Model of Occupational Performance) clearly replicated some aspects of Reed and Sanderson's (1983) work but also proposed other unique elements. This original version of the Model of Occupational Performance helped to make the theory more accessible, as it provided a background for practice. This model placed the individual in the centre of many interacting spheres. The middle sphere depicted the three areas of a person's occupational performance, which were self-care, productivity and leisure. The performance components of the individual were featured in the centre sphere. These components were spiritual, physical, sociocultural and mental. This model supported a holistic view and recognized the worth of the individual (Townsend 1993). In addition, 'the integration and execution of occupational performance is defined and shaped by the individual's social, physical and cultural environments' (Townsend et al 1990, p.71) which were joined by the political, economic and legal environments in 1993 (CAOT and Health Canada 1993).

McColl and Pranger (1994) criticized this original model, saying it was developed in an unorthodox manner. They also expressed concerns that the model was limited, as it discussed occupational performance but not occupation. No empirical support was offered for the assumptions underlying the original model (McColl & Pranger 1994). In it, 'occupational performance looked static, the environment appeared to be external and unconnected to the person, and spirituality was depicted as a performance component parallel to mental, physical and socio-cultural performance' (CAOT 1997, p.30). The model was referred to as the Canadian Occupational Performance Model but this was not an official term. However, this issue was addressed in 1997 when the model was officially named (CAOT 1997). CAOT also recognized that there were problems with this model and these were addressed in the revised version.

Revised model

To address the above issues, the name of the model was changed in 1997 to the Canadian Model of Occupational Performance (CMOP). This version is shown in Figure 7.1 and presents many new concepts. 'CMOP is a social model that places the person in a social/environmental context rather than locating the environment outside of the person' (Sumsion 1999, p.7). Occupational performance is the result of interaction and interdependence between person, environment and occupation (Townsend 1998). The revised presentation is now an interactive model showing relationships between persons, environment and occupation (CAOT 1997).

Occupation is shown as a circle overlain by a triangle representing the doing (physical), feeling (affective) and thinking (cognitive) components of the person. The points of the triangle also extend beyond the circle of occupation to interact with the environment (Townsend 1998). In reality, therapists know that the interaction between people, their roles and the environment is quite dynamic and must constantly accommodate a variety of changes. The revised model allows for change and focuses on the interaction of the elements.

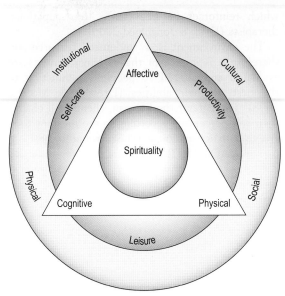

Fig. 7.1 • The Canadian Model of Occupational Performance (CMOP). Reprinted from Enabling Occupation: An Occupational Perspective (1997; 2002) by the Canadian Association of Occupational Therapists, with permission of CAOT Publications ACE, Ottawa, Ontario.

Self-care, productivity and leisure remain as performance components and are now considered to be the key components of occupation. The central sphere now focuses on the person, including their spiritual, affective, cognitive and physical components. The environments included in the outer sphere are physical, institutional, cultural and social (CAOT 1997, Sumsion 1999).

Components of the model

Occupation

The components of occupation are self-care, productivity and leisure. CAOT defines self-care as 'occupations for looking after the self' (CAOT 1997, p.37). Productivity is defined as 'occupations that make a social or economic contribution or that provide for economic sustenance' (CAOT 1997, p.37). Leisure is defined as occupations for enjoyment (CAOT 1997, p.37), which built on the definition presented by Reed and Sanderson (1983).

Performance

The 1997 CAOT document reformulated the performance components. The original four components — mental, physical, spiritual and sociocultural — could potentially be viewed in isolation from each other, and have therefore been developed into three components — affective, physical and cognitive — which facilitate interaction. The revised performance components were defined as follows:

- affective — (feeling): the domain that comprises all social and emotional functions and includes both interpersonal and intrapersonal factors
- physical — (doing): the domain that comprises all sensory, motor and sensorimotor functions
- cognitive — (thinking): the domain that comprises all mental functions, both cognitive and intellectual, and includes, among other things, perception, concentration, memory, comprehension, judgement and reasoning (CAOT 1997, p.44).

Occupational therapists are familiar with the affective, physical and cognitive performance components. However, the spiritual component, which remains central to the model, provides additional challenges and continues to lack a consistent definition (Sumsion 1999, Whalley Hammell 2001, McColl 2003). Its position is justified, as spirituality 'resides in persons, is shaped by the environment and gives meaning to occupation' (CAOT 1997, p.33), and in reality is a part of all of the components of the model and is necessary to maintain life (Sumsion 1999, Rebeiro 2001a). However, debate about the role of the occupational therapist continues through a discussion of whether occupation, rather than spirituality, should be the therapist's primary concern (Unruh et al 2002).

Environments

The original Model of Occupational Performance presented the cultural, physical and social environments and considered their impact on the person. The revised version of the CMOP (Fig. 7.1) has maintained the cultural, physical and social environments and has encompassed the economic, legal and political environments within the institutional environment (Sumsion 1999).

Everyone encompasses a number of different cultures, which may explain why the *cultural environment* fluctuates and is different for each individual (Sumsion 1997). Many issues that have an impact on a therapeutic intervention are culturally determined, including beliefs, values, customs, patterns of authority, how decisions are made and individual roles (Bonder 2001).

The *physical environment* can be seen as both a barrier and a support for individuals' participation in their community. Issues such as physical accessibility and proximity to family and support services must all be considered (O'Brien et al 2002). The physical environment is the traditional domain of occupational therapists and hence is the one with which they are most familiar (Sumsion 1999).

The *social environment* is composed of social groups such as family, co-workers and friends and their roles, as well as occupational forms such as playing cards or jogging (Sumsion 1997, 1999, Kielhofner 2008). This environment contains both people and social cues. The latter are implemented as we learn the rules and roles that govern behaviour (Hagedorn 2000). For those with mental illness, the social environment may limit engagement in occupation (Rebeiro 2001b).

The *institutional environment* includes legal elements that often overlap with the economic one as control of funds and who makes financial decisions often become legal matters (Sumsion 1997). The political and economic environments are also often connected and have the potential to expand well beyond the boundaries of this discussion. In reality, the economic environment overlaps with all other environments, including the political one, where issues such as accessible transport and buildings are of particular concern to occupational therapists (Sumsion 1997). The institutional environment has been shown to shape occupational performance,

which reinforces its importance to occupational therapists (Dyck & Jongbloed 2000).

The environment is an underused resource and therefore it is important that all environments are evaluated and altered so people can function to the best of their abilities (Dressler & MacRae 1998). Throughout the lifespan, clients will change their self-perception according to the meaning they give to both occupation and the surrounding environments (CAOT 1997). Therefore it is important for occupational therapists to remember that occupational performance is where the unique being, the environment and occupation overlap and that all environments are of equal importance in therapeutic considerations (Law et al 1996).

Current model

In 2007 the CAOT released *Enabling II* as a companion document to *Enabling Occupation* (CAOT 1997). This publication contained a revised version of the CMOP known as the Canadian Model of Occupational Performance and Engagement (CMOP-E). This version of the model has added increased emphasis to the concept of engagement signified by the 'E'. This is accomplished through the addition of a transverse section (Fig. 7.2) that presents occupation as 'our core domain of interest' (Townsend and Polatajko 2007,

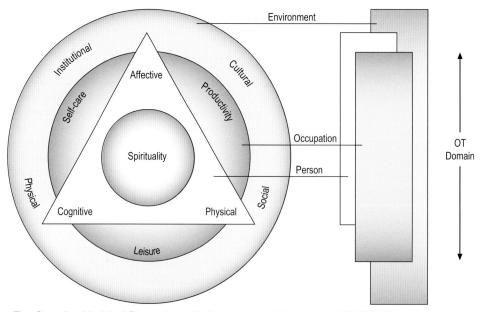

Fig. 7.2 • The Canadian Model of Occupational Performance and Engagement (CMOP-E). Reprinted from Townsend, E., Polatajko, H., 2007. Enabling Occupation II: Advancing an Occupational Therapy Vision for Health, Well-being and Justice Through Occupation, p.23, with permission from CAOT Publications ACE, Ottawa, Ontario.

p.24). The authors further state that 'we are only concerned with what is related to human occupation and its connection with the occupational person and the occupational influences of the environment' (Townsend and Polatajko 2007, p.24).

Application of the model

The CMOP and recently presented CMOP-E now truly form the basis of occupational therapy practice in Canada. Both the components and the model as a whole are the focus of research and local and national conference presentations.

At one end of the lifespan the model has been used as a framework to clarify a range of facts involved in feeding infants with congenital heart disease (Imms 2001). At the other it has been applied to work with community-dwelling older adults (Griffith et al 2007), where the application of components of the model enabled therapists to understand the person's occupational limitations and how these affected occupational performance.

Godfrey (2000) saw a clear link between the quality of a person's life and how they interact with the environment. In this discussion, the CMOP was used to illustrate how changes in one aspect of the system, such as the person or their occupation, affect all other aspects. However, concern was expressed that the model was not accompanied by a clear framework to guide practice. The need for more literature related to the application of the model in settings outside of Canada was also stressed (Clarke 2003). The CMOP-E attempts to address some of these concerns but there is still more work to be done.

Applying the model in a clinical setting

The CMOP, with a person at its centre, conveys occupational therapy's client-centred perspective (CAOT 1997). All therapists in Britain, as well as in Canada, are expected to provide services that are client-centred, as stated in the Code of Ethics and Professional Conduct (College of Occupational Therapists 2005). Therefore, any therapist committed to a client-centred approach would do well to explore this model. There are other models and associated assessments that are also client-centred (see Chapters 6 and 10); however, the appeal of the Canadian model lies in its simplicity and comprehensiveness. The Canadian model provides therapists with a simple, clear, conceptual framework for thinking about the person, with the person, throughout the occupational therapy process. Central to this model is the concept of occupational performance, which is an occupational therapist's principal domain of concern and expertise (Law et al 2005).

The link between the CMOP-E and the Canadian Occupational Performance Measure

Both the CMOP and CMOP-E are client-centred models for use in occupational therapy intervention with people with all types of health impairment across the lifespan. They look at each individual person's cognitive, affective and physical abilities within the context of the person's environment. A person's individual and unique spiritual nature is embedded within all aspects of the model.

The Canadian Occupational Performance Measure (COPM) is the outcome measure that was originally developed for use with the CMOP. It enables the occupational therapist and client to focus together on the perceived difficulties in the person's occupational performance areas of self-care, productivity and leisure. This multifunctional tool is designed for use with people of all ages and with all types of physical, cognitive and affective impairment. However, for the purposes of this chapter, the case examples will focus on how the model and the outcome measure can be used with people with a variety of mental health difficulties, at various points during the occupational therapy process.

The measure addresses the three areas of occupational performance that arise from the model (self-care, productivity and leisure) and asks the person to identify perceived difficulties in these areas. Therefore, occupational performance is presented as perceived by the individual and assessed subjectively by them. The person identifies the areas of difficulty, rates the importance of being able to perform in each area, the degree to which they feel they perform at present and their own satisfaction with their current occupational performance. Thus, the measure is truly client-centred and the person's performance can only be measured against himself or herself. In this sense the COPM is not a standardized measure, although there are specific instructions and methods for administering and scoring the test (Law et al 2005).

Description of COPM

The COPM is simple to follow and identifies perceived deficits in occupational performance. It is administered through one or more interviews in which the person is asked about problems, concerns and issues in the three areas of occupational performance, i.e. self-care, productivity and leisure.

Focusing on each area in turn, the person is asked to identify daily activities that they want to, need to or are expected to perform. The most straightforward way to do this is to ask the person to focus on a typical day or week. The problems that the person identifies are recorded on the form by the therapist. There are subdivisions for each of the occupational performance areas. For example, self-care is subdivided into personal care, functional mobility and community management. For each of these subdivisions there are additional prompts. For instance, personal care prompts are dressing, bathing, feeding and hygiene. With practice, and through working with specific groups of people, therapists will develop their own interview style and will know what prompts to use with the client. This measure is not a rigid standardized procedure, but rather a framework for thinking about the person, with the person, while remaining focused on occupational performance. It allows for a conversational style of assessment rather than a rigid question and answer approach.

Once the occupational performance problems have been identified, the person is asked to score these according to how important it is to them to be able to perform each identified task. This is a way of identifying priorities for treatment, with a client-centred focus. Once the problems have been scored for importance, the person is asked to select a maximum of five priorities and these are recorded on the form by the therapist.

Using scoring cards, which present a visual analogue scale (VAS) (1–10, with 1 meaning not able to do it at all and 10 meaning able to do it extremely well), the person is asked to rate their top five problems in terms of current performance and satisfaction with current performance. Satisfaction is rated in the same manner, i.e. a VAS 1–10 scale, with 1 indicating that the person is not at all satisfied with their performance and 10 indicating that they are extremely satisfied. Totalling these scores and dividing by the number of problems results in two overall figures. One denotes a performance score, and the other a satisfaction with performance score. At re-assessment the person scores each problem again for performance and satisfaction, and the new scores are calculated.

The following case examples provide more specific detail about how the assessment is used in a mental health setting. People's names have been changed to protect their identity and these examples are included with the express permission of the people concerned.

CASE STUDY

Sylvia

Sylvia is a 45-year-old single female diagnosed with bipolar disorder, who lives in a two-bedroom house with her 8-year-old son, Ryan. Sylvia has been involved with the outpatient mental health programme for 3 years, and recently moved to a new city where she continues to live. She had a short admission to an inpatient mental health hospital, and was referred to outpatient services after discharge from the hospital. Sylvia was referred to occupational therapy following her initial appointment with her psychiatrist and social worker. The COPM was used as an initial assessment to identify her perceived difficulties in occupational performance, and the areas she would like to address in her work with the occupational therapist.

The completion of the COPM initially identified the following concerns with Sylvia's occupational performance.

In the area of her self-care, Sylvia identified difficulties: having a shower regularly, getting up in the morning to see her son off to school and staying up after he leaves the house, budgeting her money to ensure she is paying the bills

on time, and allocating enough money to pay for groceries.

Obstacles identified in productivity included returning to competitive part-time employment, cooking for herself and her son, and completing household chores such as vacuuming, and cleaning the bathroom and kitchen environments.

Problems identified in Sylvia's leisure pursuits included participating in quiet recreation, such as flower arrangement, and active recreation, such as swimming, and socializing with her family and peers. Specifically, Sylvia reported that being involved in social situations is 'hard for me and can be very stressful'.

The therapist asked Sylvia to identify the five areas she would like to address in intervention. As shown below, Sylvia did not include all issues identified from the initial sections of the COPM as being important to address (Table 7.1). Being client-centred enables the client to identify the problems that are the most important to address in intervention and setting future goals.

Table 7.1 Sylvia's initial COPM scores

Sylvia's occupational performance problems	Importance rating	Performance rating	Satisfaction rating
1. Having a shower daily	7	5	4
2. Budgeting money, ensuring bills are paid and paying for groceries	9	5	4
3. Working part-time	8	4	3
4. Completing daily household chores	6	3	3
5. Socializing with family and peers	6	3	3
TOTAL SCORE		20/5 = 4	17/5 = 3.4

The COPM then asks the client to rate each identified occupational performance issue and reflect on their current performance and satisfaction with their performance in relation to that issue. Sylvia identified that she is not doing well in her performance as regards completing household chores and socializing with family and peers (scores of 3), nor is she satisfied with her progress in changing these occupational performance issues (scores of 3). Sylvia's perceived performance in working part-time was one point higher (score of 4), but she remains unsatisfied about attaining this goal (score of 3). Finally, Sylvia's perceived performance in showering daily and money management was in the middle of the spectrum (scores of 5); however, she remains unsatisfied with the progress she is making in these areas (scores of 4). Baseline scores of Performance = 4 and Satisfaction = 3.4 were obtained by adding the performance and satisfaction ratings and dividing by the five identified occupational performance issues.

After completion of the initial COPM assessment, intervention opportunities were discussed with Sylvia. The goal of participation in the interventions was to address her occupational performance problems.

SELF-CARE

To address showering, Sylvia identified that showering daily may be too difficult, but agreed that showering 3 days a week would be achievable. The occupational therapist and Sylvia prepared a monthly schedule to refer to and prompt her on the day she is required to complete her shower.

Interventions to address money management focused on budgeting Sylvia's monthly income and prioritizing her expenses. A weekly record was used to record her spending. This information was gathered each month and then discussed with the occupational therapist to identify when and where unnecessary spending was taking place. At the end of each month, Sylvia and the occupational therapist discussed what bills required payment, and money was

allocated to ensure the bills were paid. With regard to grocery shopping, Sylvia was encouraged to prepare grocery lists in preparation for shopping, review weekly flyers for specials, and look at use of coupons. Sylvia had also allocated a specific amount of money in her budget for grocery shopping.

PRODUCTIVITY

To address obtaining competitive part-time employment, Sylvia and the occupational therapist explored various jobs that may be of interest to her. Sylvia also identified that she would update her CV (résumé).

In addressing household chores, Sylvia agreed that having cues such as a schedule identifying exactly what to clean on a specific day will enable her to be motivated to pursue the tasks. The use of the schedule enabled Sylvia to complete small achievable cleaning tasks.

LEISURE

To address leisure, Sylvia was encouraged to attend the outpatient centre and participate in groups that promote socialization and support as well as participation in meaningful occupations. She agreed to participate in a support-based group that addressed current issues and their effect on one's mental health, and a task-based group that promoted socialization with peers through completion of a meaningful activity.

RE-ASSESSMENT

Re-assessment took place 2 years later, after intervention addressing Sylvia's occupational performance issues. At this time her identified problems were re-evaluated and scored using the same scale as at the initial assessment. There was improvement in Sylvia's score in showering daily, money management and budgeting, and household chores. By comparing Table 7.1 and Table 7.2, the reader can see that there was a one-point improvement in performance and satisfaction in socialization. At the time of re-assessment, Sylvia identified the fact that obtaining competitive part-time employment was no longer important to her and she decided not to pursue this goal at this time.

Table 7.2 Sylvia's re-assessment scores

Sylvia's occupational performance problems	Importance rating	Performance rating	Satisfaction rating
1. Having a shower daily	9	7	9
2. Budgeting money, ensuring bills are paid and paying for groceries	8	7	7
3. Working part-time	0	–	–
4. Completing daily household chores	8	7	6
5. Socializing with family and peers	8	4	4
TOTAL SCORE		25/5 = 5	26/5 = 5.2

Table 7.3 Sylvia's new occupational performance issues

Sylvia's occupational performance problems	Importance rating	Performance rating	Satisfaction rating
1. Child care (*new*)	10	8	5
2. Budgeting money, ensuring bills are paid and paying for groceries	8	7	7
3. Scheduling day to participate in meaningful activities (*new*)	9	6	7
4. Cleaning house	8	7	6
5. Socializing with family and peers	6	3	3
TOTAL SCORE		31/5 = 6.2	28/5 = 5.6

CONCLUSIONS

A client's occupational performance issues and goals are constantly being adjusted and changed as a result of intervention, and the client's perception of the importance of addressing the original occupational performance issues. As a result of completing the re-assessment 2 years after the initial COPM assessment, some original occupational performance issues were no longer relevant, new occupational performance issues were identified, and some original issues were still problems for Sylvia.

As a result of new occupational performance issues that arose and issues that still remained (Table 7.3), intervention continued to address the original issues as well as the development of a client-centred plan to address the newly identified occupational performance issues.

The use of the COPM allows the occupational therapist and client constantly to evaluate the client's occupational performance problems, identify the client's ratings related to importance, performance and satisfaction, and develop an intervention plan.

The use of the COPM is a valuable measure to identify individual occupational performance problems, develop a client-centred intervention plan, and evaluate outcomes post-intervention.

CASE STUDY

Maggie

Maggie is a 46-year-old woman diagnosed with schizoaffective disorder. She also has several medical conditions such as type 2 diabetes, hypertension and hypercholesterolaemia. All of these conditions are treated with medications. She lives in the community with two housemates and receives support from an intensive community mental health programme. Maggie was transferred to her current support programme from another community-based group 4 years ago, when local mental health services were restructured. At the time of the transfer

Maggie required high-level support to develop basic self-care skills. She did not have the attention or concentration required to address any further skill development. Maggie's finances were managed by a relative to ensure payment of bills and to help Maggie make her money last. Her spending money was administered to her daily by her trustee.

Approximately 2 years ago Maggie underwent a full re-evaluation of her medications and several adjustments have been made over time. Maggie's energy level increased and her ability to attend to and concentrate on tasks has dramatically improved. As Maggie's cognitive abilities increased, she began to develop new interests and add activities into her daily structure. She has begun to volunteer at a local nursing home with support from her service providers. Additionally, Maggie has developed new insight into the health risks associated with type 2 diabetes.

The COPM was used to assist Maggie to further define her goals and to provide direction for future occupational therapy intervention. Upon completion of the COPM, the following difficulties in Maggie's occupational performance were identified.

SELF-CARE

Maggie identified difficulties in establishing and monitoring her diabetes routine (monitoring blood sugars, identifying trends with diet and exercise with respect to her blood sugars), managing money on a day-to-day basis and independence with public transport.

PRODUCTIVITY

In the area of productivity Maggie identified challenges including maintaining her role as a volunteer at a local nursing home, looking for a part-time job, completing her household chores each week, and learning new recipes appropriate for a diabetic diet.

LEISURE

Maggie identified obstacles in developing quiet recreation activities to occupy her 'down' time and increasing her active recreation. She specifically identified difficulties establishing a walking routine that she can incorporate into her overall diabetes management plan.

OCCUPATIONAL PERFORMANCE ISSUES

After identifying the most important challenges in each of the areas of self-care, productivity and leisure, Maggie then identified which five occupational performance issues were of greatest significance to her. This process allowed Maggie to name her most important priorities and set goals for future intervention. The ratings of Maggie's occupational issues are summarized in Table 7.4.

Once Maggie had rated her occupational performance issues, the total scores for performance and satisfaction were tallied. This is accomplished by adding the scores in each column (i.e. performance rating and satisfaction rating) and dividing these by the number of issues identified. These total scores can be used as a baseline for comparison during re-assessments in the future, and to help identify changes in Maggie's challenges and goals.

Upon completion of the COPM, Maggie and her occupational therapist engaged in several sessions of problem-solving to develop intervention strategies for each of her identified goals.

SELF-CARE

Maggie highly valued the importance of establishing a routine to monitor her blood sugars. She and her occupational therapist designed a binder in which she could record her blood sugar levels from her glucometer, as well as note any remarks about diet or exercise that may have influenced her blood sugars. Maggie decided to start recording her blood sugars twice daily at the times of her morning and afternoon medication deliveries so that staff could prompt her to take them. Maggie's long-term plan is to reduce the number of prompts required until she is taking her glucometer readings independently. Together with her occupational therapist, Maggie will also review any comments about diet and exercise to identify any emerging trends, and structure intervention as needed.

The development of money management skills was less valued by Maggie than the establishment of a diabetes monitoring routine. She decided to maintain her system of having a relative pay her routine expenses at this time while she focused on managing her day-to-day spending. Maggie and her occupational therapist developed

Table 7.4 Maggie's COPM scores			
Maggie's occupational performance issues	**Importance rating**	**Performance rating**	**Satisfaction rating**
1. Establishing a routine to monitor blood sugars	8	7	6
2. Developing money management skills	5	5	4
3. Maintaining volunteer position	9	8	8
4. Learning new diabetic recipes	6	4	4
5. Establishing a walking routine	8	3	3
TOTAL SCORE		27/5 = 5.4	25/5 = 5

a list of her routine day-to-day expenses and identified strategies that can help her prioritize the division of monies amongst these expenses. Over time Maggie plans to assume increased responsibility for her spending, with the long-term goal of receiving her spending money weekly rather than daily.

PRODUCTIVITY

Maggie's most highly valued occupational performance issue was to maintain her current volunteer position at a local nursing home. She identified that she was highly satisfied with her current performance in this area, and would like to maintain this level of performance. Maggie will continue to monitor her performance in this position and seek feedback, both from her occupational therapist and from the volunteer coordinator at the nursing home, to verify her self-evaluation. With time Maggie hopes to be able to develop the skills to self-evaluate her performance with confidence, and to expand her role at the nursing home.

Although she rated it less important than maintaining her volunteer position, Maggie also identified her goal of learning new diabetic recipes. She decided to pay a visit to the local library with her occupational therapist to find diabetic cookbooks. She and her therapist found several recipes that interested Maggie, and together will try them out at home. Maggie feels that she is able to try one new recipe per week. She would like to take the recipes she likes and put them into a binder to create a personal diabetic cookbook. This activity will also provide an opportunity to reinforce the role of diet in managing type 2 diabetes, and a venue to discuss any of Maggie's concerns regarding her current diabetes management plan.

LEISURE

A clear theme running through Maggie's occupational performance issues was the management of her type 2 diabetes. This theme was visible in the areas of self-care and productivity, and also emerged in the category of leisure. Maggie wished to establish a daily walking routine to increase her physical activity with the purpose of stabilizing her blood sugars. In consultation with her occupational therapist, Maggie joined a local walking group that meets once per week, and has discussed ways of adding more exercise to her routine. Although Maggie would like to walk daily, she recognized that this is not currently a reasonable goal for herself. Instead, she aims to walk two or three times per week in addition to her walking group. Initially, Maggie and her occupational therapist will walk together while they discover walking routes that are interesting and that can also be graded to increase in duration and difficulty as Maggie improves her strength and endurance. Maggie and her occupational therapist also discussed the possibility of using specific destinations as targets (e.g. library, grocery store and so on) so that Maggie remains motivated to walk. Maggie wants to walk independently throughout her community in the future.

RE-ASSESSMENT

Maggie and her occupational therapist have agreed on re-assessment in 1 year to monitor Maggie's satisfaction with her performance in her selected areas. This re-assessment will also provide the opportunity for Maggie to decide if she still has the same goals or if she would prefer to alter the course of her occupational therapy intervention.

Summary

This chapter has discussed the importance of basing client-centred interventions on a theoretical framework or model. The CMOP and the CMOP-E provide that base. The COPM arose from the CMOP and is a most useful addition to the toolkit of measures used by occupational therapists in a variety of clinical settings. The timing of the intervention is key to its usability and success, and, as has been shown here in the case examples, it can be used at different stages of engagement with a person. The COPM provides only a framework for assessment and intervention, and thus the therapist using it needs to be a skilled interviewer in order to guide each person along in thinking about their own occupational performance.

Reflective learning

- How does the CMOP-E support client-centred practice?
- How could the COPM be used with other client groups?
- How would you use the COPM in your re-assessment session with Maggie?
- Was the COPM an appropriate tool to use with both Maggie and Sylvia?
- How would the components of the CMOP influence your work with Sylvia and Maggie?

Acknowledgement

Alison Blank is acknowledged through her work on the sections of this chapter related to the CMOP and COPM that appeared in the previous edition and that form the core of those sections in this edition.

References

Bonder, B.R., 2001. Culture and occupation: a comparison of weaving in two traditions. Canadian Journal of Occupational Therapy 65 (5), 310–319.

Canadian Association of Occupational Therapists, 1997. Enabling Occupation: An Occupational Therapy Perspective. CAOT Publications ACE, Ottawa.

Canadian Association of Occupational Therapists and Health Canada, 1993. Occupational Therapy Guidelines for Client-Centred Mental Health Practice. CAOT Publications ACE, Ottawa.

Clarke, C., 2003. Clinical application of the Canadian Model of Occupational Performance in a forensic rehabilitation hostel. British Journal of Occupational Therapy 66 (4), 171–174.

College of Occupational Therapists, 2005. Code of Ethics and Professional Conduct for Occupational Therapists. College of Occupational Therapists, London.

Dressler, J., MacRae, A., 1998. Advocacy, partnerships and client centered practice in California. Occupational Therapy in Mental Health 14 (1/2), 35–43.

Dyck, I., Jongbleod, L., 2000. Women with multiple sclerosis and employment issues: a forum on social and institutional environments. Canadian Journal of Occupational Therapy 67 (5), 337–346.

Godfrey, A., 2000. Policy changes in the National Health Service: implications and opportunities for occupational therapists. British Journal of Occupational Therapy 63 (5), 218–224.

Griffith, J., Caron, C., Desrosiers, J., Thibeault, R., 2007. Defining spirituality and giving meaning to occupation: the perspective of community-dwelling older adults with autonomy loss. Canadian Journal of Occupational Therapy 74 (2), 78–90.

Hagedorn, R., 2000. Tools for Practice in Occupational Therapy. Churchill Livingstone, Edinburgh.

Imms, C., 2001. Feeding the infant with congenital heart disease: an occupational performance challenge. American Journal of Occupational Therapy 55 (3), 277–284.

Kielhofner, G., 2008. A Model of Human Occupation: Theory and Application. Lippincott Williams & Wilkins, Baltimore.

Law, M., Baptiste, S., McColl, M.A., et al., 1990. The Canadian Occupational Performance Measure: an outcome measure for occupational therapy. Canadian Journal of Occupational Therapy 57 (2), 82–87.

Law, M., Cooper, B., Strong, S., et al., 1996. The Person–Environment–Occupation Model: a transactive approach to occupational performance. Canadian Journal of Occupational Therapy 63 (1), 9–23.

Law, M., Baptiste, S., Carswell, A., et al., 2005. Canadian Occupational Performance Measure. CAOT Publications ACE, Toronto.

McColl, M.A., 2003. Spirituality and Occupational Therapy. CAOT Publications ACE, Toronto.

McColl, M.A., Pranger, T., 1994. Theory and practice in the occupational therapy guidelines for client-centred practice. Canadian Journal of Occupational Therapy 61 (5), 250–259.

O'Brien, P., Dyck, I., Caron, S., Mortenson, P., 2002. Environmental analysis: insights from sociological and geographical perspectives. Canadian Journal of Occupational Therapy 69 (4), 229–238.

Rebeiro, K.L., 2001a. Client-centered practice: body, mind and spirit resurrected. Canadian Journal of Occupational Therapy 68 (2), 65–69.

Rebeiro, K.L., 2001b. Enabling occupation: the importance of an affirming environment. Canadian Journal of Occupational Therapy 68 (2), 80–89.

Reed, K.L., Sanderson, S.N., 1983. Concepts of Occupational Therapy. Williams & Wilkins, Baltimore.

Sumsion, T., 1997. Environmental challenges and opportunities of client-centred practice. British Journal of Occupational Therapy 60 (2), 53–56.

Sumsion, T., 1999. A study to determine a British occupational therapy definition of client-centred practice. British Journal of Occupational Therapy 62 (2), 52–58.

Townsend, E., 1993. Muriel Driver Memorial Lecture: Occupational therapy's social vision. Canadian Journal of Occupational Therapy 60, 174–184.

Townsend, E., 1998. Using Canada's 1997 guidelines for enabling occupation. Australian Occupational Therapy Journal 45, 1–6.

Townsend, E., Brintnell, S., Staisey, N., 1990. Developing guidelines for client-centered occupational therapy practice. Canadian Journal of Occupational Therapy 57 (2), 69–76.

Townsend, E.A., Polatajko, H.J., 2007. Enabling Occupation 11: Advancing an occupational therapy vision for health, well-being and justice. CAOT Publications ACE, Ottawa, ON.

Unruh, A.M., Versnel, J., Kerr, N., 2002. Spirituality unplugged: a review of commonalities and contentions, and a resolution. Canadian Journal of Occupational Therapy 69 (1), 5–19.

Whalley Hammell, K., 2001. Intrinsicality: reconsidering spirituality, meaning and mandates. Canadian Journal of Occupational Therapy 68 (3), 186–194.

The Person–Environment–Occupational Performance (PEOP) Model

8

Charles Christiansen   Carolyn M. Baum   Julie Bass

OVERVIEW

This chapter summarizes the history and evolution of the Person–Environment–Occupational Performance (PEOP) Model, a model for practice first conceived during the 1980s in the USA. As a guide to occupational therapy intervention, the PEOP Model can be considered a transactive systems model. The model focuses on the client and on relevant intrinsic and extrinsic influences on the performance of everyday occupations. It can be applied to individuals, groups (or organizations) and populations. The PEOP Model has characteristics that are similar to other social ecological models, in that it identifies three relevant domains of knowledge for occupational therapy practice:

- the person (intrinsic factors)
- the person's situation or context, including the relevant physical and social environment (extrinsic factors)
- the occupations of importance to the client's well-being (activities, tasks and roles).

It is transactive in that it views everyday occupations as being affected by, and affecting, the client and the client's context. It is client-centred in that it values and requires the active involvement of the client in determining intervention goals. It is different from other models because it makes the intrinsic, extrinsic and occupational factors explicit and applies them at the person, organizational and population levels.

Key points

The PEOP Model:
- is client-centred
- applies to individuals, groups and populations

Key points—cont'd

- is intended to be top-down, focusing first on the situations of clients
- allows the practitioner to organize current knowledge of the intrinsic and extrinsic factors in their interventions
- uses a systems perspective
- serves as a guide to creating a complete occupational profile of the client
- values collaboration with the client, with important others within the client's social circle, and other professionals concerned about the client's well-being
- works to achieve a match between the client's goals and the goals of occupational therapy intervention
- believes that outcomes must be related to well-being and quality of life
- incorporates the three components of evidence-based practice: the best evidence from research, professional and clinical expertise, and the client's unique values and circumstances.

Introduction: origins and aim of the PEOP Model

In 1985 work began in the mountains of Colorado on what was to become the PEOP Model. At the time, there was a growing awareness that it was necessary to organize the knowledge that was being used by occupational therapists in a manner that would identify, clarify and emphasize the unique contribution of occupational therapy to the health and well-being of individuals, groups and populations. We knew that occupational therapy could provide practical and relevant interventions that enabled people to preserve or improve the quality of their lives. Yet, at that time, the most influential textbooks in the field were continuing to organize their content using a bio-medical approach that resembled the diagnosis and pathology-focused approach of allopathic medicine. Influenced by writers from medicine who were calling for more health-oriented approaches (e.g. Engel 1977), as well as writers from occupational therapy who openly lamented the field's apparent divergence from ideas central to its founding (e.g. Shannon, 1977), we set about reframing the organizing structure for knowledge relevant to occupational therapy theory and practice. We intended to propose a model that would provide practitioners with an intuitive and organized way to understand the areas relevant to supporting people's ability to perform or do the activities, tasks and roles necessary for everyday living. Through creating such a framework, we aimed to facilitate thinking in ways that would guide assessment, planning and the delivery of interventions. Our goal was to have a model that would be relevant, regardless of the settings in which occupational therapists worked, the types of client they served, or the ages, life stages or diagnoses of those clients. We also felt that creating such a model would encourage a more balanced approach to care that would encourage therapists to plan intervention with a focus on the life situations of their clients. This focus, we surmised, would require that therapists consider the person-related and environment-related resources and barriers relevant to a full understanding of how to enable their clients to perform or accomplish the particular occupations necessary to live satisfying lives.

The PEOP Model is now in its third generation (Christiansen & Baum, 1991; Christiansen & Baum, 1997; Baum et al, 2005) and continously being updated. During the years since its inception, the knowledge generated from occupational science, neuroscience, environmental science and other biological and social sciences has enabled us to refine and extend our original ideas and to provide a more solid scientific basis for the constructs we believe are central to understanding the occupational performance of humans. Throughout this process of elaboration, we have been influenced by many emerging ideas and innovations in healthcare, disability, social policy, technology, rehabilitation and public health. Although some terminology has changed, definitions have been revised, and new concepts have been added, the basic philosophical orientation of the model and its central features have remained consistent. This,

we believe, indicates that we were successful in achieving a model that was not only conceptually sound, but straightforward in its ability to organize a knowledge base of information useful for practice.

The PEOP Model values collaboration

Because occupational therapy is based on a cooperative approach toward care (Meyer 1922), the PEOP Model was designed to facilitate the development of a collaborative intervention plan with the client and with other professionals. Use of the term 'client' is meant to apply, whether the intervention is directly with a patient, a well community-dwelling child or adult, or a family, or done in consultation with a physician, a social worker, a student, an architect, an employee, an organization or an entire community. Each of these 'clients' would seek the knowledge and skills of the occupational therapist to address issues that influence occupational performance or the ability of people to participate fully in their lives. Occupational therapists provide a unique knowledge and skill set that bridges the world of the client and the world of healthcare and includes other important social services in communities. A core assumption is that people cannot truly be well if they cannot participate fully in their lives.

Occupational performance

The concept of occupational performance has become the mainstay of the development of most models of occupational therapy. Occupational performance operates as a means of connecting the individual to roles and to the sociocultural environment (Reed & Sanderson 1999, p.93). We define occupational performance as the complex interactions between the person and the environments in which they carry out activities, tasks and roles that are meaningful or required of them (Baum & Christiansen 2005).

A systems perspective

The PEOP Model is a systems model, recognizing that the interaction of the person, environment and occupational performance elements is dynamic and reciprocal, and that the client must be central to the care-planning or intervention process. Only the client (whether person, family, organization or community) is able to determine what outcomes are most important and necessary.

Client-centred

In the traditional medical model it is the practitioner who determines the approach to care. The PEOP Model provides a bridge from the biomedical model to a sociocultural model and provides students and clinicians with a tool to organize evidence for use in practice. That is, it recognizes impairments when they limit performance participation but also views the client in context, including a consideration of the abilities and strengths that a client can use to enable performance, as well the environmental characteristics that provide support, whether those include places, people, policies or technologies. Ultimately, the comprehensive assessment of a client, what that client needs and wants to do, and the environment clients will inhabit collectively determine the interventions aimed at enabling the client to perform valued roles, activities and tasks that are central to living, whether these pertain to management of self and others, work or community engagement. A central theme of the PEOP Model is that, ultimately, the client determines the performance goals toward which therapy is targeted.

The PEOP Model is used as a guide to creating a complete occupational profile of the client, which includes information about the client's perception of the current situation, and includes consideration of the client's roles, interests, responsibilities and/ or mission and values. The assessment and planning phase of care is grounded in evidence. We believe that clients should enter into the intervention phase with a clear understanding of the outcome that should ultimately result. Intervention must be a collaborative endeavour, with effort and commitment contributed through the partnership of the practitioner and the client.

Description of the model

Figure 8.1 provides a graphic representation of the model. This representation is intended to convey that occupational performance is determined not only by the nature of the activity, task or role to be performed, but also by the characteristics of the person or client

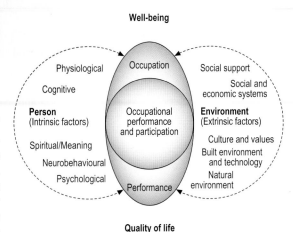

Fig. 8.1 • The Person–Environment–Occupational Performance Model. Reprinted with permission from SLACK Incorporated. Christiansen, C.H., Baum, C.M., Bass, J., 2005. Occupational Therapy: Performance, Participation and Well-being, third ed. Slack Inc. Thorofare, NJ.

(depicted as intrinsic factors) and the environment (depicted as extrinsic factors). Performance and participation always occur in context, and ultimately determine well-being and quality of life. It should be noted that, for a given situation or context, the applicability or importance of given intrinsic and extrinsic factors will vary. The model presupposes that a complete assessment to plan intervention will include a consideration of each of the factors.

Using the PEOP Model to plan care

The PEOP Model visually represents the constructs that must come together to support both the practitioner and the client in developing a realistic and sequenced plan of care. Success in this process depends on the practitioner's skills in forming a relationship with the client, asking the right questions, and being able to access the knowledge necessary to understanding the issues and options presented by the client's occupational performance issues and goals. Using the PEOP Model involves a 'top-down approach', in that it first considers the individual in context, identifying the client's roles, occupations and goals. The model requires the occupational therapist to use this context to address the personal performance capabilities/constraints and the environmental performance enablers/barriers that are central to the occupational performance of the individual.

Intrinsic factors

Intrinsic factors in the PEOP Model that are central to occupational performance are:

- physiological, including strength, endurance, flexibility, inactivity, stress, sleep, nutrition and health
- cognitive, including organization, reasoning, attention, awareness, executive function and memory, all necessary for task performance
- neurobehavioural, including somatosensory, olfactory, gustatory, visual, auditory, proprioceptive and tactile, as well as motor control, motor planning (praxis) and postural control
- psychological and emotional, including emotional state (affect), self-concept, self-esteem and sense of identity, self-efficacy and theory of mind (social awareness)
- spiritual: that which brings meaning.

Extrinsic factors

Extrinsic factors in the PEOP Model that are central to occupational performance are:

- social support, practical or instrumental support and informational support
- societal, including interpersonal relationships (groups), social and economic systems and their receptivity (policies and practices) to supporting participation, laws
- cultural, including values, beliefs, customs, use of time
- the built environment, including physical properties, tools, assistive technology, design and the natural environment, covering geography, terrain, climate and air quality.

Situational analysis

In order to incorporate key elements of planning, the occupational therapist completes a situational analysis. This analysis seeks information from the client by interview and by employing assessments that give the practitioner a clear understanding of constraints and/or barriers that may limit the person's activity and participation. As well, the practitioner will gain insight into barriers and environmental enablers that will limit or support the individual in doing the things he or she wants and needs to do.

There are a number of key elements of a plan of care in the PEOP Model. These client-centred elements change, depending on whether the client is a person, an organization, or the community, as reflected in a population approach. Each will be discussed.

The following situational analyses were designed to help the practitioner organize information to address the issues of individuals, of organizations and of communities. In each situational analysis, evidence underpins the practitioner's decisions as to what measures to include and which interventions to employ. All professionals are held to a standard — the expectation of competent practice using methods that have been objectively shown to be effective. Evidence thus becomes the filter through which clinical decisions about the type of evaluation or assessment and the interventions that will support the client in achieving their goals will be made.

Planning person-centred interventions

The following elements describe the steps necessary for gathering and analysing client-related information (Fig. 8.2).

The collection of client information

The occupational history

It is during the process of obtaining a history that the practitioner learns what the person has done previously and how culture impacts on their everyday life. An occupational history should include a description of leisure interests and social activities, and provide a clear understanding of the responsibilities clients have for work and for self- and home management tasks.

Client's perception of the current situation

Another key element is the client's perception of the current situation. People (and groups) vary in the level of knowledge or understanding they have of their medical or health conditions. Thus, it is important to know what the client thinks has happened, how the situation is appraised, and what the client knows about a likely course of intervention. It is also important to estimate the impact that the current situation is having on a client's life experience(s).

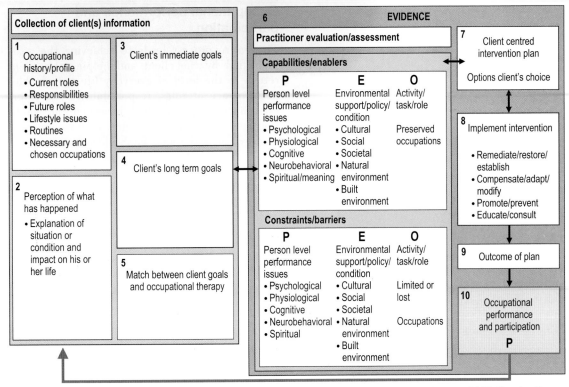

Fig 8.2 • A situational analysis: using the PEOP Model for planning person-centred interventions. © 2005. Carolyn Baum, Julie Bass & Charles Christiansen. Used with permission.

The client's immediate and long-term goals

What are the client's goals? It is important to determine the client's long-term goals so that, as discussions emerge about short-terms goals, the practitioner can help the client plan the necessary goal-related steps. It is always easier to establish goals if the therapist has completed an occupational history. By knowing about the client's interests, skills, values, roles, traditions, habits and routines, it is possible to help formulate goals that not only will be achievable, but also will be meaningful. Current practice encourages therapists to avoid applying cultural stereotypes and to focus on the particular narrative of a given client.

Match between the client's goals and occupational therapy

The final step in the client information section of the analysis is to determine the match between the person's goals and the occupational therapy approach. If there is no match, the occupational therapist should make an appropriate referral to another professional or to other resources to address the client's goals. When there is a match, the practitioner should begin the second section of the situational analysis to determine the person's capabilities and enablers, and to identify barriers and constraints that will need to be overcome.

The evaluation and assessment of intrinsic (person) and extrinsic (environmental) factors that will impact on or support occupational performance

Selection of measures/assessments to understand the intrinsic and extrinsic factors

The person factors (intrinsic) include physiological, psychological, cognitive, neurobehavioural and spiritual characteristics. The environmental (extrinsic) factors include cultural, social and economic, natural environment, built environment, and social and societal influences on performance. Assessments are chosen that will allow the therapist to understand the person's capabilities and what might be limiting the individual's performance of activities, tasks or occupations that are central to fulfilling valued roles or expectations.

Client-centred intervention plan

With the client's information and the practitioner's assessment of the client's capacity and constraints, a client-centred plan is constructed. The practitioner uses their skill to help the client understand what is possible, and also helps the client understand the issues involved in helping to achieve identified goals. The client has the right and the practitioner has the responsibility to review and share available evidence that a given intervention will be able to help the client achieve their goals in the most effective and efficient manner. Identifying and communicating the evidence used to formulate a given intervention plan not only promotes sound reasoning, it also reflects the highest principles of ethical practice.

Implement intervention

Several interventions can and should be employed to meet the client's goals. These interventions range from remediation strategies designed to restore function to compensation, including promoting health, preventing secondary problems, and educating the client and their support network to be able to self-manage the situation. One additional intervention is advocating for change to remove societal barriers that limit occupational performance. These interventions are discussed throughout the interventions section of the book.

Outcome of the plan

Following the implementation of the plan, the client (hopefully) will be able to achieve their goals. Outcomes should be measured, not only to demonstrate the progress to the client, but also to demonstrate the effectiveness and efficiency of the occupational therapy interventions to the referral source, to other appropriate stakeholders and to the public. The effectiveness of occupational therapy must be public in order to shape the policies of institutions and payment sources.

Occupational performance and participation

The entire process leads to achieving the goals identified by the client and helping the client return to the level of everyday life that enables performance of roles, responsibilities and interests. Since many individuals have a chronic condition or a disability that requires a self-management strategy, part of the outcome should include the possibility of additional services from an occupational therapist, if an occupational performance issue emerges that would benefit from or require occupational therapy expertise.

Addressing the occupational performance issues of communities/populations

The process described above fits well when the occupational therapist is working with individuals or small groups of people such as families. However, an emerging area of practice for occupational therapy addresses the occupational issues of communities and populations (Fig. 8.3). Population-based care may theoretically range from as large as all of the people in the world who fit some characteristic (e.g. people with AIDS, children who are homeless) or may reflect a small group of people or a community with issues of concern (e.g. mid-life women with family issues that affect their work for a company, or older people who have become isolated in a neighbourhood because of transport issues). Sometimes, these issues are identified within a more obvious or defined organizational structure, such as within a community group, business, or a group of people within a designated government category (e.g. people over 65 within a designated political or geographic jurisdiction). One might guess that the situational analyses conducted will look different in these different situations. Population-/community-centred situational analyses may serve as the starting point for occupational therapists who are interested in improving the health of populations or communities in general or working within specific organizations.

Consider a hypothetical situation where an occupational therapist who has worked with older people in long-term care settings for several years wants to continue to work with older people but

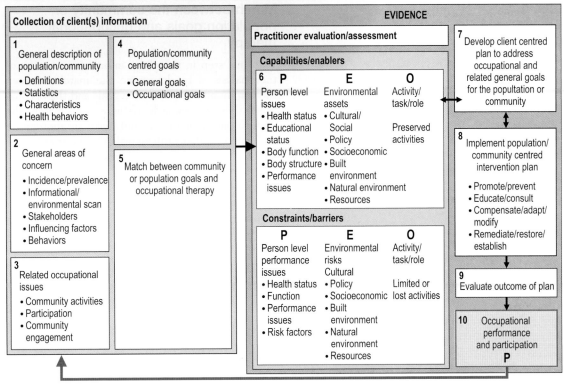

Fig 8.3 • A situational analysis: using the PEOP Model for planning population- or community-centred interventions. © Carolyn Baum, Julie Bass and Charles Christiansen, 2005. Used with permission.

would like to work with well elders to enable them to remain at home and improve their quality of life. How does the therapist begin? Does one already have the background and knowledge that will enable success in this new practice arena? Is one ready to begin immediately to promote these services to organizations that work with this population or in these communities? Such a possibility may occur, but is it likely?

In this situation, a population/community situational analysis may better prepare the therapist to understand the general characteristics and issues of the older population, the community in which clients live, and, most importantly, to plan interventions that will meet the needs and goals of specific organizations.

This example can be followed through a situational analysis. Although the therapist has worked with elders who have health conditions and diminished abilities in the long-term care setting, they do not have a clear understanding of well elders. So the therapist begins a population-/community-centred situational analysis by acquiring general information and conducting a broad assessment. What things should the therapist examine?

The collection of client information

General description of the population/community

This will help the therapist define the population/community (e.g. age, gender, ethnicity, income, education, employment, religion, geographic area), obtain statistics of interest (e.g. risk factors), and identify characteristics that are associated with people who are part of this population/community (e.g. knowledge, attitudes, beliefs, habits, preferences, sensitivities). This exercise may also support some of the therapist's assumptions and/or dispel any myths that may be commonly believed.

Identification of general areas of concern

For a given population/community, this requires the therapist to look outside of occupational therapy to gain a broader understanding of the pertinent array of critical issues (e.g. barriers, policy, supports, services, motivators for change). The therapist will often find these areas identified by local, national and international agencies and organizations, census information, and even reports from the popular press. In a sense the therapist is conducting an environmental/informational scan to learn more about the prioritized areas of concern for a population/community, the incidence/prevalence of the issues, and the major stakeholders (e.g. transport has been identified as a major issue for older people living in communities).

Related occupational issues

It is important to identify an occupational therapy role for this population/community. Some groups may not have significant occupational issues associated with them; however, others will. This step may require the therapist to explore occupational therapy literature that can help identify potential occupational performance-related issues. It is more likely, however, that such identification will result from using strong critical thinking skills coupled with the therapist's knowledge of factors that support (or limit) occupational performance (e.g. transport issues may limit engagement in all occupations that are typically done outside the home — shopping, financial matters, socialization and so on).

The population/community — general goals

It is important to identify areas of concern; these often come from the same sources, as noted two sections above. These goals may be broken into immediate goals and long-term goals, or they may be overall general objectives. Knowledge of these goals will help the practitioner in communications with stakeholders for this population/community. The population/community's occupational goals are developed from one's consideration of this and the previous two sections, and identification of how the general health of the community is understood by the stakeholders.

Match between the community or population goals and occupational therapy

The final step in the client information section of the analysis is to determine the match between the community or population goals and the occupational therapy approach. If there is no match, the occupational therapist should make an appropriate referral to another professional or to other appropriate resources qualified to address the client's goals. When a match is identified, the practitioner should begin the second section of the situational analysis to determine the community or popuation's capabilities and enablers, and to identify barriers and constraints that will need to be overcome.

The evaluation and assessment of intrinsic (person) and extrinsic (environmental) factors that will impact on or support occupational performance

Selection of measures/assessments/methodologies to understand the intrinsic and extrinsic factors

The occupational therapist selects appropriate tools to understand the intrinsic and extrinsic factors that are enabling as well as constraining the occupational performance of the community population. The person factors (intrinsic) include physiological, psychological, cognitive, neurobehavioural and spiritual influences on performance. The environmental factors (extrinsic) include cultural, social, natural environment, built environment and societal influences on performance. Clinical reasoning supports occupational therapists in applying their knowledge of the person, environment and occupational factors to the activities and tasks that are central to the community roles. At the community level many of the factors will be environmental. For example, the lack of an accessible playground for children, inadequate public transport to support older adults' community independence, and poor or confusing signage at the health centre would each represent environmental factors. However, there are also community problems that can affect the person (or intrinsic factors). Examples would include air quality, water quality, limited access to fresh food, and housing with lead paint.

Developing a client-centred plan to address occupational and related general goals for the population or community

With the client's information and the practitioner assessment of the client's capacity in hand, a client-centred plan can be developed. The client has the right to know and the practitioner has the responsibility to share the evidence that the interventions will be able to help the client achieve identified goals. Evidence will help the therapist understand the approaches that have already been tried to meet general and/or occupational goals and the outcomes of these various interventions. This step is important in determining strategies that work for this population/community, discarding ideas that do not have evidence to support them, and identifying intervention plans that have not yet been evaluated in the literature. If an untried strategy will be used, it is important for the client to understand the principles on which the therapist will base the intervention. The client must agree to the use of interventions proposed under such conditions.

Implementing a population-/community-centred intervention plan

If a therapist's work entails broad population/community initiatives and responsibilities (e.g. public health, labour, legislation), one may work with others to implement these strategies as part of an overall plan. If one's work involves developing partnerships with organizations and agencies, these overall strategies may serve as the foundation for a new situational analysis designed for organization-centred interventions.

Outcome of the plan

Following the implementation of the plan, the client hopefully will be able to achieve their goals. Outcomes should be measured, not only to demonstrate the progress to the client, but also to document the effectiveness of the occupational therapy interventions to the referral source, to other appropriate stakeholders, and to the public. The effectiveness of occupational therapy must be public in order to shape policies of institutions and payment sources.

Occupational performance and participation

The entire process leads to achieving the goals identified by the client and helping them achieve the goals that will improve the occupational performance of the population in their communities. Since many communities are facing new problems with an emerging population of older adults and many persons living with chronic diseases and disabling conditions, they need to provide the infrastructure to enable full participation of all members of the community. Part of the outcome should include the possibility of additional help from an occupational therapist if occupational performance issues emerge in the future that could benefit from an occupational therapist's expertise.

Planning organization-centred interventions

An organization situational analysis begins with an analysis of those served by the organization (Fig. 8.4). This step in the process enables the occupational therapist to approach the organization with a level of credibility that will open doors of opportunity. After developing expertise with regard to a specific population, an occupational therapist may not need to do this step in an explicit manner. Rather, the knowledge base of the professional includes this foundational information. Entry-level practitioners, however, would likely need to begin by determining an understanding of the population served by the organization as a preliminary step and prior to any discussions with a specific organization.

The collection of client information

Description of the organization

Once there is an understanding of the population and of its needs, its resources and its goals, the next step in an organization situational analysis is a full description of the organization. An understanding of the organization's mission, history, focus, values, activities, funding, clients and stakeholders is essential for assessing their need and potential for occupational therapy services. Some of this information may be obtained in publications about the organization. Other information may be acquired through initial conversations with a contact person in the organization.

The organization's area(s) of concern

The occupational therapist begins to explore the organization's areas of concern and unmet needs for the clients they serve. Many of these concerns

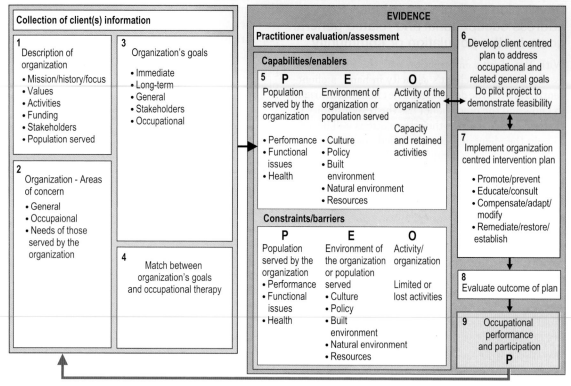

Fig 8.4 • A situational analysis: using the PEOP Model for planning organization-centred interventions. © 2005. Carolyn Baum, Julie Bass, and Charles Christiansen. Used with permission.

may be expressed in terms of general issues. For example, a community agency might be concerned about the adaptation of recent immigrants to the expectations of the larger culture. A school district may be concerned about the social and emotional health of some student groups. A corporation may be concerned about retention of workers who are mothers or caretakers. In this step, the occupational therapist also uses critical reasoning skills to identify and communicate the occupational issues that may be influencing the general areas of concern for the organization. For example, recent immigrants may have vocational backgrounds that are different from the work opportunities currently available, adolescents may only have access to extracurricular activities that are sport-related, and workers may not have sufficient support systems to solve parenting or caretaking problems as these arise.

The organizational goals

The goals of the organization and its stakeholders are considered next in the process. The occupational therapist enquires about the organization's immediate and long-term goals as they relate to general and occupational areas of concern. The practitioner also asks for information that will allow them to determine the organization's commitment and ability to achieve these goals.

The match between the organization's goals and occupational therapy

The final step in the first stage is to evaluate the match between the organization's goals and the occupational therapy services one can provide. The therapist will use population/community situational analysis, all the information gathered about the organization, and discussions with people in the organization to decide whether to continue the process. At this point, the therapist's personal investment in the organization has been limited. However, if one continues the process, the therapist and the organization may make a considerable commitment of personnel and resources for client assessment and interventions.

The evaluation and assessment of intrinsic (person) and extrinsic (environmental) factors that will impact on or support occupational performance

Selection of measures/assessments/methodologies to understand the intrinsic and extrinsic factors

The occupational therapist selects appropriate tools to understand the intrinsic and extrinsic factors that are enabling as well as constraining the occupational performance of the organization. The person factors (intrinsic) include physiological, psychological, cognitive, neurobehavioural and spiritual influences on the occupational performance of the organization's members. The environmental (extrinsic) factors include cultural, social, natural environment, built environment and societal influences on occupational performance. Clinical reasoning supports the occupational therapist in applying knowledge of the person, environment and occupational factors to the activities and tasks that are central to a community's roles. At the organization level many of the factors will be environmental. Examples might include the lack of training that fosters full participation of children in a mainstreamed classroom, managers who do not understand how to make accommodations for workers who wish to return to work after an accident or injury, or bus drivers' poor attendance related to lack of training. However, there are organizational problems that affect the person or intrinsic factors. Examples would be work practices that foster poor posture or repetitive motion injuries.

Developing a client-centred plan

With the client's information and the practitioner's assessment of the client's capacity, a client-centred plan can be constructed. The client has the right and the practitioner has the responsibility to share evidence that the interventions will be able to help the client achieve their goals.

Implementing an organization-centred plan

The therapist is now ready to develop an organization-centred intervention plan that can help the organization achieve its general and occupational goals. The therapist will want to consider initial population-/community-centred plan, variations of this plan that are appropriate for the organization, and the current evidence that is available. It also may be important to pilot any interventions, especially if this represents a new of area of occupational therapy practice. Pilot studies are a way to establish relationships with organizational clients, as initial outcomes can pave the way for additional work and funding. The organization will use the time to evaluate a therapist's capacity to help them achieve their goals. Implementation of the occupational therapy intervention plan may include any of the strategies identified in the person-centred situational analysis. However, promotion/prevention and education/consultation strategies are probably most common and effective when the target of an intervention involves an organization and its clientele.

Evaluating the outcome of the plan

The therapist's success with this organization can only be verified and documented if an evaluation of the effectiveness of the interventions is conducted, based on attainment of identified goals. This step is important in helping the therapist solidify their relationship with the organization. Additionally, it serves as a useful step in preparing a therapist to work with other related organizations. Disseminating the outcomes of interventions to the broader community is also essential for expanding practice into new arenas.

Occupational performance and participation

The entire process leads to achieving the occupational performance goals identified by the organization, with the possibility that such outcomes extend benefits to other clients they serve. Since many organizations are experiencing new problems with an emerging population of older adults, many of whom may be faced with chronic diseases and disabling conditions, they need to provide the infrastructure necessary to enable successful participation by clients in their organizations. Again, part of the outcome summary for the organizaton should include the possibility of providing additional help from an occupational therapist if occupational performance issues emerge in the future.

Summary

Three templates are provided to make explicit the activities that must come together to apply the PEOP Model effectively and appropriately. Occupational therapists have a widespread reputation for 'doing good work'; however, because that work often employs 'commonsense' strategies, it is not always obvious that there is a systematic and complex thought process underlying intervention and that various sources of knowledge converge during decision-making to lead to specific recommendations. By using these templates, the practitioner is provided with appropriate language to use in reports and recommendations that will communicate the complexity of the process and the care that has gone into the resulting plan. In the end, we are confident that the templates provide a convenient means for applying the PEOP Model, so that individuals, communities and organizations can accomplish goals related to improved well-being and quality of life, despite the presence of conditions that otherwise limit or restrict occupational performance.

Reflective learning

- How does the process of determining interventions differ between application to individual clients and application to groups?
- Reflect on the distinction between intrinsic and extrinsic factors as they apply to an individual client and groups or organizations.
- Consider your own life. Given the activities that are important to your health and well-being, what intrinsic and extrinsic factors most influence your ability to participate in them?

References

Baum, C., Bass, J., Christiansen, C., 2005. Person-environment-occupational performance: A model for planning interventions for individuals and organizations. In: Christiansen, C., Baum, C., Bass, J.D. (Eds.). Slack Inc, Thorofare, NJ, pp. 373–392.

Baum, C., Christiansen, C., 2005. Person-environment-occupational-performance: An occupation-based framework for practice. In: Christiansen, C., Baum, C., Bass, J.D. (Eds.), Occupational Therapy: Performance, Participation and Well-being, 3rd ed., Slack Inc., Thorofare, NJ, pp. 242–267.

Christiansen, C., Baum, .C., 1991. Occupational Therapy: Overcoming Human Performance Deficits. Slack, Thorofare, NJ.

Christiansen, C., Baum, C., 1997. Person-environment occupational performance: A conceptual model for practice. In: Christiansen, C., Baum, C. (Eds.), Occupational Therapy: Enabling Function and Well-being, 2 ed. Slack, Thorofare, NJ, pp. 46–71.

Engel, G.E., 1977. The need for a new medical model: A challenge for biomedicine. Science, 196 (4286), pp. 129–136.

Meyer, A., 1922. The philosophy of occupational therapy. Archives of Occupational Therapy 1 (1), 1–10.

Reed, K., Sanderson, S., 1999. Concepts of Occupational Therapy, 4th ed., Lippincott Williams & Wilkins, Baltimore, MD.

Shannon, P.D., 1977. The derailment of occupational therapy. American Journal of Occupational Therapy, 31 (4), 229–234.

The Functional Information-processing Model

9

Jackie Pool

OVERVIEW

This chapter describes the work of Claudia Kay Hoover Allen, an American occupational therapist, who developed the Cognitive Disability Model, which was later refined and renamed as the Functional Information-processing Model (FIPM). This is an occupational therapy model that is used when working with people with cognitive impairments, including those caused by dementia, developmental delay, mental health problems, such as depression or schizophrenia, and acquired brain injury. The FIPM proposes that there are six cognitive levels, each of which can be described in terms of limitations associated with the medical condition and remaining abilities, as seen in patterns of behaviour in everyday tasks. The levels range from level 6, where functioning is normal and no intervention is required, to level 1, where the person is profoundly impaired. An analysis of the results aids understanding of the patient's behaviour when carrying out everyday tasks. Optimum environmental stimulation and support can then be planned and implemented to decrease confusion, maximize functional capacities and help the person retain a sense of competence despite impairment.

The theoretical basis of the FIPM and its relevance to occupational therapists are explored and the levels of cognitive ability within the model are defined. A battery of assessments based on the model are outlined and information about their reliability and validity is provided. The chapter explores the application of the FIPM to practice.

Key points

- The Functional Information-processing Model (FIPM) is an occupational therapy model, developed by

Key points—cont'd

Claudia Allen, which is used when working with people with cognitive impairments.

- The FIPM proposes that there are six cognitive levels, known as Allen's Cognitive Levels. Each level is described in five modes of performance.
- Allen's Cognitive Levels define cognitive functioning in the way that it affects the person's engagement in occupation and with others.
- Allen has developed a range of reliable and valid assessment tools that can be used to determine the cognitive level of an individual.
- The role of the therapist is to interpret the assessment results in order to plan interventions for rehabilitation and using adaptation and compensatory approaches in order to enable the person to engage meaningfully in occupational performance.

Introduction

The Allen Cognitive Battery was pioneered in the 1970s in Los Angeles by a small group of occupational therapists led by Claudia Allen. It was developed in an occupational therapy department for patients with psychiatric disorders as a quick assessment, designed to be not culturally biased or language-based, and which could be sensitive to small changes in how medication alters a patient's day-to-day functioning. The first publication was in 1982 (Allen 1982) and the 'test' materials first distributed in 1985. Since that time, the procedure for administering the testing has been formalized and inter-rater reliability has been established among patients in psychiatric, acute and long-term care facilities.

In the USA the FIPM has been adopted for use to meet the requirements of Medicare. In 1965, the Social Security Act established Medicare as a prepaid medical insurance plan extending health coverage to almost all Americans aged 65 or older. Medicare requires that rehabilitation goals be functional, practical, sustainable and completed in a reasonable period of time. For the people with longer-term needs, goals must establish safe and effective maintenance programmes that will be sustained after therapy is discontinued. Allen proposed that the battery of assessments help occupational therapists to meet the Medicare requirements with rehabilitation goals that are relevant, reasonable and possible.

Historically, the cognitive and physical components of people have been assessed and treated separately. While there are many assessments for determining cognitive disability, the Allen's Cognitive Levels constitutes one that defines cognitive functioning in the way that it affects the person's engagement in occupation and with others. It is useful to all disciplines in the rehabilitation department, and in both the USA and the UK is used by occupational therapists to contribute to the findings of multidisciplinary teams. Although the FIPM and the battery of assessments have been developed for use by occupational therapists, they are also viewed by Allen as appropriate for use by other therapists, such as physiotherapists, who have an understanding of neuropsychology and experience in working with people having impairments of information-processing.

In May 2001, the World Health Organization (WHO 2002) endorsed the use of the International Classification of Functioning, Disability and Health (ICF). The ICF is a multi-purpose classification of health and health-related domains that helps to describe changes in body function and structure, and what a person with a health condition can do in a standard environment (their level of capacity), as well as what they actually do in their usual environment (their level of performance). These domains are classified from body, individual and societal perspectives by means of two components: body functions and structure, and activity and participation. The ICF also lists environmental factors that interact with all of these components (WHO 2002). Allen's FIPM fits well with the ICF, as the assessments aim to identify both level of cognitive capacity and level of performance. Interpretation of the assessment findings guides the occupational therapist to create a helping, therapeutic environment that meets the individual's needs and at the same time enables the individual to use their existing abilities to engage with their world.

The Allen assessment battery is now used widely in the UK by occupational therapists in a variety of clinical settings. The main users are those working with older people with dementia, because this has been the field where information about the FIPM has been most widely disseminated. The older persons' specialist section of the UK College of Occupational Therapists (COTSS-OP) has created a dementia clinical forum where information and workshops about Allen's model and materials have been featured. Increasingly, occupational therapists from other fields, including forensic psychiatry, adult psychiatry and learning disability, are also beginning to use the FIPM in practice.

In the USA, there are two websites dedicated to Allen's modules. Allen's Conferences, Inc. (http://www.allen-cognitive-levels.com/) is the official website of Allen's Cognitive Levels and information about their products and some research is available. More recently a website, the Allen Cognitive Network (http://www.allen-cognitive-network.org/), has been developed by an association of Allen Cognitive Level advisors, whose aim is to network about the Allen Cognitive Battery and applications in various practice arenas.

Theory

Cognition may be defined as the full range of processes and mechanisms that support thinking, as well as the thoughts themselves, which can be viewed as the products of those processes. This definition encompasses cognitive skills, such as attention, concentration, memory, comprehension, reasoning and problem-solving, as well as the cognitive processes, including styles of thinking, interpretations, judgements and assumptions (O'Neill 2002). Allen proposes that cognition is the processing capacity that defines what a person pays attention to, their motor response and their verbal performance. This processing capacity determines how a person engages in everyday activities and with their environment.

The clinical reasoning of the FIPM is based on the scientific assumption that human functioning is a general qualitative capacity to use mental energy to guide motor and verbal performance. Cognitive and physical components are intrinsically related since the brain guides physical behaviour. Allen suggests that cognitive disability is viewed as 'a restriction in voluntary motor action originating in the physical or chemical structures of the brain and producing observable limitations in routine task behaviour' (Allen 1985, p 31). These motor actions are the movements that a person makes as they are carrying out their everyday activities. Allen is therefore proposing that an individual's cognition can be assessed by observing their engagement in everyday activities.

Allen's early work was influenced by Piaget's theory of cognitive development and she attributes the idea that there are six possible levels of cognition to Piaget's sensorimotor period (Allen 1985). She later developed her theory to include the influence of the Soviet psychologist Vygotsky, whose work also focused on activity (Vygotsky 1978).

Allen describes a patient's cognitive progress as a continuum along two paths, motor performance and verbal performance, which are linked by attention. Attention is defined as the way that information is noticed and used. Use of information can be expressed in motor and verbal performance, in isolation or simultaneously. In order to understand a person's ability to function, Allen proposes that the therapist must first have an understanding of cognitive processing. Because the variation in human behaviour is so diverse, and there are so many variables resulting from unique experiences and personality, Allen bases FIPM on the structuralism of Piaget. Structures are the mental components used to organize thinking and learning processes; the selection of these components is influenced by the purpose for thinking and learning. Allen has defined the structures in broad, general terms that are intended to be universal and therefore free from gender and cultural bias. These structures, or processes, guide the qualitative differences in the actions and activities of individuals, and can be organized as observations, speed, visual spatial, verbal prepositional and memory.

- *Observations* include attention to cues or external stimuli and making sense of cues. The understanding of actions and activities as producers of primary and secondary effects may also be viewed as observations.
- *Speed* refers to the rate at which the information-processing system operates.
- *Visual spatial* processes of working memory that are applied to understanding objects and space include sensation, perception, topographical orientation and imagination.

- *Verbal propositional* processes of working memory that are applied to understanding communication, social order and time include non-verbal communication, verbal communication, cause and effect relationships where relationships are transferred into sounds, classifications of objects by perceptual properties, functional use or abstract concepts, and orientation to time and social rules.
- *Memory* processes are divided into declarative (explicit) intentions to learn, and non-declarative (implicit) learning that occurs without being aware of storing or retrieving knowledge.

The conceptual framework of Allen's FIPM is based on an understanding of these cognitive structures and the remaining abilities of the information-processing system. The model is designed to clarify remaining capacities in a disabled brain and is therefore an abilities-focused model.

Allen's Cognitive Level Scale

Claudia Allen proposed six cognitive levels ranging from 'coma' (0.8) to 'normal' (6.0) (Allen et al 1992, Katz 1998). Each level has three components: attention, motor control, and verbal performance. Table 9.1 summarizes the components of cognitive performance and the resulting impact on functional ability at each of these levels.

Allen (1996) summarizes the functional implications of the cognitive levels as:

- *Level 0*. The individual is alive but in a coma or under general anaesthesia. No conscious control of movement is evident.
- *Level 1*. The individual responds to an external stimulus. A general response, like a change in heart rate, usually precedes a specific response to noxious stimuli, followed by additional stimuli like bells, voices, pictures and mobiles.
- *Level 2*. The individual controls gross body movements to sit up, stand up, walk and do push/pull exercises. Adaptive equipment that protects the individual from hazardous postural movements or supports functional position is indicated.
- *Level 3*. The hands are used to reach for and grasp objects. Repetitive manual actions are common, but the effect produced on the object is not judged. Constant supervision is required to protect the patient from harm. Activity that requires repetitive actions may sustain attention.

Table 9.1 Cognitive performance and impact on functional ability

	Level 1	Level 2	Level 3	Level 4	Level 5	Level 6
Sensory cues	Subliminal	Proprioceptive	Tactile	Visible	Related	Symbolic
Information-processing	Reflex	Effect on body	Effect on environment	Several actions	Overt trial and error	Covert trial and error
Motor actions	Automatic	Postural	Manual	Goal-directed	Exploratory	Planned
Reason for response	Arousal	Comfort/movement	Interest Touching	Compliance Seeing	Self-control Reasoning	Reflection Reasoning
Perception of objects	Penetrate subliminal state	Own body	Exterior surfaces	Colour Shape	Space and depth	Intangible
Setting of objects	Reflex zones	Range of motion	Arm's reach	Visual field	Task environment	Potential task environment
Use of objects	Stimulated body part	Spontaneous use of body part	Chance use of found objects	Hand tools as a means to an end	Hand tools used to vary means and ends	Tool-making
Verbal directions	Verbs	Pronouns Names of body parts	Names of material objects	Adjectives Adverbs	Prepositions Explanations	Conjunction Conjectures
Demonstrated directions	Physical contact	Guided movements	Action on an object	Each step in a series	Each step and precautions for errors	Not required

Surprise at having produced an end result may occur.

- *Level 4*. Actions are goal-directed to complete a familiar activity. The routine activities of daily living can be done independently. Assistance is required to solve any problems presented by changes in the environment and to protect from unseen hazards. Simple projects, with rules to follow, are preferred. Striking visual cues, like primary colours and familiar shapes, are matched according to a sample project.
- *Level 5*. New actions are learned by doing an activity. The novelty presented by new products is explored. Hazards are not anticipated, and supervision in using dangerous or expensive products is advised. Aesthetic judgements about less striking visual cues are made, but with difficulty.
- *Level 6*. The individual anticipates the consequences of his or her actions. An effective and efficient course of action is planned. The creation of an individual design can be

premeditated and accomplished with ease. The fun of discovery and creativity is blended with discipline of good craftsmanship.

The difference between levels 1 and 2 is the ability to attend to and grasp moving objects. Between levels 2 and 3 there is a difference in the ability to manipulate objects in a meaningful way.

In order to discriminate further between the levels, five modes of performance have been added to each cognitive level to allow the therapist to locate the patient's function level more precisely. The five modes are each in a scale that increases by 2 points, i.e. 1.0, 1.2, 1.4, 1.6 and 1.8. At mode .0 the patient is likely to be functioning in only some of the described manner; at mode .2 the person is characteristically more likely to have problems of orientation in time and place. Mode .4 is a consolidation and the classic description of the level, whereas at mode .6 the person is likely to be open to the next level as thought orientation shifts up. At mode .8 the person is working at a composite level by adding information from the next level.

Allen states that an interval scale, which assumes equal distances between all points on the scale, is inappropriate when dealing with all the variables of human behaviour. Some abilities to function have a greater meaning to some individuals than others, and this will affect individual performance as much as will the integrity of the cognitive structures and the ability to process information. Allen's Cognitive Level Scale is therefore ordinal. This means that there is not an equal distance between each mode, there is a larger distance in ability between point 4 and point 6 of a mode, and between point 8 and point 0 of a mode, than between any of the others.

To use this ordinal scale to predict performance, two evaluations must be made by the therapist. Firstly, the best ability of the person must be assessed. Then the cognitive demands of the activity must be analysed. Successful performance in the activity occurs when the person's cognitive structures match the demands of the activity. Assessment in the FIPM is undertaken using the Claudia Allen Diagnostic Module.

The Claudia Allen Diagnostic Module

Allen has developed a range of tools that can be used to evaluate the best ability of the person to use the cognitive structures in order to function. The instruments for use within the FIPM are referred to as the Allen Diagnostic Module and include the Allen Cognitive Level Screen (ACLS), the Large Allen Cognitive Level Screen (LACL), the Routine Task Inventory (RTI), the Cognitive Performance Tests (CPT), the Allen Diagnostic Module projects and the Sensory–Motor Stimulation kits. Therapists who use the Allen Diagnostic Module establish a numerical score for each client in order to predict that client's best ability to function, as well as their optimal learning conditions, rather than to establish a label focusing on their impairments or problems. Each evaluation should be used to reduce the burden of care, to improve the quality of life, and to establish measures to protect each person with cognitive difficulty and their caregiver(s).

Allen Cognitive Level Screen (ACLS)

This is a tool for the evaluation of problem-solving and new learning ability. It is based on the premise that in a situation of 'new learning' the therapist is

more readily able to ascertain true cognitive ability rather than testing ability to remember older, learned skills.

The screening tool is designed to provide an initial estimate of cognitive function. The score from the screen should be validated by further observations of performance. However, Allen states that the score from the screen is 90% accurate in determining an individual's level of cognitive ability and predicting occupational performance. In most cases, administration of further assessments in the module confirms the screen outcome.

The ACLS is quick and easy to administer. It consists of an oval piece of heavyweight leather punched with holes around the edge. Three laces are spaced around the perimeter of the leather, each formed into a different stitch. The person being assessed is asked to do the stitches. They begin with the simplest and, if successful, progress through to the hardest. Errors are built in to the task and the person is asked to identify and solve these. Standardized instructions for administering and scoring the screen are included in the commercially available test (Allen 1996) and are also available from the website of Allen's Conferences, Inc. (http://www.allen-cognitive-levels.com/acls.htm). The large version of the screen was developed for use with older people and those with visual impairments. There is no significant difference between scores on the ACLS and the LACL (Conroy 1998).

The test is a visuo-motor test and assumes that learning is required to complete all of the stitches successfully. Some people are frightened by tests and may refuse to cooperate. However, the apparent lack of face validity of the ACLS, in that it does not appear to be able to predict occupational performance in routine tasks, causes most patients to find it non-threatening. As with the administration of all assessments, any refusals to participate should be accepted graciously and the therapist may try to elicit the person's cooperation in performing an appropriate Allen Diagnostic Module activity.

Reliability and validity of the ACLS

The ACLS has been used in a number of studies that explored its reliability and validity. Inter-rater reliability, congruent validity and predictive validity were all significant (Conroy 1996).

The ACLS screens only ACL modes 3.0 to 5.8. At levels 1 and 2 people do not work with objects, and level 6 is concerned with attention to symbolic cues.

The ACLS is designed to access the middle of the ACL range, where the most important questions about ability to function occur.

Routine Task Inventory (RTI)

The anticipated discharge environment determines the selection of further observations of performance. When the anticipated discharge setting is a stable home environment or an institution, activities of daily living (ADLs) can form the basis for further observation. ADLs use procedural memories to follow habitual routines in an environment that is not changing. The most common ADLs are analysed in the RTI (Allen et al 1992, 1995).

In the RTI, performance of eight activities is evaluated within each definition of four disabilities: self-awareness, situational awareness, occupational role and social role. Performance is evaluated by either self-report, caregiver report or observation. The inventory makes statements about the pattern of behaviour for each activity and enables a record to be made of the corresponding cognitive level to be scored. Analysis of performance actions (Allen et al 1992) reveals differences of behaviour in modes for each of the routine tasks. The record can be used to highlight differences in carer perception and actual performance of the client from direct observation by the therapist, and between enabling and disempowering environments. This information can be used to help to create enabling environments.

Reliability and validity of the RTI

A study to explore the relationship between observed cognitive performance using the ACLS and a caregiver's report using the RTI revealed significant test–retest reliability and a positive correlation with the ACLS (Wilson et al 1989). Studies have also demonstrated an acceptable degree of test–retest and inter-rater reliability and have found the RTI to be an internally consistent instrument (Conroy 1996).

Cognitive Performance Tests (CPT)

When the anticipated discharge environment is the community or other changing environment, working memory must be assessed. Working memory processes new information in order to adapt to a changing environment. One effective method of assessing working memory is with the CPT.

The CPT was initially conceived as a research instrument to be used in longitudinal studies of functional change over time. It is also used for serial assessment to detect change in response to pharmacological and environmental intervention.

For each task, a set of verbal instructions is initially given. The tester then performs the standardized interactions that correspond to the specific behaviours of the patient. In essence, the tester changes the task demands in response to deficit behaviours by controlling or simplifying the information-processing requirements of the task.

The tasks comprise shopping, using the telephone, travel, getting dressed, making a piece of toast and washing hands. Each task is standardized and the instructions are described elsewhere (Burns 1992).

The CPT do not tap the full range of abilities associated with level 6 functioning, as some tasks do not require functioning above level 5. Therefore a person may perform the CPT without error but still be limited in more cognitively demanding tasks such as the management of their own finances.

Reliability and validity of the CPT

The validity of the CPT as an instrument to predict global performance decreases as tasks are eliminated. Administration of all six tasks offers a valid representation of global ability. Individual tasks offer specific ability. Inter-rater and test–retest reliability, and congruent, internal and predictive validity have all been established for the CPT (Conroy 1998).

Allen Diagnostic Module Projects

Another effective method of assessing working memory is with the 24 craft projects in the Allen Diagnostic Module (ADM). In the UK, the use of crafts as an occupational therapy assessment method has become unpopular, but it is still highly regarded in the USA. The craft project kits are available commercially, together with an instruction manual (Earhart et al 1993) that provides the observations of performance for each craft project in the battery.

The projects have been standardized to control the new information presented to individuals. They are selected to match the ACL score. The project that an individual completes must have meaning and value to that individual. The ADM contains extensive rating criteria for the modes of performance and is sensitive to small degrees of change in ability to function that can be objectively monitored.

Sensory–Motor Stimulation Kits

The Sensory–Motor Stimulation Kits provide the possibility of observing the performance of individuals whose cognitive impairment is severe and who are only able to engage with objects using reflex responses. The diagnosis may include traumatic brain injury, cerebrovascular accidents, the end stage of Alzheimer's disease and other progressive brain diseases, profound developmental delays and severe psychosis.

There are two portable kits available commercially, one for people operating at modes 1.0–2.2, and the other for modes 2.2–3.2. The kits contain a variety of stimulation materials for the five senses and for mobility, and the user is encouraged to add to these with media of their own choice. A manual accompanies each kit, which provides a philosophy and rationale for use and guidelines for presenting the stimulants, together with precautions and considerations. A rating sheet is also included (Blue & Allen 1992).

Interpreting the results

Allen's Cognitive Levels are based on theories of cognitive development and memory function. An understanding of these is essential when interpreting the test scores, so that the way in which a person is able to engage with their world, including objects and other people, can then form the basis for treatment-planning and interventions. For example, at level 5, a person will be able to use their working memory for reasoning in order to plan their engagement in activities, although they may not be able to use abstract ideas to reason through concepts. At level 4, a person is engaging with their world with a much heavier reliance on procedural memory in very familiar activities, and will find it difficult to use reasoning skills to solve problems and to work in unfamiliar environments.

Use of cognitive development theory guides the therapist to consider a range of skills and processes, including attention to sensory cues, motor actions, perceptibility of media, use of objects, and communication. Allen developed a computer program for occupational therapy documentation (available from Allen Conferences, Inc.), and from this a helpful handbook was produced which gives a short description of each mode, the best ability to function by a person in this mode, functional goals applicable to the mode, treatment methods and safety precautions (Allen et al 1995). The list for each mode follows the same format, beginning with a general description that includes percentages of cognitive and physical assistance. These seem a little prescriptive and do not allow for individual variables. However, the UK-based therapist should realize that the percentages are based on US Medicare guidelines, which are useful to the US therapist. UK-based therapists should use their own clinical reasoning skills to benefit from what is meaningful to their own client and practice.

As with all other treatment approaches, a treatment programme can be developed that focuses on the client's prioritized needs and aims to facilitate an improvement in occupational performance. The emphasis is on discovering what the person needs and wants to do, assessing how the person processes information in order to function, and analysing the activities that the person has chosen to do, in terms of the Information-processing Model. The role of the therapist is then to explain to carers and other professionals what alterations need to be made to tasks so that the person can meaningfully engage in the occupations (Pool 1997). The person's best ability to function takes place in the least restrictive environment. When the environment corresponds to the person's Allen Cognitive Level, the person can function at their best ability to function. Guidance is given for the redesign of environments to compensate for limitations and to encourage the use of remaining abilities (Allen & Bertrand 1999). Caregiver education is a major part of the use of the Allen Diagnostic Module, so caregivers can understand the level of ability of the person being cared for and not only focus on disability. Caregivers can also be assisted to increase the safety of self and others.

The therapist's role is not only to maintain the current levels of ability of a client, but also to probe for a higher level of cognitive performance. Treatment plans should identify interventions that facilitate a gradual increase in an individual's level of cognitive ability, by grading activities so that the demands of the performance of the activity are carefully increased. The FIPM focuses on the cognitive structures of the brain and therapists must also take into consideration the physical, social and psychological components of each individual. Because there is a complex interaction between these components, individuals whose social psychology is undermined may have a correspondingly lowered level of cognition. Therapists may find that, by addressing these social psychological needs, the cognitive structures of a person can be raised and a person's level of occupational performance can improve (Pool 2001).

Understanding the difference between working memory and procedural memory is key to interpreting the cognitive levels and identifying how the person needs help to engage as fully as possible within their environment. There are many good texts on memory (Kluwe, Luer, Rosler 2003, Baddeley 2004). For people with progressive organic conditions that cause impairments of cognitive structures, the view has traditionally been that new learning is not possible. However, when the concept of procedural memory is applied, it is possible for a person to re-learn implicitly using errorless learning and the repetitive performance of an activity. Consideration needs to be given to the time and effort this will take. For some individuals, if performance of a particular task has high importance to them, it may be well worth the effort; for others, it may not.

CASE STUDY

Richard

BACKGROUND

Richard Wilson is a quiet and gentle man who lives at home with his wife, Joan, and attends Parklands Day Hospital twice weekly for assessment and the introduction of a therapeutic programme.

Richard worked as a clerk in the County Council offices before his retirement. When he was not working, Richard enjoyed gardening and DIY. Soon after his retirement, Richard seemed to become forgetful. He would go out into the garden to do a task and then return to the house unable to remember why he had gone out. Initially, Richard and Joan laughed this off as being a part of growing older, but one day Richard went to a local shop and was unable to find his way home again.

A visit to the doctor confirmed their fears and Richard was diagnosed as having Alzheimer's disease. Luckily, Richard and Joan made contact with their local Alzheimer's Society, which was able to offer them some useful information. Additionally, Richard's calm and contented personality together with the close, supportive relationship he has with his wife enabled him to live at home despite his limited ability to plan and do things. Even so, Richard gradually became less able to carry out tasks and relied on Joan to help him in most areas. Most of their time was taken up with the daily chores and there was no time left for enjoying leisure activities. Richard was particularly frustrated by not being the 'chief gardener' and was beginning to refuse to go into the garden any more, saying 'there is no point'.

Two weeks ago Richard began to attend Parklands Day Hospital so that an assessment of his level of cognitive and functional disability could be made and appropriate therapeutic activities could be planned, which would probe for a higher level of function and enhance his well-being.

ASSESSMENT

Staff at Parklands observed that, when in a group situation, Richard was aware of others but acted as though the group task was an individual one and concentrated only on his particular part of it. Joan confirmed that, at home, Richard was unable to work through a task and that, without her guidance, he would keep repeating the same step. The occupational therapist at Parklands used the Allen Cognitive Level screening tool to determine that Richard's cognitive level was 3.6. When carrying out the functional performance tests of making a piece of toast and hand-washing, Richard's baseline cognitive level was 4.0, which supports these observations. Completion of the Routine Task Inventory 2 with Richard and his wife reveals the pattern of Richard's activity performance to be within levels 3–4.

The occupational therapist arranged to visit Richard at the couple's bungalow. She found that Richard follows Joan around the house and seems to want to engage in the chores with her, but Joan is unsure how to help him to do this. When Joan is preparing meals in the kitchen, Richard keeps coming in, even though Joan keeps sending him back out to lay the table in the dining room. Joan also reports that Richard is often up at night and has begun to urinate in the waste bin in the sitting room. The therapist notices that the hall is central in the house, with identical doors leading off to all of the other rooms.

INTERPRETATION OF ALLEN'S COGNITIVE LEVEL SCORE

At level 3.6, Richard's best ability to function will be that he is able to:

- pay attention to the effects of his actions on objects
- have motor control of placing and sorting objects
- imitate demonstrated activity
- carry out repetitive activities that have a predictable outcome.

At level 3.6, Richard will be limited in his ability to:

- initiate an action to produce a planned result
- follow a sequence of stages in an activity
- notice mistakes and solve problems.

In addition to interpreting the cognitive level, the therapist also noted, as an ability, the strong relationship between Richard and his wife and the patient's high level of psychological well-being.

TREATMENT PROGRAMME

Richard identified his priorities as needing to feel useful again, not wanting to be a burden to his wife, and being able to find the toilet at night. The therapist advised Richard and his wife to leave the bathroom door open at night and to leave a small light on in the bathroom, so that the toilet could easily be seen.

Joan was shown how to involve her husband in the daily domestic chores so that he could carry out the single-step activities, such as wiping the table, dusting and doing the washing-up, while she carried out the more complex activities close enough to be able to give him guidance should he need it. Joan also agreed that it would be helpful if a home carer assisted Richard with dressing in the morning and undressing in the evening, and Richard was happy with this arrangement.

Gardening and DIY activities were agreed to be important to Richard, and he and his wife were shown how to break these down into manageable stages of no more than two or three steps at a time. Joan was advised to stand by to assist and to give directions one at a time if needed. For Richard to regain independence in some activities, he was advised to take charge of the single-step activities such as sweeping and raking in the garden, and sanding and polishing in DIY activities.

Richard continued to attend the Parklands Day Hospital for 12 weeks while his treatment programme was implemented. The aim was for him to achieve a higher level of occupational performance, by grading the activities and introducing higher cognitive demands. Richard chose to complete a woodwork project of making a bird table for his garden. The therapist set this up in the woodwork room, so that Richard was cued to the activity. Tools for the task were initially placed on the woodwork bench, in Richard's visual field. As the project progressed, the tools were left in their usual familiar cupboards and shelves, and Richard was encouraged to seek them out. The therapist assisted Richard at the start of the project by giving directions one at a time and gradually increased the complexity of these. She also encouraged Richard to make choices and decisions and to initiate the actions required to complete the stages of the woodwork task.

As the treatment programme progressed, Richard became more confident in his own ability. A further interview with Richard and his wife revealed that the difficulty with his night-time visit to the toilet had resolved and that he had returned to spending more time in the garden. However, his wife reported that sometimes Richard tries to do the weeding and pulls out the wrong plants. Even though Richard still had difficulties, they both felt that their situation had improved.

This improvement and Richard's success in increased occupational performance at the day hospital were reflected in the re-assessments of his cognitive level at the 6th and 12th weeks. The therapist re-administered the LACL, which revealed that Richard's cognitive level had risen to 3.8 and then to 4.0.

Richard then moved to a local Alzheimer's Society day centre, where he continued with his gardening interests and also chose to participate in a news group. As his condition progresses, he and his wife will need further guidance about assisting him to engage in activity.

Outcome measurement

Because the ADM consists of tools that have been scientifically tested for their reliability and validity, they are also useful as outcome measures using a single-case experimental design. In other words, the instruments can be used to gain a baseline cognitive level and then can be re-administered following therapeutic intervention to measure the effectiveness of the programme.

The scores can be shown in a variety of ways: for example, in table form or as a graph (Fig. 9.1).

Clinical application — treatment planning and interventions

Allen's earliest work was with people who had mental health problems. Conditions such as depression and anxiety are viewed as being linked to some degree of cognitive impairment. Therefore, the ADM is viewed as being very appropriate for these client groups. The potential for application of the FIPM and the diagnostic module has now broadened to include other clients with cognitive disability.

Therapists who use the diagnostic modules must also use activity analysis and environmental adaptation. When they have determined the level of an individual's cognitive ability, they will have guidance from within the manuals and books as to what this means for the client in functional and practical terms.

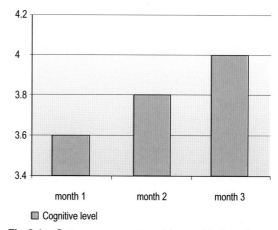

Fig 9.1 • Outcome measurement in graphic format.

Summary

The FIPM and ADM are useful as part of the process of occupational therapy intervention with any client who has cognitive impairment. The onus is on the occupational therapist to apply clinical reasoning skills to the measures and to use the handbooks for interpretation of the results as a guide to treatment planning.

Allen's application of the FIPM and diagnostic module seems to suggest that the role of the occupational therapist is to determine the current level of an individual's occupational performance and to aim to maintain the person at that level by making maximum use of residual abilities while preventing or minimizing limitations. This attitude may be viewed as disregarding the belief that it is possible for an individual to influence the state of their health by engaging in meaningful activity (Keogh 1998). Furthermore, there is a major conceptual shift for occupational therapists from attempting to help the person to change, to changing the demands of the activity. This is a valid role for the occupational therapist once clients have reached a plateau in terms of their potential for improved cognitive ability and occupational performance. However, the therapist must first probe for an improved level of ability and performance, and assist the client to reach that plateau through careful treatment planning and intervention.

Perceived disadvantages of the module seem to be associated with its American origins and its craft-oriented assessment tools. In addition to the use of the module being driven to some extent by Medicare requirements, some of the language used in the standardized directions is different from that used in the UK. However, Allen gives permission for therapists to deviate from the instructions in the interests of client understanding. In the past, it has been difficult to obtain the books and assessment tools in the UK, but this is easier now with the availability of the website.

The biggest deterrent to acceptance seems to be the emphasis on associated crafts (Conroy 1998). Allen defends this, explaining that craft projects were selected because they can be standardized to present new information that is meaningful to disabled people most of the time (Allen & Reyner 2002). Activities that are not familiar present new learning opportunities, so the therapist can observe performance that is more likely to be using working memory and less likely to be relying on procedural memory. Occupational therapists in the UK who have moved away from an association with crafts may be deterred from using the craft activities in the ADM and the ACLS, which is a leather lacing activity. They are often concerned about the stereotypical image that they may be presenting to their colleagues. However, a therapist who is confident in the underlying philosophy and principles of the FIPM and the ADM will be able to draw on the existing evidence base to justify its use.

Reflective learning

- How might the development of the WHO International Classification of Function have contributed to the renaming of Allen's Cognitive Disability Model as the Functional Information-processing Model (FIPM)?
- How is the generally held scientific assumption that human functioning is a qualitative capacity to use mental energy to guide motor and verbal performance applied in the FIPM?
- Can cognitive impairments be inferred from observing limitations in routine task performance?
- What are the strengths and weaknesses of Allen's Cognitive Level Screen (ACLS)?
- Does Allen's model raise questions about the role of the occupational therapist with individuals with cognitive disabilities?

References

Allen, C.K., 1982. Independence through activity: the practice of occupational therapy (psychiatry). American Journal of Occupational Therapy 36, 731–739.

Allen, C.K., 1985. Occupational Therapy for Psychiatric Diseases: Measurement and Management of Cognitive Disabilities. Little Brown, Boston.

Allen, C.K., 1996. Large Allen Cognitive Level Screen Test Manual. Allen Conferences, Ormond Beach, FL.

Allen, C.K., Bertrand, J., 1999. Structures of the Cognitive Performance Modes. Allen Conferences, Ormond Beach, FL.

Allen, C.K., Earhart, C.A., Blue, T., 1992. Occupational Therapy Treatment Goals for the Physically and Cognitively Disabled. American Occupational Therapy Association, Bethesda, MD.

Allen, C.K., Blue, T., Earhart, C.A., 1995. Understanding Cognitive Performance Modes. Allen Conferences, Ormond Beach, FL.

Allen, C.K., Reyner, A., 2002. How to Start Using the Allen Diagnostic Module. Allen Conferences, Ormond Beach, FL.

Baddeley, A., 2004. The Essential Handbook of Memory Disorders for Clinicians. John Wiley, Chichester.

Blue, T., Allen, C.K., 1992. Sensory Motor Stimulation Kit I and II. Allen Conferences, Ormond Beach, FL.

Burns, T., 1992. Cognitive Performance Test. In: Allen, C.K., Earhart, C.A., Blue, T. (Eds.), Occupational Therapy Treatment Goals for the Physically and Cognitively Disabled. American Occupational Therapy Association, Bethesda, MD, pp. 69–84.

Conroy, M.C., 1996. Dementia Care: Keeping Intact and In Touch. Avebury, Aldershot.

Conroy, M.C., 1998. Allen's cognitive levels with people who are dementing. British Journal of Therapy and Rehabilitation 5 (1), 21–26.

Earhart, C.A., Allen, C.K., Blue, T., 1993. The Allen Diagnostic Module Instruction Manual (ADMIM). Allen Conferences, Ormond Beach, FL.

Katz, N., 1998. Cognition and Occupation in Rehabilitation. American Occupational Therapy Association, Bethesda, MD.

Keogh, C., 1998. Cognitive disability model: moving to an informed position. Irish Journal of Occupational Therapy 28 (2), 2–7.

Kluwe, RH, Lüer, G, Rösler, F (Eds.), 2003. Principles of Learning and Memory. Birkhauser Verlag, Basel.

O'Neill, H., 2002. Cognitive — cognitive what? British Journal of Occupational Therapy 65 (6), 288–290.

Pool, J., 1997. Helping carers change their role. Journal of Dementia Care 5 (3), 24–25.

Pool, J., 2001. Making contact: an activity-based model of care. Journal of Dementia Care 9 (4), 24–26.

Vygotsky, L.S., 1978. The Development of Higher Psychological Processes. Harvard University Press, Boston.

WHO, 2002. Towards a Common Language for Functioning, Disability and Health. ICF, World Health Organization, Geneva.

Wilson, D.S., Allen, C.K., McCormack, G., et al., 1989. Cognitive disability and routine task behaviours in a community based population with senile dementia. Occupational Therapy Practice 1 (1), 58–66.

Resources

Allen Cognitive Network, www.allen-cognitive-network.org.

Allen's Conferences, Inc., www.allen-cognitive-levels.com.

The *Kawa* (River) Model

10

Kee Hean Lim   Michael K. Iwama

OVERVIEW

In the pursuit of providing meaningful and relevant occupational therapy with an increasingly diverse global clientele, occupational therapists are being challenged to examine the relevance, construct and content validity of their contemporary models and practice frameworks. The *Kawa* Model, infused with its naturalistic and contextual philosophy, provides a radically different perspective of how occupation and the self are conceptualized. The *Kawa* Model recognizes the uniqueness, dynamic nature and diversity of each client's occupational narrative and provides a framework within which occupational therapists can appreciate each client in the unique context of their day-to-day realities and circumstances, thereby gaining a greater appreciation of their complex occupational world.

Key points

- Each person's experience of and meanings they attach to daily life are unique. Clients and occupational therapists alike carry diverse interpretations of occupation and of occupational therapy.
- Context and experience are important and central to understanding and shaping one's occupational world and daily life narratives.
- Professional culture, standard practice frameworks and prescriptive assessments based on universal criteria can exclude as well as reinforce power differentials between client and professional.
- In the current climate of evidence-based practice there can be an over-emphasis on standardized clinical assessment and measurement, at the expense of appreciating clients' lived experiences and wellness narratives.

Key points—cont'd

- Client-centred occupational therapy begins, is based on, and ends with the client's narrative of daily life experience.
- To be meaningful and relevant, occupational therapy must be both person- and context-focused, inclusive, enabling and culturally safe.

Introduction

The great promise of occupational therapy, to enable people from all walks of life to engage/participate in activities and processes that have value, is simple yet profoundly complex and challenging to fulfil for the diverse clientele that typifies an increasingly global, postmodern world (Iwama 2007). Occupational therapists the world over have been challenged to provide occupational therapy that is relevant and responsive to the day-to-day realities of their diverse clientele. An examination of current occupational therapy models reveals that the values and meanings of *occupation*, like other socially situated constructs, have been ascribed mainly by people situated in the English-speaking Western world, who have a common context of shared experiences (Iwama 2006, Lim 2008a). The meanings of human occupations are uniquely tied to socio-cultural contexts, varying from group to group, from person to person and from situation to situation. Given this degree of diversity and cultural relativity in occupation's fundamental meaning, a single or universal interpretation of this core construct of occupational therapy is virtually impossible to maintain. How, then, will specific conceptual models in occupational therapy, largely constructed on such universal premises, explain, describe and guide occupational therapy approaches and processes for a diverse clientele in diverse contexts? How well do the learned and tacitly held ideas that essentially reflect middle-class, middle-North American and Western European ideals of self-determinism, competence, individual agency and autonomy explain the day-to-day realities and meanings of occupation for clients that do not fit these socio-cultural ideals?

Though many aspects of contemporary occupational therapy and its locations of practice have aligned with biomedicine, diehard occupational therapists have endeavoured to keep occupational therapy focused on occupation, preferring to shift occupational therapy's focus and location of practice into the realm of clients' day-to-day living issues and experiences (Iwama 2005a). Instead of focusing on pathology, symptoms and functional limitations, occupational therapists have maintained an interest in and focus on the consequences of these medically defined factors, on the day-to-day circumstances and needs of a diverse clientele. This is where the power of occupational therapy lies: in the relevance to the client's day-to-day circumstances to enable people from all walks of life to engage and participate in activities and processes that have personal meaning and value (Lim & Iwama 2006).

Occupation-based occupational therapy is challenging to deliver, especially when diversity and cultural relativity are brought into the equation. Cultural variation and the challenges of diversity were not such strong concerns for the pioneering occupational therapy scholars when they first embarked upon constructing their practice models. Theoretical materials created in the past century in occupational therapy and rehabilitation appear to have been largely constructed on the premise of a relatively homogeneous clientele, whereby a one-size-fits-all worldview or single framework seeks to explain the experience of human occupation and occupational therapy practice for all (Iwama 2005a, Lim 2008b). What may work well for clients whose experiences fall within minor deviations from the norm/mean for a particular conceptual phenomenon may possess limitations for those 'other' clients who stand as outliers in the demographic mean curve, who may be either excluded or disadvantaged by the same standard. What happens when norms and imperatives of autonomy, personal causation and self-determinism are also foisted on to 'outlier' clients who come from a sphere of shared learning and experience that idealizes dependency, group harmony and collective determinism? How does the single-parent client of four young children, a young man with mental illness, and others who have survived circumstances of abject poverty and social marginalization relate to occupational therapy's middle-class, Western principles and ideals of competence, self-agency and self-reliance (Whalley Hammell & Carpenter 2004, Iwama 2006)?

Delivering an occupation-based service for a diverse client population that makes sense of the value of activities and processes of daily life (occupation) in unique and diverse ways remains a daunting task for occupational therapists. Catering to the uniqueness of each client's day-to-day occupational issues is difficult to enact when conventional theory and the approaches that this theory guides and explains are based on a questionable premise of homogeneity of clientele, their needs and universality of a given occupational therapy model.

Emerging issues of culture and cultural safety in occupational therapy theory and practice

Culture is more than individual-embodied features of ethnicity and race. It is broadly defined here as spheres of shared experience and the ascription of meaning to phenomena and objects in the world (Iwama 2007, Lim 2008a). A broader definition that takes in social context qualifies the profession of occupational therapy as a sphere of shared experience, or cultural entity, as much as 'Western' or 'Japanese' might. Occupational therapy has its own unique sphere of shared experiences, a developing specialized language, tacit rules of professional conduct and acceptable rules for knowledge production, including theory development. For many occupational therapists, the cultural features and imperatives buried within conventional occupational therapy theory may go problematically unnoticed (Iwama 2005a). The preference for individual-centric views of daily life occupations, the imperatives of autonomy and independence in daily living skills and de-emphases on contexts that shape occupational meanings are often taken for granted and accepted as 'normal' — especially by those who have shared experiences in Western contexts of daily living (Lim 2008b). Unwittingly, occupational therapists find themselves enquiring about and filtering clients' unique and rich narratives of their daily living contexts and circumstances through predetermined (and often sophisticated) concepts and principles belonging to someone else's (unfamiliar) world view and interpretation of human occupation. Problems are identified and plans for intervention are then determined that can potentially stray or diverge from what the client actually regards to be meaningful, valued, worth knowing and worth doing. Often, the ideals of client-centred occupational therapy do not extend far enough into the rich, contextual cultural world of the client (Iwama 2005c, Lim 2006).

For many occupational therapists and their clients who fall outside of such mainstream cultural norms, universal models that have risen out of a dominant mainstream culture, infused with its own tacit standards and ideals of what is considered 'normal', 'acceptable' and 'good', can be regarded in some instances as being *culturally unsafe* (Lim & Iwama 2006). Ramsden (1990) highlights the importance and principles of cultural safety: a framework by which power relationships between health professionals and the peoples they serve are critically considered. The impact of historical, social and political processes on minority health groups holds important implications for equity wherever health issues of a particular group are being described, explained, mediated and evaluated by other people within their own standards (Jungerson 1992). This idea of cultural safety is especially pertinent to occupational therapists when taking their ideas and processes into new cultural domains, including into the lives of their diverse clients and contexts (Gray & McPherson 2005, Iwama 2006). Often the recipients may be in weaker, disadvantaged positions and are discriminated against further by being compared and evaluated against standards and norms belonging to a different cultural context (Lim 2005, 2008a). Further, they may also lack the experience, knowledge and means to examine critically the veracity, utility and cultural safety of the procedures and materials imposed upon them.

There are also relevant issues of cultural safety in the interface between theory construction and theory application. When critical questions are asked about where the ideas have come from, on what realities these materials and ideas have been based, and who has participated in the production of such knowledge, valuable insight is gained into the cultural features of the epistemology and theory of a profession. Theories and models, often developed in academic settings, can be far removed from the very people, situated in diverse, dynamic and changing practice contexts, for whom these theoretical materials and models are universally intended and considered appropriate (Lim & Iwama 2006).

Empowering occupational therapy clients — the way forward

Reconfiguring client-centred practice may be difficult for both the seasoned therapist and conditioned client to come to terms with, as the current way of top-down delivery of occupational therapy often privileges the professional as 'knowing best' and the client submitting to the role of 'patient'. The reliance on certain (universal) frameworks and the standardized tests that reify and accompany them can take some of the guesswork out of professional decision-making and enhance the efficiency of occupational therapy processes, but the occupational therapist must ultimately understand whether the client and their 'story' of day-to-day living and circumstances are being comprehended and that the ensuing occupational therapy is being truly client-centred and based on factors that are meaningful to the client.

Occupational therapists stand to benefit from theory, instruments, methods and approaches that enable clients to translate their real experiences of daily living into the therapeutic process, to form the basis on which occupational therapy is fashioned. Ideally, the client's 'story' of their day-to-day occupational issues, constructed and told by the client, in their own words, ought to be enabled and centralized to form the basis to the occupational therapy process (Lim & Iwama 2007). Achieving this to any degree is not an easy or a simple undertaking, for it involves a series of difficult transitions for the professional therapist. Firstly, a change in power relation between the therapist and client is required. The familiar hierarchical power structure of professional and client is upended, and the heterogeneity and diversity of clients and their 'stories' become *normal*. The skills necessary for those engaged in occupational therapy will change from being technical experts capable of delivering standard procedures of assessments and interventions, to health professionals who are able to apply their knowledge and skills effectively according to the unique and diverse clients and their contexts that emerge in each complex therapeutic instance.

Achieving this will move occupational therapy further towards becoming client-centred and more equitable with regard to the power differential that commonly exists in therapeutic relationships, where the occupational therapist is situated as expert and the client is regarded as 'patient' (Ramsden 1990, Lim 2005). Rather than forcing and fashioning the client to adapt to some standard requirements of occupational therapy, such an approach requires occupational therapy and occupational therapists to adapt and fashion their occupational therapy to the unique needs and specific requirements of the client. Imagine a process whereby the client 'names' the concepts of their occupational therapy model and explains the principles that tie these highly personal concepts together, in which the occupational therapy process is transformed into a collaborative one in which it is bound by the client's occupational narrative. The client is now (acknowledged and respected as) the 'expert' of their own occupational narrative and the therapist becomes a partner or facilitator to enable better life flow.

The *Kawa* (River) Model

Such a significant departure from the tacit ways in which theory is normally structured and translated into occupational therapy practice, the empowering of client and their occupational narratives to form the basis of the occupational therapy processes and interventions to follow, represents a revolutionary breakthrough in conventional occupational therapy practice. For conventional practice until now has been to take a set of predetermined concepts and principles that tie these concepts into some plausible, standard narrative and impress these upon the client, assuming that the model was valid and unassailable.

Recently, a group of Japanese occupational therapists, grappling with the issues of incongruent occupational therapy theory and practice forms, embarked on a project that aimed to develop an alternative approach that would transform their occupational therapy and bring it more in line with their client's day-to-day realities and experiences of disablement (Iwama 2006). The qualitative research processes they engaged in also unearthed the fundamentally overlooked issue of culture, theory construction and practice. These Japanese therapists with the aid of a Canadian therapists

endeavoured to develop a conceptual framework that would not impose a universal narrative of occupation on every client but would actually reverse this process and value each client's unique occupational narrative, reflecting a rich comprehension of the client in the context of their experiences and explanations of day-to-day realities. The qualitative research processes that gave rise to the *Kawa* Model and its fuller description can be studied in greater detail in *The Kawa Model: Culturally Relevant Occupational Therapy* (Iwama 2006).

Philosophical underpinnings

A social constructionist perspective

The primary philosophical orientation underlying the *Kawa* Model is one of *social constructionism*. Burr (1995) highlights the fact that, from a social constructionist perspective, knowledge and the meanings of phenomena and their explanations (theory) are understood to be created between people who share common experiences and agree on interpretations of those phenomena. This is in opposition to the dominant view in the scientific and empirical traditions that truth and reality are singular (universal) and material, lie external to (or outside of) the self and are knowable through rational enquiry (Gergen 1999).

Burr (1995) argues that our current accepted ways of understanding the world are a product not of objective observation of the world, but of the social processes and interactions in which people are constantly engaged with each other. The implication of this alternative way of conceptualizing phenomena is that people's understandings of issues, such as occupation and occupational performance, are said to be historically and culturally situated. Occupation and its enactment will therefore mean different things to different people situated in differing spheres of experience and circumstances (Iwama 2006, Lim 2008b).

Ontological views: self in relation to context, environment and time

Culture can be identified at the core of most contemporary conceptual models of rehabilitation, and is particularly observable in how the 'self' is socially constructed and situated in relation to the surrounding environment or context. The interpretations and meanings we derive through what we do in the world may vary according to how this dualism of self vis-à-vis the environment is regarded and understood. These models construe the *self* as being not only focally situated in the centre of all concerns, but also understood to be rationally separate and superior in power and status to the environment and nature. Well-being is constructed to be contingent on the extent to which the *self* can act on and demonstrate its ability to control one's perceived circumstances located in the environment. Failure or compromise in controlling the environment is construed with such terms as *dysfunction* and *disability*. These terms are often pejorative in a sociocultural context in which the self is required to be competent, able and in control (of one's environment and circumstances). In these worldviews, dependency can often represent an undesirable state of disability.

An independent self, centrally situated and agent upon a separate and subordinated environment, also appears to coincide with a particular sensation of time. When the self is centrally located in relation to the environment at large, one's sense of entitlement to *doing* in the present (here and now) can also extend temporally into one's future. The relation between intention, one's immediate action on the environment, and some specific (future) objective is often rationally connected. It is not uncommon for people situated in the Western world to believe that they carry primary responsibility for their own destinies. 'You make your bed and lie in it' and 'you get what you pay for' are familiar adages, particularly in Western social contexts. It should come as little surprise, then, to see that independence, autonomy, equality and self-determinism are celebrated ideals that point to a common worldview and value pattern shared between mainstream rehabilitation ideology and the broader Western social contexts from which they emerged (Iwama 2006).

Lying in contrast to this worldview is the East Asian and Aboriginal one. In the primitive cosmological myth (Bellah 1991), the 'self' is not central nor unilaterally empowered but rather construed to be just one of many parts of an inseparable whole (Bellah 1991, Gustafson 1993). In this view of reality, one does not need to *occupy* or wrest control of anything because in an integrated view of self and nature, one is already *there* amongst others. In this view of reality, health and disability states are also not imagined nor believed to be an individual-centred matter. Life circumstances are dependent on a broader whole,

determined by a constellation of factors and elements located both within and outside of the physically defined body (Shakespeare 1994). The self is decentralized and not accorded an exclusive privilege to exercise stewardship, nor unilateral control, over one's environment or circumstances. Hence, conceptual models in occupational therapy that are based on a tacit understanding of a central individual separate from a discrete environment are often incongruent with experiences of disability and well-being for many who are situated outside of mainstream Western social norms.

The *Kawa* Model follows the more 'primitive' ontological view of people and nature, drawing no clear distinctions or separations between selves and their contexts of reality. This is a dynamic view of human experience and meanings. The self and surrounding context share an inseparable co-existence in which changes to any one aspect of the self-context complex will affect the entire frame. *Kawa* is the Japanese term for 'river', and is employed as a metaphor for 'life flow'. The river's rocks, configuration of the river banks and driftwood in the *Kawa* Model combine uniquely, from instance to instance, to shape and determine the quality of the ensuing river flow. Such is the flow of life, as self and context fluidly change from instance to instance. Problems, the social and physical environments, one's own personal attributes, strengths and limitations all combine to render a particular quality of one's life flow. This is the *Kawa* Model, and occupational therapy's subsequent mandate is to help the client enhance and balance the flow within their lives.

The power of metaphor

A metaphor can be understood to be a figure of speech in which an expression or symbolic image is used to refer to something that it does not literally denote, in order to suggest a similarity. 'Life is a river' or 'people are complex machines' are just two common examples of metaphors. Models can also be seen as metaphors, whether they be of 'systems' like machines, or 'rivers' of nature. Lakoff and Johnson's seminal work in *Metaphors We Live By* (1980) illuminates the degree to which metaphor plays a fundamental role in matters of self-identity and one's relation to the world. We not only communicate through metaphors but we also think through them. The occupational therapeutic relationship is structured and mediated through metaphor (Iwama 2006), and the *Kawa* Model serves as one particular metaphor through which the powerful processes of occupational therapy can be enacted.

When the *Kawa* Model was first developed, there was a tendency to situate the model in Japanese culture, and therefore it was assumed to be applicable to 'Eastern' clients and others located in East Asian contexts. Since its development, the metaphor of the river, used to depict life flow or the life journey, has been found to resonate with people beyond Asian societies. When the *kawa* metaphor is found to be a common link spanning the therapist's and client's spheres of shared experience, it can be exploited as an effective medium through which the process of occupational therapy can *flow*. The authors speculate that the explanatory power of conceptual models in occupational therapy has much to do with the power and resonance of the metaphor that underpins the model, in relation to the spheres of shared experience (culture) of the client and occupational therapist. The resonance of the river metaphor to diverse occupational therapy practice contexts, in a relatively short period of time since its publication, has been remarkable. The *Kawa* Model is currently being translated into six languages and utilized by occupational therapists located across six continents.

Original rendition of the model

The qualitative research process engaged in by a group of occupational therapists in Japan initially yielded a rather cumbersome, linear representation of their model along conventional, linear box and arrow structures (Fig. 10.1A). At that early stage, it became readily apparent that there were fundamental differences in how self and environment were imagined and represented in established (Western) models and actually *lived* and *experienced* by the group participants. For a model purposely to explain self and context, the central placement of a distinctly defined self, adjacent to a separate but distinct environment commonly seen in conventional (Western) models, was non-existent. Further consideration revealed comprehensions of self and environment or context that were more diffuse and inseparably integrated by the Japanese than by their Western counterparts. Consistent with a worldview that imagined self and the world with all of its elements as integrated parts of an all-encompassing whole, phenomena as complex as well-being and disability

could not be adequately described and explained by linear diagrams that connect rationally defined categories through logical principles. These Eastern perspectives of wellness and disability states could not be readily contained in and explained by boxes/categories set in a logical sequence, familiarly observable in rational formulae or continua.

In this initial diagram, the interconnectedness of all elements and phenomena in the frame of life experience, the fact that states of well-being and disability are neither internally (in the body) nor externally (in the environment) isolated, is conveyed. The self and environment are inextricably connected in a manner in which changes in one or more components effect changes in the greater whole. The four fundamental categories of concept were life flow, health and occupations; life circumstances and difficulties; personal assets and liabilities; and environment.

Currently, occupational therapists leaning towards a more rational representation and use of the *Kawa* Model prefer to use this initial framework over the metaphorically graphic river in the following manner. Briefly explained, the four concepts are treated as categories of occupational therapy factors of enquiry (Fig. 10.2). The occupational therapist makes appropriate enquiries of the client to draw relevant and pertinent subjective and objective information about each of the conceptual categories. Therapists can determine what components need further clarification and understanding, and choose both standard and non-standard instruments to yield a relevant, comprehensive occupational profile of the client. Through an active interaction between therapist and client, intervention plans can be set, executed and eventually evaluated.

Emergence of the river metaphor of the *Kawa* Model

In order to capture and represent better a conceptualization of a diffuse self, unified, interdependent with and inseparable from other elements in the environment, this initial box and arrow diagram was augmented by the addition of an alternate, complementary image. The research participants decided to employ a metaphor of nature (a river, or *kawa* in Japanese) to explain the dynamic and fluid nature of the model better. The use of such a metaphor contrasted substantially with more familiar mechanical and 'system' metaphors often seen in contemporary

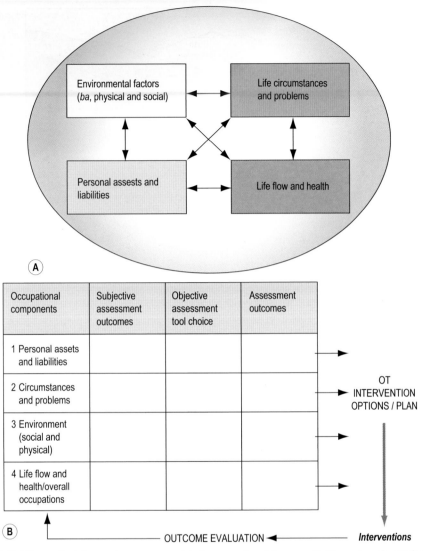

Fig 10.1 • A. Initial figure depicting a Japanese model of occupational therapy. B. Example schema for applying the original rendition of the *Kawa* Model.

occupational therapy conceptual models. With the Japanese word *kawa* translated as 'river', the former box and arrow diagram was transformed into a more dynamic, fluid and integrative image to represent the complexity and *harmony* of the client's occupational life flow.

Each individual is perceived to have their own unique 'personal river' that symbolizes their life journey, flowing through time and space (Fig. 10.3). An optimal state of well-being in one's life or *river* can be metaphorically portrayed by an image of strong, deep, unimpeded flow. Aspects of the environment

and phenomenal circumstances, like certain structures found in a river, can influence and affect that flow. Rocks (life circumstances), walls and bottom (environment), and driftwood (assets and liabilities) are all inseparable parts of a river that determine its boundaries, shape and flow (Fig. 10.4). Occupational therapy's purpose in this metaphorical representation of human being, then, is to enable and enhance *life flow*. The upstream of one's river represents the past, the lower stream represents the future, and personal health and well-being are expressed by the free and unrestricted flow of one's river.

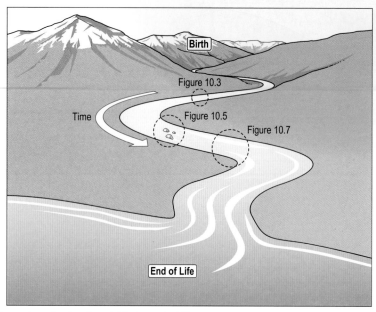

Fig 10.2 • Life is like a river, flowing from birth to end of life.

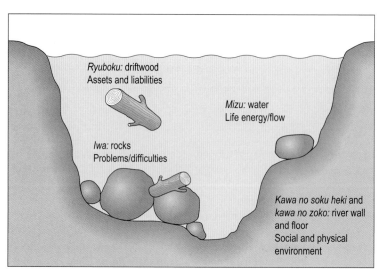

Fig 10.3 • At any given point along its continuum, a cross-section view of the river can be considered as understanding life's condition from the client's vantage point. The quality of water flow is affected by the river walls and bottom, and by rocks and driftwood. Wherever there is a need to enhance life flow, there is a need for occupational therapy.

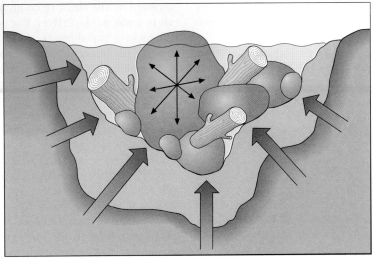

Fig 10.4 • The shape and status of water, or life flow, are determined by the compounding interplay of rocks (problems), driftwood (assets/liabilities) and the river walls and floor (environment). Rocks increase in size, shape and number, and exist in a dynamic, enclosing environment, trapping driftwood. Life flow is compromised, indicating a need for occupational therapy.

Components of the *Kawa* Model

The four basic (categories of) concepts outlined in the initial rational depiction of the *Kawa* Model and their metaphorical counterparts, listed in both the original Japanese concepts and their English equivalents, are explained in the following section.

Mizu (water)

Mizu, Japanese for 'water', metaphorically represents the individual's *life energy* or *life flow*. Fluid, pure, spirit, filling, cleansing and renewing are only some of the meanings and functions commonly associated with this natural element. Just as people's lives are bounded and shaped by their surroundings, people, experience and circumstances, the water flowing as a river touches the rocks, sides and banks and all other elements that form its context. The volume, direction and rate of flow can reflect the state of one's health; that is, when life energy or flow weakens, the individual may be said to experience a state of ill health or disharmony. Just as water is fluid and adopts its form from its container, people in many collective-oriented societies often interpret the social as a shaper of individual self. There is greater value in 'belonging and 'interdependence' than in unilateral agency and

individual determinism (Nakane 1970, Doi 1973, Lebra 1976). In such experience, the interdependent self is deeply influenced and even determined by the surrounding social context, at a given time and place (Iwama 2006, Lim & Iwama 2006).

Kawa no soku-heki (river side-wall) and *kawa no zoko* (river bottom)

The river's sides and bottom, referred to in the Japanese lexicon respectively as *kawa no soku-heki* and *kawa no zoko*, are the structures/concepts from the river metaphor that stand for the client's environment. These are perhaps the most important determinants of a person's life flow in a collectivist social context because of the primacy afforded to the environmental context in determining the construction of self, experience of being and subsequent meanings of personal action. In the *Kawa* Model, the river walls and sides represent the subject's social context/ frame or *ba* (Nakane 1970). This comprises mainly those others who share a direct relationship with the subject. Depending upon which social frame is perceived as being most important in a given instance and place, the river sides and bottom can represent family members, workmates, friends in a recreational club, classmates and so on. In certain non-Western societies like those of Japan, social relationships are regarded to be the central (Nakane 1970) determinant of individual and collective life flow.

Aspects of the surrounding social frame on the subject can affect the overall flow (volume and rate) of the *kawa*. Harmonious relationships can enable and complement life flow. Increased flow can have an agent effect upon difficult circumstances and problems, as the force of water displaces rocks in the channel and even creates new courses through which to flow. Conversely, a decrease in flow volume can exert a compounding, negative effect on the other elements that take up space in the channel (Fig. 10.5). If there are obstructions (rocks and driftwood) in the watercourse when river walls and bottom are constricting, the flow of the river is especially compromised. The rocks in this river can directly butt up against the river walls and bottom, compounding and creating larger impediments to the river's usual flow. When applying the *Kawa* Model in collectivist-oriented populations, these components and the perceptions of their importance are paramount.

Iwa (rocks)

Iwa (Japanese for 'large rocks') represent discrete circumstances that are considered to be impediments to one's *life flow*. They are life circumstances perceived by the client to be problematic and difficult to remove. Most rivers, like people's lives, have such rocks or impediments, of varying size, shape and number. The impeding effect of rocks by themselves or in combination with other rocks, jammed against the river walls and sides (environment), can profoundly impede and obstruct flow. The client's rocks may have been there since the beginning, such as with congenital conditions. They may appear instantaneously, as in sudden illness or injury, and even be transient (Lim & Iwama 2006).

A person's bodily impairment becomes disabling when interfaced with the environment. For example, the functional difficulties associated with a neurological condition can change according to the environmental context. A (physically) barrier-free environment can decrease one's disability, as can social and/or political/organizational environments that are accepting of people with disabling conditions. Once the client's perceived rocks are known (including their relative size and situation), the therapist can help to identify potential disabling circumstances and areas of intervention and strategies to enable better life flow. Occupational therapy intervention can therefore include treatment strategies that expand beyond the traditional patient, to their social network and even to policies and social structures that ultimately play a part in setting the disabling context.

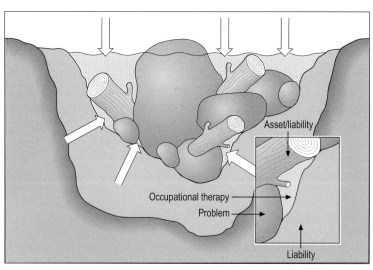

Fig 10.5 • *Sukima*/spaces: potential focal points for occupational therapy. Intervention can be multi-faceted and include breaking or eroding away the (medical) problem, limiting personal liabilities and/or maximizing personal assets, as well as intervening on elements of the greater environment (including the social and physical). Focusing water on these objects to erode or move them is metaphorical of the client using their own abilities or 'life force'.

The subject, be it an individual or a collective, ideally determines specific rocks and their number, magnitude, form and situation in the river. As with all other elements of the model, if the client is unable to express their own river, family members or a community of people connected with the issue at hand may lend assistance.

Ryuboku (driftwood)

Ryuboku is Japanese for 'driftwood', and represents the subject's personal attributes and resources, such as values (e.g. honesty, thrift), character (e.g. optimism, stubbornness), personality (e.g. reserved, outgoing), special skill (e.g. carpentry, public speaking), and immaterial (e.g. friends, siblings) and material (e.g. wealth, special equipment) assets that can positively or negatively affect the subject's circumstance and life flow.

Like driftwood, they are transient in nature and carry a certain quality of fate or serendipity. They can appear to be inconsequential in some instances and significantly obstructive in others, particularly when they settle in amongst rocks and the river sides and walls. On the other hand, they can collide with the same structures to nudge obstructions out of the way. A client's religious faith and sense of determination can be positive factors in persevering to erode or move rocks out of the way. Receiving a grant to acquire specialized assistive equipment can be the piece of driftwood that collides against existing flow impediments and opens a greater channel for one's life to flow more strongly. Driftwood is a part of everyone's river and often resembles intangible components possessed by each unique client of occupational therapy. Effective therapists pay particular attention to these components of a client's or community's assets and circumstances, and consider their real or potential effect on the client's situation.

Sukima (space between obstructions): the promise of occupational therapy

In the *Kawa* Model, spaces are the points through which the client's life energy (water) evidently flows, and these spaces represent 'occupation'. When the metaphor of a river depicting the client's life flow becomes clearer, attention turns to the *sukima* (spaces between the rocks, driftwood, and river walls

and bottom). These spaces are as important to comprehend in the client as are the other elements of the river when determining how to apply and direct occupational therapy. For example, a space between a functional impairment such as arthritis (an *iwa*/rock) and a social group or person (in the river sides and walls) may represent a certain social role, such as parent, company worker, friend and so on.

Water coursing naturally through these spaces can work to erode the rocks and river walls and bottom, and over time can transform them into larger conduits for life flow (Fig. 10.6). This effect reflects the latent healing potential that each subject naturally holds within themselves and in the inseparable context. Thus occupational therapy in this perspective retains its hallmark of working with the client's abilities and assets, and seizing upon opportunities to bring about change and promoting health. It also directs occupational therapy intervention toward all elements (in this case, a medically defined problem, various aspects and levels of environment) in the context (see inner image, Fig. 10.6).

Spaces, then, represent important foci for occupational therapy. They occur throughout the context of the self and environs, between the rocks, walls and bottom, and driftwood. *Spaces* are potential channels for the client's flow, allowing client and therapist to determine multiple points and levels of intervention (Fig. 10.6). In this way, each problem or enabling opportunity is bounded by and appreciated in a broader context.

Rather than attempting to reduce a person's problems (i.e. focusing only on rocks) to discrete issues, isolated from their particular contexts, similar to the way in which rational processes in which client problems are identified and discretely named/diagnosed in conventional Western health practice, the *Kawa* Model framework compels the occupational therapist to view and treat issues within a holistic framework, seeking to appreciate the clients' identified issues within their integrated, inseparable contexts. Occupation is therefore regarded in wholes, to include the meaning of the activity to self and to the community to which the individual inseparably belongs, and not just in terms of biomechanical components or individual pathology and function. Indeed, phenomena and life circumstances rarely occur in isolation. By changing one aspect of the client's world, all other aspects of their river change. The river's spaces represent opportunities to problem-solve and to focus intervention on positive opportunities, which may have little direct relation to the person's medically defined condition.

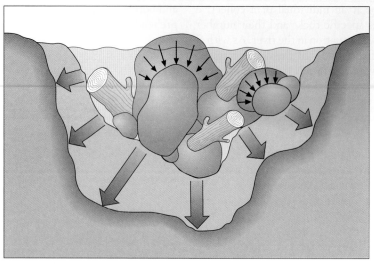

Fig 10.6 • Occupational therapy helps to identify spaces where water (life force) can still flow, and directs water through the spaces, over rocks (problems/obstacles), driftwood (resources, liabilities and assets) and walls/sides of the river (environmental context), eroding the surfaces and thus increasing life flow.

By using this model, occupational therapists, in partnership with their clients, are directed to stem further obstruction of life energy/flow and look for every opportunity in the broader context, in order to enhance it (Fig. 10.7). Through the vantage point of the *Kawa* Model, a subject's state of well-being coincides with life flow. Occupational therapy's overall purpose in this context is to enhance life flow, regardless of whether it is interpreted at the level of the individual, institution, organization, community or society. Just as there are constellations of inter-related factors/structures in a river that affect its flow, a rich combination of internal and external circumstances and structures in a client's life context inextricably determine their *life flow*.

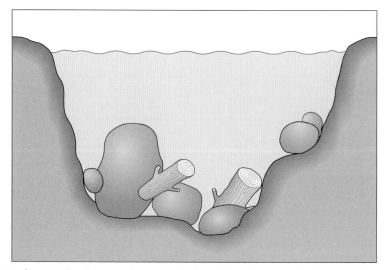

Fig 10.7 • The power of occupational therapy: increased life flow. All obstacles may not have been completely eliminated; some may have even remained unchanged. However, *life* flows more strongly, despite obstacles and challenges.

CASE STUDY

Joan

This case vignette and the following one illustrate the use of the *Kawa* Model in practice.

Joan is a 78-year-old lady who has recently had a stroke. She is optimistic and has led an active life.

She can walk slowly using a cane but needs to use a wheelchair for longer distances. She has some difficulties with her personal activities of daily living (ADLs) and her mobility. She enjoys socializing, gardening and swimming.

Joan currently lives in her own ground-floor flat, which would need adapting. She has a good network of friends and family. She is currently attending the inpatient rehabilitation unit and is due for discharge in 2 weeks.

The focus of Joan's occupational therapy intervention is shown in Figure 10.8 and Table 10.1.

Fig 10.8 • Cross-section of Joan's river before occupational therapy.

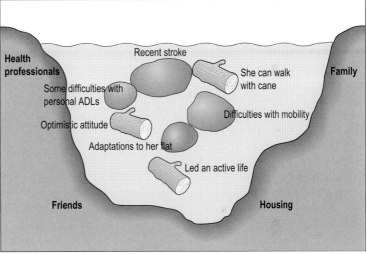

Spaces: She likes socializing, gardening and swimming

Table 10.1 Joan's occupational therapy intervention

Element	Therapy
Break the rocks	Remove the obstacles by providing ADL skills, working on gait and balance Tackle housing adaptation
Maximize the spaces	Promote the inner strength, interest and skills that Joan possesses (gardening, swimming and socializing, active lifestyle etc.)
Utilize the driftwood	Enhance the positive aspects of her character and attributes (optimism, desire for independent living, ability to walk with cane etc.)
Widen the river walls and bed	Assist with housing through home adaptation or looking at alternative housing Provide wheelchair to promote independence Engage with her friends and family to help in her recovery and in achieving her goals Involve the multidisciplinary team in her discharge planning and return home

CASE STUDY

Stewart

Stewart is 32-year-old white male. He lives on his own, in a rented flat in a suburb of London. He has a long-term mental health condition and is preoccupied with his benefits situation. He does not cope well with change and was bullied at school. His strengths are as follows. He is friendly and sociable, has supportive friends and brother, has an interest in football, is involved in art classes and is a local volunteer. His difficulties are poor concentration affecting his reading ability and low self-esteem. He has some interest in seeking work but is concerned about whether he would manage.

The focus of Stewart's occupational therapy intervention is shown in Figure 10.9 and Table 10.2.

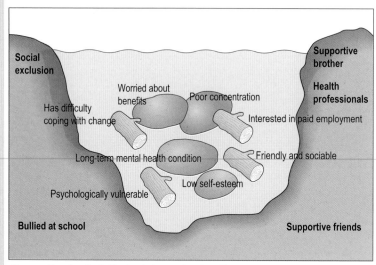

Fig 10.9 • Cross-section of Stewart's river before occupational therapy.

Spaces: He enjoys football, art, volunteer work and reading

Table 10.2 Stewart's occupational therapy and recovery process

Element	Therapy
Water	The aim of occupational therapy is to maximize Stewart's life flow and thereby support his personal recovery. This involves reducing and removing elements that impede his river flow and maximizing existing channels where his water currently flows, thereby promoting his health and well-being
Rocks	Identify the difficulties (rocks) and work towards reducing these obstacles. This involves enhancing Stewart's concentration through him engaging in regular focused adult education art and pottery sessions, which also promotes his self-esteem whilst supporting his health and recovery Work with his anxiety positively through exploring his concerns and arranging for him to see a benefits adviser who can answer his questions, whilst teaching him techniques for coping with stress and anxiety Provide psycho-education sessions so that Stewart understands his condition better, how the medication and other therapies can help and also how his existing lifestyle and occupations may support his recovery
River bed and sides	Widen the river's walls and deepen the river bed, through supporting Stewart in his relationships with his brother and friends and involving them more in supporting his goals, interest and recovery Ensure that the health professionals involved with Stewart are aware and supportive of his goal of engaging in adult education classes, football sessions and exploring the opportunities for paid employment Work with the adult education institutions and course leaders to ensure support and inclusion for Stewart in the art, pottery and voluntary work sessions

(Continued)

Table 10.2 Stewart's occupational therapy and recovery process—cont'd

Element	Therapy
	Offer Stewart the opportunity to be referred for psychological help to explore his experience of being bullied at school Examine his socio-cultural context to understand such factors as his educational experience, personal beliefs and values, family relationships, and cultural perspectives that may influence his health, recovery and well-being
Driftwood	Identify positive aspects of Stewart's character and attributes that may enhance his life flow and recovery, like his friendliness, sociability and potential interest in paid employment Work on areas like his psychological vulnerability and difficulties with change to equip him with more confidence, skills, knowledge and coping strategies to manage his anxiety and negative ideas
Spaces/ channels	Identify potential spaces and the context of Stewart's river, whilst determining the areas most important to him Maximize spaces through supporting his engagement in art and pottery classes and exploring opportunities for him to join a book club Maximize the support of his friends in helping him to continue with voluntary work in his local charity shop and to engage in fortnightly five-a-side football to enhance his physical health

Client feedback on the *Kawa* Model

Joan mentioned that she liked the simplicity of the *Kawa* Model and could relate to its naturalistic qualities, having lived near a river for many years. She found the concepts easy to grasp and was able to sketch her recent journey to the point she was admitted to hospital. She mentioned that by looking at the wider context, as highlighted within the *Kawa* Model, she could see how the various individuals and groups around her, i.e. family, friends and health professionals, could support her rehabilitation and return home.

Stewart mentioned that he found the *Kawa* Model really helpful as a framework in assisting him to visualize and understand his recovery journey. He was able to identify with and relate to the metaphor of his life journey, represented as a river. Stewart felt that the depictions within his own river indicated that, despite his health condition, he did lead an active life, meeting up with friends, attending football games and community art classes, visiting his brother and helping as a volunteer, and that all these occupations of meaning contributed to and supported his personal journey of recovery through mental health.

Qualities of the *Kawa* Model

The *Kawa* Model represents a novel addition to conventional occupational therapy conceptual model development in a number of ways. To begin with, the *Kawa* Model was developed by occupational therapy practitioners representing a broad scope of practice. These occupational therapists wanted a guiding framework that could be easily understood and put to use by both client and therapist. Because the model exploits the use of a common metaphor, there is a refreshing simplicity to the key concepts and features of the *Kawa* Model, enabling it to be easily understood by many.

The *Kawa* Model provides a radically different perspective on how occupation and the self are conceptualized and how the client's perspective can be understood. If the model represents one idea more than others in its emphases, the importance and centrality of *context* to an occupation-based occupational therapy would be it. By ascribing an ontological basis of viewing the 'self' as inextricably embedded in the environment rather than as a discrete, centrally situated concern, users of this model are enabled to appreciate better the complexities and transactional qualities of the client in occupational context. Harmony and balance in this fluid, comprehensive integration of person(s) in context are not based on individual determinism or causation but on all elements that share the complex. The individual within the framework of the *Kawa* Model is visualized within a wider context, inclusive of their family, community and socio-cultural, economic and political environments (Lim & Iwama 2006). A change in any part of this complex will affect its entirety. Importantly, the *Kawa* Model can potentially assist the clinician and client to focus on the holistic interplay of strengths, difficulties, assets, circumstances, pressures and so on that may have an impact on the individual (Lim 2006).

Such a framework, which harmonizes the status of self vis-à-vis context, is also mirrored in the *Kawa* Model's view of client-centred occupational therapy. The conventional top-down, hierarchical pattern to therapeutic interactions is upended to enable the client to be the 'expert' in their own occupational narrative. Although certain categories of concern (life flow, environment, assets and liabilities, difficulties and circumstances) are suggested, ultimately the client names (in their own words) the concepts of the model and explains the principles that relate these concepts. The occupational therapist acts as a facilitator and looks for ways in which their skills and knowledge can contribute toward enabling the client's life to flow better. The quality of this framework and philosophical leanings encourages the occupational therapist to 'come alongside the client' (Lim 2008b). This represents a stark difference from the usual practice of 'expert professional knows best' and forcing clients' occupational narratives through (universal) frameworks/instruments containing predetermined sophisticated concepts and principles that are likely to have originated in a different sphere of experiences. How many clients of occupational therapy can readily understand the concepts of occupational therapy models? The *Kawa* Model challenges the existing, hidden power relations embedded in occupational therapy model structures and applications.

The representation of a pictorial image that includes the client not only as a stand-alone individual who has difficulties or needs to be addressed, but also as one who possesses strengths, assets and the innate potential to recover. It also helps in focusing attention beyond the individual to include the collective strengths of the individual within their wider context. The visual qualities of the *Kawa* Model are another asset. They promote greater understanding of the model for those who might otherwise be unable to understand the concepts of existing occupational therapy models that require the mastery of a series of technical terms and professional jargon and terminology understood by few clients or carers that we encounter.

All universal assumptions and proprietary interpretations of the model and its applicability are discouraged, permitting and encouraging occupational therapists to alter and adapt the model in conceptual and structural ways to match the specific social and cultural contexts of their diverse clients. Although the *Kawa* Model may appear to favour Japanese cultural contexts, it should not be viewed as culturally exclusive. The utility and safety of this model for varying populations depend on the river metaphor's familiarity and relevance to its users. The *Kawa* Model has been introduced to groups of practitioners in a variety of cultural settings spanning six continents, with encouraging results (Okuda et al 2000, Iwama et al 2002, Hibino et al 2002, Fujimoto et al 2003, Iwama et al 2005b, Iwama 2006, Lim 2008a&b).

Occupational therapists should view the *Kawa* Model as a tool for better understanding and appreciation of their clients' complex occupational worlds. This model is only as powerful as the metaphor that represents it in the client's own cultural context of meanings. The authors of the model wish that it never be used as a universal framework brought to bear on compliant, subordinated clients. Therapists applying the *Kawa* Model in new or unfamiliar settings are best advised to refrain from transferring their own views of the metaphor on to the client.

Research and ongoing development

Research and development into the use of the *Kawa* Model have increased tremendously over the last few years, and more and more case studies have been collected of the model's application reflected across the spectrum from neonate to end of life, from individuals to organizations and communities, and across the medical categories of rehabilitation and mental health (Hatsutori et al 2003, Iwama 2006).

Since its appearance in the 4th edition of this book, the *Kawa* Model has appeared in a number of publications, spanning peer-reviewed journals and textbooks of occupational therapy and rehabilitation. *The Kawa Model: Culturally Relevant Occupational Therapy* was published in 2006 (Iwama 2006). The *Kawa* Model textbook is currently being translated into five languages and the model has been featured in peer-reviewed journal articles in German, French and Spanish, in addition to English and Japanese. The *Kawa* Model's presence across electronic resources has also flourished. An English language website (www.kawamodel. com) is available. A healthy and lively discussion forum connected to the website is also attracting worldwide dialogue, discussion and critique around the utility, limitations and innovative use of the *Kawa* Model within research, practice and education. Research into the utility of the *Kawa* Model has also extended across several fields including education, clinical practice, academia and research studies involving diverse client groups (Carmody et al 2007, Iwama et al 2008).

Discussion

The *Kawa* Model was introduced to provide occupational therapists with an alternative perspective aimed at understanding the experiences of their patients and clients. It recognizes the uniqueness, dynamic nature and diversity of each client's occupational narrative and provides a framework within which occupational therapists can appreciate each client in the unique context of their day-to-day realities and circumstances.

Hagedorn (2001) highlights how important it is for occupational therapists to be educated in learning how to think, as opposed to being told what to think or what to do. The *Kawa* Model fulfils this objective, as it encourages exploration, debate and discussion, and does not prescribe a fixed and predominant view or way of understanding the situation in hand. Ultimately, the model seeks to empower the client by giving credence to their occupational life and issues in the context of the client's perspective of reality rather than imposing a prescribed framework of concepts and principles raised out of another experiential context (Iwama 2006, Lim & Iwama 2006).

As occupational therapy continues its foray into new cultural frontiers, the diversity of contexts in which people define what is important and of value in daily life in relation to their states of well-being will continue to broaden. Beyond race and ethnicity, conditions of poverty, limited access to technology, a global economy, diversity in health policy, continuation of population migration, and deprivation of meaningful participation in society, to name but a few, represent some real-world contexts for the lives of millions of people. These increasingly familiar contexts will challenge the meaning and efficacy of occupational therapy in this era.

Occupational therapy proceeds when the client privileges the occupational therapists to develop an interest in their day-to-day circumstances and world of meaning. To appreciate the complex dynamic of people's lives and to deliver meaningful interventions that support a better state of harmony, occupational therapists require approaches that are guided and informed by theories and conceptual models that are culturally responsive and safe for their clients. Existing occupational therapy theories and methods of application must be adequate to meet these diverse societal conditions, and blindly applying social–theoretical precepts with universal intent may result in compromising the client's capacity to participate fully in their unique social context and requirements of everyday life.

The *Kawa* Model challenges the therapist to recognize and respond to the uniqueness of each subject's situation/context. The structure and meanings of the river metaphor take shape according to the subject's views of their circumstances, in an appropriate cultural context (Lim & Iwama 2006). The *Kawa* Model facilitates an examination and understanding of the complex dynamic between people's day-to-day realities and their contexts, and the need to deliver meaningful interventions that support a better state of harmony in people's lives. Occupational therapists require approaches that are guided and informed by theory that is culturally relevant and *safe* for their clients. The *Kawa* Model represents one example of the kind of theoretical material that occupational therapy may need to develop if it is to retain its relevance and effectiveness as it transcends cultural borders (Iwama 2003).

Along with the acknowledgement of the primacy of nature in human experience, the *Kawa* Model also serves as a prototype for a new way of regarding and employing theoretical material in our profession. In this postmodern era of recognizing cultural relativity, and variation in worldviews and interpretations of life, the notion of one rigid explanation of occupation and well-being will be increasingly difficult to maintain. That notion would limit occupational therapy's cultural relevance and meaning to a narrower exclusive scope of practice. In many cases, occupational therapists have grown accustomed to wielding their professional licence to enforce clients to abide by their own culturally bound assumptions for normal occupational performance. Occupational therapy, in an ideal sense, should be as unique as its clients — changing its form and approach according to the clients' diverse circumstances and meanings of well-being. To move closer to that ideal, conceptual models and theory should be better informed and drawn, at least in part, from diverse social landscapes and profound contents of the occupational therapist–client practice context. Unless occupational therapists themselves acknowledge and understand the cultural boundaries of their occupational therapy — in particular theory — they may never know with confidence if their profession is truly useful and meaningful to the world they endeavour to serve.

Reflective learning

- What socio-cultural norms are embedded in occupational therapy models and frameworks? Do these theoretical materials privilege one cultural group or individual profile over another?
- To what extent are current occupational therapy models and practice frameworks sensitive and relative to the actual, unique, day-to-day contexts and lived realities of your clients?
- Can occupational therapy models, practice frameworks and professional culture end up excluding certain client groups?
- How do we address issues of diversity, cultural safety and power differentials between professionals and their clients when examining issues of the socio-cultural context, interpretations of occupation, assessments and interventions?
- How do the power relations and dynamics between client and therapist as depicted in the *Kawa* Model differ from other contemporary models?
- How might implementing the *Kawa* Model into my practice affect my understanding of my client's occupational world, narrative and lived experience?

References

Bellah, R.N., 1991. Beyond Belief: Essays in a Post-Traditionalist World. University of California Press, Berkeley.

Burr, V., 1995. An Introduction to Social Constructionism. Routledge, London.

Carmody, S., Nolan, R., Chonchuir, N., et al., 2007. The guiding nature of the Kawa (River) Model in Ireland: creating both opportunities and challenges for occupational therapists. Occupational Therapy International 14 (4), 221–236.

Doi, T., 1973. The Anatomy of Dependence. Kodansha International, Tokyo.

Fujimoto, H., Yoshimura, N., Iwama, M., 2003. The Kawa (River) Model Workshop Addressing Diversity of Culture in Occupational Therapy. 3rd Asia Pacific Occupational Therapy Congress, Singapore.

Gergen, K.J., 1999. An Invitation to Social Construction. Sage, Thousand Oaks.

Gray, M., McPherson, K., 2005. Cultural safety and professional practice in occupational therapy: a New Zealand perspective. Australian Occupational Therapy Journal 52 (1), 34–42.

Gustafson, J.M., 1993. Man and Nature: A cross-cultural Perspective. Chulalongkorn University Press, Bangkok.

Hagedorn, R., 2001. Foundations for Practice in Occupational Therapy. Churchill Livingstone, Edinburgh.

Hatsutori, T., Hibino, K., Iwama, M., et al., 2003. Applications of the Kawa (River) Model: Findings from Case Studies and Discussions. 3rd Asia Pacific Occupational Therapy Congress, Singapore.

Hibino, K., Tanaka, M., Iwama, M., 2002. Applying a New Model of Japanese Occupational Therapy to a Client Case of Depression. 13th International Congress of the World Federation of Occupational Therapists, Stockholm.

Iwama, M., Hatsutori, T., Okuda, M., 2002. Emerging a Culturally and Clinically Relevant Conceptual Model of Japanese Occupational Therapy. 13th International Congress of the World Federation of Occupational Therapists, Stockholm.

Iwama, M., 2003. The issue is . . . toward culturally relevant epistemologies in occupational therapy. American Journal of Occupational Therapy 57 (5), 582–588.

Iwama, M., 2005a. Situated meanings: an issue of culture, inclusion and occupational therapy. In: Kronenberg, F., Algado, S.A., Pollard, N. (Eds.), Occupational Therapy Without Borders — Learning from the Spirit of Survivors. Churchill Livingstone, Edinburgh.

Iwama, M., 2005b. The Kawa (River) Model: nature, life flow and the power of culturally relevant occupational therapy. In: Kronenberg, F., Algado, S.A., Pollard, N. (Eds.), Occupational Therapy Without Borders — Learning from the Spirit of Survivors. Churchill Livingstone, Edinburgh.

Iwama, M., 2005c. Meaning and inclusion: revisiting culture in occupational therapy. Australian Occupational Therapy Journal 51, 1–2.

Iwama, M., 2006. The Kawa Model: Culturally Relevant Occupational Therapy. Churchill Livingstone, Edinburgh.

Iwama, M., 2007. Culture and occupational therapy: meeting the challenge of relevance in a global world. Occupational Therapy International 14 (4), 183–187.

Iwama, M., Higman, P., Lim, K.H., et al, 2008. The Kawa (River) Model: The power of Culturally Relevant Occupational Therapy. European Occupational Therapy Congress Extended Workshop, Hamburg.

Jungerson, K., 1992. Culture, theory and the practice of occupational therapy in New Zealand/Aotearoa. American Journal of Occupational Therapy 46, 745–750.

Lakoff, G., Johnson, M., 1980. Metaphors We Live By. University of Chicago Press, Chicago.

Lebra, S., 1976. Japanese Patterns of Behavior. University of Hawaii Press, Honolulu.

Lim, K.H., 2005. Partnerships, Involvement and Inclusion. Mental Health Occupational Therapy 10 (1), 22–24.

Lim, K.H., 2006. Case studies in the application of the Kawa Model. In: Iwama, M.K. (Ed.), The Kawa Model: Culturally Relevant Occupational Therapy. Elsevier, Edinburgh.

Lim, K.H., 2008a. Cultural sensitivity in context. In: McKay, E.A., Craik, C., Lim, K.H. et al (Eds.), Advancing Occupational Therapy in Mental Health Practice. Blackwell, pp. 30–47 Oxford.

Lim, K.H., 2008b. Working in a transcultural context. In: Creek, J., Lougher, L. (Eds.), Occupational Therapy and Mental Health, fourth ed. Churchill Livingstone, Edinburgh, pp. 251–274.

Lim, K.H., Iwama, M., 2006. Emerging models — an Asian perspective: the Kawa (River) Model. In: Duncan, E. (Ed.), Foundations for Practice. Elsevier, Edinburgh.

Lim, K.H., Iwama, M., 2007. The Utility of the Kawa 'River' Model in Exploring the Recovery Journey of Mental Health Service Users. 4th Asia Pacific Occupational Therapy Congress, Hong Kong.

Nakane, C., 1970. Tate shakai no ningen kankei [Human Relations in a Vertical Society]. Kodansha, Tokyo.

Okuda, M., Iwama, M., Hatsutori, T., et al., 2000. A Japanese model of occupational therapy. One: the 'river model' raised from the clinical setting. Journal of the Japanese Association of Occupational Therapists 19 (Suppl.), 512.

Ramsden, I., 1990. Kawa Whakaruruhau — Cultural Safety in Nursing Education in Aotearoa: Report to the Ministry of Education. Ministry of Education, Wellington.

Shakespeare, T., 1994. Disability, Identity, Difference. In: Barnes, C., Mercer, G. (Eds.), Exploring the Divide: Illness and Disability. The Disability Press, Leeds.

Walley Hammell, K., Carpenter, C., 2004. Qualitative Research in Evidence-based Rehabilitation. Churchill Livingstone, Edinburgh.

Section 3

Frames of reference

The client-centred frame of reference

11

Davina M. Parker

OVERVIEW

Client-centred practice is a fundamental element of occupational therapy, and studies to define its parameters have done much to name and frame our current practice.

Occupational therapists have always held, as a core value, the client as the primary focus of occupational therapy intervention, but when faced with the theory of client-centred practice and the reality of working-day pressures, there is little to ensure that this occurs.

Theory-based models have done much to provide occupational therapists with a rationale for their thinking, but little has been done to explore the application of client-centred practice as a frame of reference with which to mould and shape practice. This chapter guides the therapist and aspiring practitioner through the occupational therapy process to enable the theory of client-centred practice to link clearly with the reality of practice.

Key points

This chapter:
- describes what being client-centred means in practice
- emphasizes the role of each therapist's personal values
- explores how to be client-centred throughout the occupational therapy process
- emphasizes respect and partnership
- discusses how best to work together to achieve goals.

Introduction

Client-centred care is considered the optimum way of delivering healthcare, as clients' perspectives are regarded as important indicators of quality in healthcare (Gan et al 2008). Client-centred practice is increasingly encouraged and advocated as the way ahead for occupational therapy internationally (Falardeau & Durand 2002, Palmadottir 2003, Conneeley 2004). The reality of being a client-centred therapist can, however, be a demanding and sometimes bewildering, but for many also a rewarding, way to practise. It requires a true understanding of how to deliver client-centred practice and a recognition that it permeates all aspects of interactions with people.

So what is client-centred practice all about? Put simply, client-centred practice is a process in which occupational therapy revolves around the client as the focal point of intervention (Maitra & Erway 2006). This chapter will help you to understand and use a client-centred frame of reference in practice. The chapter aims to:

- define the client-centred frame of reference
- describe the context of client-centred practice
- explore the principles of a client-centred frame of reference
- provide examples of the application of the client-centred frame of reference in practice.

A case study is presented throughout the chapter to illustrate ways in which client-centred practice can be achieved by applying this frame of reference. This should assist both students and therapists to link theory with practice more readily. Throughout this chapter, the task for you, the reader, is to examine your own working style for evidence of client-centred practice. Reflective questions at the end of the chapter will help you achieve this.

Historical roots of client-centred practice

Client-centred practice is firmly rooted in the work of Carl Rogers, who used the term 'client-centred practice' in his book, *The Clinical Treatment of the Problem Child* (Rogers 1939, 1951, Law et al 1995, Corring & Cook 1999). In this text he described and emphasized a variety of factors including:

- the importance of individuality
- holism
- the sense of self
- the influence of the environment
- values development
- self-actualization
- goal-directed behaviour, both in relation to the development of the individual and as part of the client–therapist relationship.

Two of the most important points he made in the articulation of client-centred practice were the skill of listening and the exploration of the quality of the therapist–client interaction (Law et al 1995).

Rogers, along with other theorists such as Abraham Maslow, tried to separate the humanistic approaches of human interaction from the more mechanistic and biological approaches favoured by Freud, Skinner and others at the time (Simon & Daub 1993). His approach stressed the importance of some key elements: empathy, respect, active listening and an understanding of the person's self-actualization. These themes echo the structures underpinning a client-centred frame of reference in occupational therapy.

Background to client-centred practice

Much of the development of client-centred practice in occupational therapy has taken place in Canada. During the 1980s the Canadian occupational therapists explored and described the links between the theoretical framework of occupational performance and the core values of client-centredness. In the *Guidelines for the Client-centred Practice of Occupational Therapy* (Canadian Association of Occupational Therapists &

Department of National Health and Welfare 1983, 1991), the acknowledgement of the worth of, and the holistic approach to, the individual was explicit. Law et al (1995) presented a detailed discussion of the fundamental issues of client-centred practice, in their pursuit of a definition and a greater understanding of its application in practice. They described the key concepts of client-centred practice as:

- autonomy/choice
- partnership/responsibility
- enablement
- contextual congruence
- accessibility
- respect for diversity.

These concepts are now described in greater depth to aid understanding of how to apply a client-centred frame of reference in practice.

Autonomy/choice

It is well recognized that clients are unique and bring their own perspective to the therapeutic relationship (Canadian Association of Occupational Therapists & Dept of National Health and Welfare 1991). As the experts in their own occupational functioning, they uniquely understand how their condition affects their everyday life. As such, only clients can relate to their experiences, know their own needs and be able to make choices that affect them individually. However, to enable them to make informed choices and set achievable goals, clients have the right to be given information in a manner they understand. They should expect to have their opinions considered and their values respected (Polatajko 1992). Providing choice means that client-centred care should address individual needs and values (Rebeiro 2000b).

Partnership/responsibility

Client-centred practice is about partnership. The assessment and intervention process is about relating the client's needs to the constraints of their environment and the roles that the client assumes. The therapist becomes a facilitator rather than a director of intervention. The shift in power occurs as the result of the client taking on greater responsibility for their own health and welfare and directing more of the intervention process (Sumsion 1993). However, a person's desire and ability to participate will be influenced by their diagnosis and the phase of their illness. Despite this, client participation is the ideal method for decision-making in healthcare (Larrson-Lund et al 2001). With partnership comes responsibility, for both the client and the therapist, with the client articulating their needs as goals and the therapist negotiating expected outcomes. Clients may be exposed to risks to individual safety when defining their own problems and seeking solutions. Risks and failure can be a valuable learning experience, but the client must be competent to recognize the risks cognitively and to seek necessary safety factors (Hobson 1996). The therapist should not support actions that are unethical, could lead to harm or be deemed as malpractice (Law et al 1995). Therapists have an ethical and moral responsibility to ensure that clients are informed about risks and to advise them on techniques and activities that may support risk avoidance (Moats & Doble 2006). They should be explicit with the client when they do not support them following an action plan that would otherwise cause harm, and should document this accordingly (Canadian Association of Occupational Therapists 1993).

Enablement

Historically, occupational therapists have used remedial activities to gain improvement in functional performance. Client-centred care means intervention is structured by the goals and expected outcomes agreed between client and therapist. Achievement of these goals may come about as a result of changing roles or environment, skills or occupations rather than pure remediation. The emphasis throughout is on listening to the client and enabling them to achieve their goals. Enabling is a process that involves clients as active participants in occupational therapy (Townsend et al 1999).

Contextual congruence

Contextual congruence is about understanding the situation within which a client lives and recognizing the individual nature and circumstances of each person, their roles, interests, culture and environments. It is about seeing people as individuals, rather than as a medical diagnosis. Protocols for assessments and interventions for diagnostically identified clients are not supported within client-centred practice, as this directs intervention from a medical or mechanistic approach rather than a client-centred one. Finally, recognizing the influence that the environment has on the outcome of intervention is vital.

Accessibility and flexibility

Services should be constructed to meet the needs of clients rather than clients fitting the service. Therapists should work with the client to enable them to access services smoothly and efficiently, with honesty and realism. A service defined as client-centred should also be client-friendly; it should be welcoming and focused on clients' needs rather than service issues. Clients should be able to select appointment times to suit them rather than the therapist. In the UK, for example, Choose and Book is a national electronic system that gives people the choice to select their outpatient appointment times and dates (NHS Connecting for Health 2004). Information regarding waiting times and therapeutic procedures should be publicly available.

Respect for diversity

Intervention based on the client's expressed goals and values demonstrates respect for the diversity of the values held. Therapists must be aware of the potential influence that their own values may have on the client and should not impose them. Differences will occur, but client-centred practice is all about sharing and listening, as well as recognizing the strengths and resources that a client brings to the therapeutic encounter (Law et al 2001).

A definition of client-centred practice

Research and practice development has evolved since Law et al first defined client-centred practice in 1995; in particular, work carried out by Sumsion (2000) on a revised British definition has expanded our understanding. Client-centred practice is embedded in the Code of Ethics and Professional Conduct for Therapists (College of Occupational Therapists 1995, 2000) and in professional standards (American Occupational Therapy Association 1998), where we are reminded that services should be client-centred and needs-led. These documents remind therapists that each client is unique and brings an individual perspective to the occupational therapy process (College of Occupational Therapists 1995, 2000).

In 2000 Sumsion redefined client-centred practice by recognizing the need to relate the client-centred approach to the realities of clinical practice.

In the preamble to the definition, success was placed firmly on knowing who the client was and recognizing the impact of resources on the process. This also reinforced some key elements of client-centred practice: namely, partnership, empowerment, engagement, participation and negotiation, all processes supported by active listening to, respect for and meeting the needs of clients to enable them to make informed decisions about their care.

This definition clearly shaped client-centred practice within the context of resource-limited health services but which still aspired to a working respect for and real partnership with people, whilst recognizing that many factors influenced its successful implementation.

To be comfortable using a client-centred frame of reference, the therapist should identify their own values and assumptions (Rebeiro 2000b) and check that they match the core values of client-centred practice: namely, respect, partnership and the ability to listen to the client. Essentially, the foundation of client-centred practice is the capacity of the therapist to view the world through the client's eyes (Jamieson et al 2006). In order to achieve this, it is vital that therapists understand the key elements of this frame of reference.

Key elements of a client-centred frame of reference

The individual

The client-centred nature of occupational therapy acknowledges the individual as the central element of treatment (Donnelly & Carswell 2002). However, who is the client? The client is usually the individual who is referred to the service, but a contemporary view suggests that the client may also be carers, family, support groups or others (Sumsion 1997). It is important, therefore, always to be clear about the real client in a therapeutic encounter and keep focused on their needs.

Partnership

The importance of engaging in an effective partnership with an individual is vital. Understanding the meaning of partnership requires the therapist to recognize that to achieve the end goal requires working together. Several studies have noted the dissonance

that occurs when the therapist's and client's expectations of the results of therapy are at odds (Law et al 1995, Banks et al 1997, Blank 2004, Sumsion & Smyth 2000). These studies found that the client's perception of the problem was usually much more relevant than that of the therapist. Partnership is about working together to achieve goals — goals that are focused on what the client wants to achieve. Those that are important to them and are framed within an agreed clear intervention plan are more likely to succeed. A practical way of achieving this is for the client to have a copy of their goals and intervention plan. Another is to use a client-centred outcome measure: for example, the Canadian Occupational Performance Measure (COPM) (Law et al 1990) (see Chapter 7). Clients whose views on intervention and service issues are sought are likely to experience increased confidence about engaging in a working partnership with therapists.

Respect and listening

Listening is vital to understand truly what is and what is not said (Whalley Hammell 2002). Bibyk suggests that a client-centred therapist is welcoming, that they are non-threatening and non-authoritarian (Bibyk et al 1999). By being non-judgemental, they are in a better position to listen to the client and engage in conversation. Respect is about demonstrating value for a person's views and opinions, not imposing your views on others. A client-centred therapist accepts a client for who and what they are and where they are at (Bibyk et al 1999). Falardeau & Durand (2002) suggest that respect of the individual goes beyond their opinions, choices and values; it includes their limitations and capabilities. Individual abilities and understanding may set limits on client interaction and in some circumstances it may be helpful to intervene against a person's will, especially when issues of risk and safety have been identified. Being able to show respect for an individual, to listen and to demonstrate empathy provides the basis for a trusting relationship with a client. Such respect makes sense of this suggested definition, 'client-centred care means I am a valued human being' (Corring & Cook 1999).

Empowerment

Bibyk et al (1999) suggest that the absence of a struggle for power and control is one of the most tangible indicators of how it feels to be with a client-centred therapist. Client-centred practice shifts power in the therapeutic relationship from the therapist as the expert to the client as a partner (Townsend 1998, Canadian Association of Occupational Therapists 2002). Clients are experts in their own condition and hold a wealth of knowledge about their own unique circumstances. Enabling the client to recognize this knowledge base and use it to aid recovery is what makes the client-centred approach so unique (Lane 2000).

Goal negotiation

One of the challenges of applying a client-centred frame of reference to practice is recognizing the shift from therapist-created goals to client-led ones. Many studies reinforce the need for clients and therapists to work together at defining, clarifying and achieving goals (Peloquin 1997, Rebeiro 2000b). Negotiation can only start once a relationship has been forged with the client and when listening to and communicating with each other are comfortable. Active engagement in problem identification and planning is a fundamental part of working in a client-centred way (Law et al 1997). The therapist should use clinical reasoning skills to evaluate performance and match client skills with potential to achieve goals (Mew & Fossey 1996). Negotiation about how to achieve established goals, the risks involved and an agreed time frame demands constant attention and much sharing of information between therapist and client. The biggest barrier that prevents client-centred practice taking place occurs as a result of a therapist and client having different goals (Sumsion & Smyth 2000). This barrier can often be resolved through effective communication.

Language

The use of language in communication is vital but do we speak the same language? In modern healthcare our client population is diverse and varied, and comes from many ethnic backgrounds. It is inevitable that a therapist may not share the mother tongue of the clients with whom they work. Therapists may need to access interpreters to assist, but that in itself may create a barrier to true client-centred working. The use of language is equally important: in other words, what and how things are said. Too often we as therapists hide behind our 'professional' language both to protect and to preserve a sense of our authority and knowledge. If we are really

to apply a client-centred frame of reference to our practice, then we must consider the language we use when working with our clients. Clear information and simple explanations can go a long way to ensuring equality in the way we communicate with clients. The way that language is used is also important. Check out this example:

- 'You must use your delta walker in the house or else you will fall and end up in hospital' — a non-client-centred approach
- 'You have told me you do not want to use your walking aid at home and I understand why, but I have concerns about your risk of falling. Have you thought about that?' — a client-centred version.

Informed decision-making

It is unrealistic to expect anyone to make decisions about their lives if they do not have relevant information or do not understand how to interpret that information to inform their decision-making. As clients acquire more knowledge of their condition, this promotes self-esteem (Christiansen 1991), but Parker (1995) suggests that this in turn may pose a threat to therapists, especially those who fail to understand about partnership in client-centred working. Honest and factual explanations about risk and safety are another way of informing clients and helping them to make safe and appropriate decisions about their care. The way we communicate is also important, backing up verbal explanations with clear and easily understandable written information, or clearly signposting clients to other sources of information, e.g. the Worldwide Web.

Definition of a client-centred frame of reference

A client-centred frame of reference is a framework that *guides* practice where the client is the *focus* of *needs*-led occupational therapy, delivered with *respect* and in *partnership*. In short: *Think Person, Plan Practice*.

Core beliefs of this frame of reference are:

- assumed values of respect, partnership and enablement
- a shared belief that the client is the centre of all therapeutic activity

- the client's needs and goals directing how the occupational therapy process is delivered
- clinical reasoning and practice delivery structured to reflect those needs.

Applying the client-centred frame of reference in practice

In order to understand how to apply a client-centred frame of reference in practice, it is necessary to appreciate the complexity and challenges of such practice and demonstrate this with confidence (Rebeiro 2000a, Chen et al 2002). Given that a frame of reference is there to provide structure to practice, it makes sense to consider how a client-centred approach can be applied throughout the occupational therapy process. A case example is used to illustrate this. Each stage includes questions to assist in the development of reasoning in the application of this frame of reference. It is also important that therapists and students have support, training and the opportunity for reflection in order to grasp the challenge of client-centred practice and to develop confidence and competence in its practice (Parker 1995, Lewin et al 2008).

The occupational therapy process

For the purposes of this chapter, Foster's occupational therapy process will be used (Foster 2002), namely:

- gathering and analysing data
- planning and preparing for intervention
- implementing intervention
- evaluating outcomes.

This process is a logical sequence followed by occupational therapists in most areas of practice. Its success is dependent on the rigour of data collection and its analysis at each stage. Frequently, the occupational therapy process is not a linear event but a cyclical one, which should be sensitive to the changing health and environmental needs of the client. The client should be engaged at all times throughout the process and should be guided by their occupational therapist's clinical reasoning ability and expert knowledge of the condition (Hong et al 2000). The occupational therapist's judgement and

reasoning will, however, depend on experience, clinical expertise, data analysis and a true understanding and connection with the individual (Carpenter et al 2001, Turner 2002) (Also see Chapter 17).

Referral, data-gathering and analysis

Aim

- To provide baseline information for assessment and intervention.

Data-gathering is continuous throughout the occupational therapy process and information is gained by assessment, observation, listening and analysis, all of which contribute towards the evaluation of progress and attainment of goals.

Process

- Receiving a referral is the first information that the therapist has about a client.
- The referral itself may provide little information about the person and should act as a reason for contact rather than directing what must take place.
- Gathering of data may be indirect, noting information from the medical records, or direct, when first contact is made with the individual.
- All information gathered should be accurate and reliable, and must meet professional requirements by being documented within the records to provide an honest, contemporaneous record of the history of the client encounter.

Considerations

How are referrals received? Does the occupational therapy service dictate who, when and how people are seen for occupational therapy or are users involved in that process? Can users self-refer? Do they have a choice? Action:

- Review whether your service is clear about how people can access it.
- Change the process of referral, away from the traditional method of 'medical referral' by doctors, to a system based on client need or self-referral.
- Consult with and involve user representatives, to ensure their opinion influences how the occupational therapy service is delivered.
- Publicize how people can access occupational therapy by means of information leaflets, posters, website and audiovisual material.

When the referral is received, how do you name your client? Action:

- Always ask the client how they wish to be addressed and then note that in the occupational therapy records. This reflects respect for, and recognition of, the individual as a person in their own right and prevents the likelihood of assumed superiority by the therapist.

Does the person understand the reason for the referral? Action:

- Ask the person referred whether they know and understand the reason for a referral to occupational therapy.
- Check that they are comfortable with this and are happy to proceed.
- Check that you have told them how occupational therapy will be delivered.

Does the individual know why an occupational therapist needs to ask certain questions about their personal circumstances? Action:

- When the occupational therapist is gathering data about the individual, it is important to ensure that this is accurate and the source of that information is noted.
- Information taken from a third party may not truly reflect accuracy, may be out of date or may be biased by individual views.
- Place the client at ease in what may be a stressful and bewildering situation by explaining each step clearly.
- Be aware of how the client responds to the therapist and the therapeutic environment, as this will form part of the data-gathering that will provide the occupational therapist with useful background information to intervention planning.
- At the start of the initial interview, the occupational therapist should take the opportunity to introduce and explain about occupational therapy.
- Giving information, both verbal and written, is part of achieving the client–professional balance and will empower the client with knowledge.
- Clients may need time to reflect on the role that an occupational therapist plays in their care and so may have additional questions/issues to explore at future meetings.

Is the client able to give informed consent for occupational therapy? Action:

- Unless the client has the information about what an occupational therapy service does and what support it can give them, they will not be able to give informed consent actively to participate in a course of therapy.

Do they have capacity or is this impaired? Can they make decisions for themselves? (Department for Constitutional Affairs 2007) Action:

- Provide accurate information about your service, e.g. information leaflets.
- Consult with users of your service and invite feedback when developing service information, by establishing user focus groups.
- Take care with language, making sure the tone is 'right' without seeming patronizing and that the message is clear and accurate.
- For paediatric and learning difficulty services, a client-friendly information leaflet can be designed using characters or cartoons.
- Audiotape or CD versions of the same information can be created for those with visual impairment.
- Visual message boards can be used for the hearing-impaired.
- Check that mental capacity has been assessed if problems occur, but still include the client in all aspects of intervention even if capacity is impaired.

CASE STUDY PART 1

Sarah: referral, data-gathering and analysis

Sarah is a 36-year-old single mother with a young son aged 12 years; they live in a council flat in a new development in a large town. Up until recent months she has coped alone with her declining health problems, with limited support from family. She is self-motivated and resourceful, enjoying a good relationship with her son and taking pleasure in social interaction with others.

She has had chronic renal failure for the last 5 years and her recent spell in hospital resulted in the amputation of her left leg below the knee. She is gradually adjusting to life in a wheelchair whilst in hospital, but is determined to cope at home looking after herself and her son.

Planning and preparing for intervention

Aim

- Using all available information, to formulate an assessment of function and need and to determine goals to be achieved.

Process

- Using a semi-structured interview, explore occupational performance issues relevant to the client.

- Consider self-care, productivity and leisure issues.
- Identify and document which issues are most important to the client.
- Know the client's deficits.

The initial assessment meeting with the client is crucial in setting the scene and establishing the parameters of the therapeutic encounter. Frequency, duration of sessions and the focus of occupational therapy are important parts of this phase. Once the person's problems have been identified, the next stage is to determine what goals need to be achieved. Once this has been agreed, the method of attaining them, the approach used and the individual responsibilities for specific aspects of intervention need to be confirmed. The client-centred approach may need explanation, as it is probably unfamiliar to the individual who is more used to a traditional model of encounter with medical staff. It is crucial that the client understands the key issues of the working relationship you establish with them, as this will be built on throughout the encounter (Sumsion 1999).

It is also at this stage that the occupational therapist must explore with the client their views of the problem for which they were referred. Problems and issues need to be discussed, as well as how the individual wishes to see these changed. As the relationship with the client develops, the therapist should start to determine the individual's strengths and resources. During the assessment phase the therapist will help the client understand the reason for referral to the service and link this with an early understanding of the client's views of the problem. Out of this the client's goals should emerge. Identification of problems and goal-setting are two of the most important elements of the rehabilitation process (Wressle et al 2002). Therapists should be aware that time can be a barrier to the client-centred approach (Wilkins et al 2001, Maitra & Erway 2006), as it takes time to share information, develop the relationship and understand the outcome of the assessments before goals are agreed (Corring 1999).

Considerations

How do you introduce the assessment process with the client? Action:

- Use language that a client will understand when explaining how you are going to assess their skills and why.
- Be comfortable with your own words; if you are not, practise key phrases with peers or user focus groups.

Does the client understand and agree with the reason for referral? Action:

- Check and note in the records an understanding of this.
- An easy check is to note the actual way that the person expresses themselves.

Does the client understand what the process of assessment means? Action:

- Explain clearly the steps of assessment and what is involved.
- Be aware that some people may view assessments as a test of their ability.
- Give reassurance that there is no one correct way of doing things.
- Respect the individual way a client carries out activities.

Can the individual identify their own needs and problems? Action:

- In an unfamiliar environment, clients may require help to identify needs which relate to their home circumstances.
- Assist them by talking through their day, noting issues with which they may with or need support.
- Use this information to help the person formulate their own goals.
- Reflect back to the client an outline of their issues to ensure clarity.

Is there an issue of 'locus of control'? Action:

- Recognize the client's expert knowledge of their own condition and how it affects them.
- Listen to the way in which they explain their problems and articulate the issues of their life.
- Use a client-centred outcomes measure, like the COPM, to ensure that true client-centred intervention planning takes place.
- Encourage the client in making choices and initiating ideas.

Studies by Rotter (cited in Turner 2002) may help occupational therapists who have concerns about being client-centred. Rotter identified that people vary in their beliefs about how much control they can exert over their lives. The person who believes that control is located beyond them and is held externally by others may feel that outcomes are determined by others. Such a person may show a ready compliance with suggestions made by the occupational therapist because he/she is perceived as representing 'powerful others'. Pollock (1993) suggests that, if clients are encouraged to define their own problems, they are more likely to devise solutions to them. Individuals who see control lying within their own realm of responsibility are more likely to contribute ideas and demonstrate motivation to achieve.

What happens if the client is confused, cognitively impaired or lacking in capacity? Action:

- Clearly identify deficits through assessment.
- Explain these in simple terms to both client and carer together.
- Involve the client at all stages of intervention by not ignoring their changed mental state.
- Repeat instructions carefully and keep language simple.
- Use picture boards to remind or replicate complex directions.

The term client-centred recognizes the potential of different ways of practising with cognitively impaired clients (Hobson 1996).

CASE STUDY PART 2

Sarah: planning and preparing for intervention

The hospital occupational therapist met Sarah on the ward and set about establishing what her abilities and occupational performance issues were. Sarah told the occupational therapist that her key aim was to go home. The initial assessment and goal-setting enabled them to agree what support was required to enable her to go home and, as an initial date had been agreed for her discharge, a plan was mapped out.

Sarah needed to attend the large hospital three times a week for renal dialysis and transport would be arranged, but clearly there were long-term issues which needed addressing in the community on discharge from the hospital. Sarah wanted to stay at home and be independent as well as support herself and her son.

Talking to Sarah about her desire to go home as soon as possible, the occupational therapist helped her focus on what she needed to work on in order to be fit for discharge. Together they completed a COPM to help name and frame the occupational performance problems and to understand Sarah's priorities. The following issues were identified and it was agreed that they would form the basis for the intervention plan:

- Self-care:
  - ○ Managing to wash and shower
  - ○ Preparing meals
  - ○ Cleaning the flat
  - ○ Reaching awkward spaces
  - ○ Getting about in her wheelchair.
- Productivity:
  - ○ Being self-supporting
  - ○ Going to meetings at school
  - ○ Getting out and about.
- Leisure:
  - ○ Regaining some fitness
  - ○ Wanting to feel feminine again
  - ○ Wanting to watch her son at football matches.

The five key issues she chose to concentrate on in hospital were:

1. To be able to cook, clean and look after self and son
2. To be able to get out of the flat independently using a wheelchair
3. To be able to attend events related to her son
4. To feel positive about self and image
5. To feel fitter.

Implementing intervention

Aim

- To practise the skills necessary to achieve individual outcomes.

The intervention plan should set out how an individual's goals are to be met and in what timescale. It should be explicit about the approaches used, the activity to be carried out and the range of options available. Choices of where the intervention is to be carried out are also important. This may be at home, or in the community or therapy department; these choices may impact on performance. Intervention may not always be on a one-to-one basis; groups may provide a more suitable medium to achieve goals related to communication and social skills.

Process

- Agree a programme of intervention, negotiating time and duration.
- Be clear about what resources are and are not available.
- Provide feedback to the client on their performance.
- Identify and explain risks and explore alternative actions.
- Listen to the client's opinions on progress and concerns.

Considerations

Does the client understand how the intervention plan will meet their goals? Action:

- Explain the intervention plan to the client and check for understanding.

- Provide a copy for the client to keep.
- Negotiate times within the constraints of everyday commitments and work pressures.
- Keep the client informed of changes to the plan that may have an impact on outcomes.

Does the client understand that other agencies are involved in providing care and intervention? Action:

- Gain consent to liaise with colleagues and carers.
- Carry out home visits and specialist interventions jointly, with the client, carers or community agencies present.
- Always ensure the client's voice is heard amidst the professional ones.
- Review goals throughout the intervention stage to check against reality.

What happens if a client changes their mind about what they want to achieve? Action:

- Work in partnership with your client — then you will understand the challenges they face.
- Listen to their views and concerns.
- Point out the risks of pursuing a particular course of action if there are concerns about risk or safety.
- Suggest alternative or safer options.
- Engage the client in active problem-solving.
- Adjust the intervention plan to accommodate new goals.
- Use clinical reasoning to adjust and adapt intervention.

CASE STUDY PART 3

Sarah: implementing intervention

The occupational therapist used the Canadian Model of Occupational Performance (CMOP) to provide the theoretical underpinning to her practice and selected the client-centred frame of reference to steer her practice. The intervention plan included assessment and practice using the shower (transfers and use of equipment), meal-planning and preparation, mobility skills and activity tolerance (upper limb exercise, transfers, wheelchair mobility, managing external surfaces and pre-prosthetic strength), home care (self-organization, house care skills, shopping planning), and relaxation techniques to improve self-image and stress control.

Evaluating outcomes

Aim

- To measure and evaluate intervention in relation to the goals agreed with the individual person.

Process

- Evaluate performance.
- Carry out specific tests if indicated.
- Match performance with agreed outcomes.
- Agree an action plan if there are deficits.
- Agree on referral to other agencies to meet further needs.

At an agreed point in the occupational therapy process, the therapist evaluates progress with the client. This may be at frequent intervals throughout the therapeutic encounter, but ultimately the final evaluation of whether goals have been achieved will be made at the transition from one environment to another, usually at the point of discharge from a service. Evaluation is a means for determining continuation or change for both the therapist and the client.

The evaluation of outcomes should take the form of a meeting between the therapist and client to review goals and match intervention with progress. The most client-centred way of doing this is to use a client-centred outcomes measure, such as the COPM. This tool will ensure the client is engaged in the occupational therapy process, as client-selected goals reflect prioritized issues of occupational performance, and change in a client's perception of their performance is measured during the course of occupational therapy (Law et al 1990) (see Chapter 7).

Considerations

What happens if the client has not reached their goals? Action:

- Encourage realism throughout intervention by reminding the client of the end goal or destination.
- Check that the client understands about any changes in role or environment.
- Clarify how satisfied the client is with progress.
- Use the COPM to match performance and satisfaction.
- Share outcome results with the client.

CASE STUDY PART 4

Sarah: evaluating outcomes

Once the discharge was agreed, Sarah and the occupational therapist reviewed progress and Sarah re-evaluated herself on the COPM with the following change scores:

Change in performance score = 3.2

Change in satisfaction score = 4.6

This phase focused on her return home; however, as she had outstanding issues remaining, Sarah was referred on to the community occupational therapist, who worked with her to establish new goals, completing a new COPM and continuing intervention.

These included kitchen skills practice with intermediate care support, sorting out external access by provision of a platform lift, attending the outpatient occupational therapist for relaxation training, joining a local gym to increase social contacts, personal fitness and self-image, creating a level-access shower and attending the limb centre for mobility exercises and prosthetic advice. When Sarah and the occupational therapist agreed that she had met her goals, she reassessed her performance using the COPM and the following change scores were calculated:

Change in performance score = 2.4
Change in satisfaction score = 6.1

The client's perspective

Up to now this chapter has considered the client-centred frame of reference from a professional viewpoint, exploring values, practice and the process of delivering occupational therapy to our consumers. Bibyk et al (1999) shift this perspective quite powerfully by reminding us about the client in all of this, and challenge readers to consider the client's view of client-centred care. In the final stage of understanding and applying a client-centred frame of reference to practice, consider the issues Bibyk et al (1999) raise:

- What does it feel like to be a client-centred therapist?
- What does a client-centred therapist act like?
- What does a client-centred practice look like?

The answers may help you reflect and apply a client-centred frame of reference to your own unique circumstances. To help you reflect on how client-centred you are in practice, complete Table 11.1.

What does a client-centred therapist feel like?

- They are welcoming.
- They are non-threatening and non-authoritarian.
- They point things out but are non-judgemental.
- They listen to the client and engage in conversation.
- Conversation is built on social equity, giving importance to both parties.
- No one holds power.
- Values are discussed but not imposed.

Table 11.1 Client-centred checklist

Do I?	Yes/no
Consider my client as an individual?	
Listen to what they say?	
Inform them about what I am doing in a way they will understand?	
Educate them about occupational therapy?	
Naturally approach them in a genuine and honest manner?	
Treat them with respect and value their opinions?	
Cut down barriers to ensure they feel welcome in my service?	
Engage them actively in a partnership throughout the occupational therapy process?	
Negotiate with them about goals and outcomes?	
Treat them politely and equally?	
Respect them when they change their minds and re-focus their goals?	
Ensure they understand about risks, safety issues and resource limitations?	
Demonstrate confidence in my practice?	
Can I consider myself client-centred?	

- Caring and respect for the individual are valued.
- Conversation is open, egalitarian and spontaneous.

What does a client-centred therapist act like?

- They are approachable and authentic.
- They are genuine, can make mistakes and are perceived to be real.
- They are secure with who they are and generate security with the client.
- They are caring, they listen and they value the contribution of the client as valid and valuable.
- They are able to connect emotionally and intellectually with the client.
- Ownership and direction for change remains with the client.
- Both work towards what the client wants to be.

- They are supportive of personal growth.
- They act as an ally.

What does a client-centred practice look like?

- It provides a welcome.
- It pays attention to access, parking and other facilities.
- It provides information on occupational therapy.
- It lacks physical barriers between the therapist and client.
- The environment does not make a client feel uncomfortable and powerless.

Summary

This chapter has explained the meaning of a client-centred frame of reference, put it into context and considered its application in practice. At the heart of occupational therapy are the people for whom we train and educate each generation of occupational therapists: namely, our clients. If we adopt a client-centred approach to our practice by discussing clients' needs with our clients, then we will achieve

a higher level of agreement with them about their issues (Liu et al 2005). If we can successfully apply a client-centred frame of reference, matching our own values and beliefs plus clinical expertise and knowledge with our client's needs and expectations, in an environment that supports respect and partnership, and which provides us with a process of articulating and teaching this in the workplace, then we have achieved something worthwhile. The client-centred frame of reference should help you practise that.

Reflective learning

- What personal values are important to me as a therapist?
- How would I explain client-centred practice to a friend?
- How would I explain client-centred practice to a client?
- What role does client-centred practice have in my clinical reasoning?
- Which aspects of client-centred practice do I find easy? How can I maximize my use of these aspects?
- Which of the above items causes me most challenges? What can I do to improve them?

References

American Occupational Therapy Association, 1998. Reference Guide to the Occupational Therapy Code of Ethics: AOTA Commission on Standards and Ethics. AOTA, Bethesda, MD.

Banks, S., Crossman, D., Poel, D., et al., 1997. Partnerships among health professionals and self help group members. Canadian Journal of Occupational Therapy 64 (3), 259–269.

Bibyk, B., Day, D.G., Morris, L., et al., 1999. Who's in charge here? The client's perspective on client-centred care. Occupational Therapy Now 1 (5), 11–12.

Blank, A., 2004. Clients' experience of partnership with occupational therapists in community mental health. British Journal of Occupational Therapy 67 (3), 118–124.

Canadian Association of Occupational Therapists, 1993. Occupational Therapy Guidelines for Client

Centred Mental Health Practice. CAOT Publications ACE, Toronto.

Canadian Association of Occupational Therapists, 2002. Enabling Occupation: an Occupational Therapy Perspective. CAOT Publications ACE, Ottawa.

Canadian Association of Occupational Therapists and Dept of National Health and Welfare, 1991. Occupational Therapy Guidelines for Client Centred Practice. CAOT Publications ACE, Toronto.

Canadian Association of Occupational Therapists, Department of National Health and Welfare, 1983. Occupational Therapy Guidelines for Client centred practice. CAOT, Toronto.

Carpenter, L., Baker, G., Tyldesley, B., 2001. The use of the Canadian Occupational Performance Measure as an outcome of a pain management programme. Canadian Journal of Occupational Therapy 68 (1), 16–22.

Chen, Y.H., Rodger, S., Polatajko, H., 2002. Experiences with the COPM and client centred practice in adult neuro rehabilitation in Taiwan. Occupational Therapy International 9 (3), 167–184.

Christiansen, C., 1991. Occupational therapy for life performance in occupational therapy. In: Christiansen, C., Baum, C. (Eds.), Overcoming Human Performance Deficits. Slack, Thorofare, NJ.

College of Occupational Therapists, 1995. Code of Ethics and Professional Conduct for Occupational Therapists. COT, London.

College of Occupational Therapists, 2000. Code of Ethics and Professional Conduct for Occupational Therapists. COT, London.

Conneeley, A.L., 2004. Interdisciplinary collaborative goal planning in a post acute neurological setting: a qualitative study. British Journal of Occupational Therapy 67 (6), 248–255.

Corring, D., 1999. The missing perspective on client centred care. Occupational Therapy Now 1, 8–10.

Corring, D., Cook, J., 1999. Client centred care means that I am a valued human being. Canadian Journal of Occupational Therapy 66 (2), 71–82.

Department for Constitutional Affairs, 2007. Code of Practice Mental Capacity Act 2005. Stationery Office, London.

Donnelly, C., Carswell, A., 2002. Individualised outcome measures: a review of the literature. Canadian Journal of Occupational Therapy 69 (2), 84–94.

Falardeau, M., Durand, M.J., 2002. Negotiation-centred versus client-centred: which approach should be used? Canadian Journal of Occupational Therapy 69 (3), 135–142.

Foster, M., 2002. Theoretical frameworks in occupational therapy and physical dysfunction, principles, skills and practice. In: Turner, A. (Ed.), Occupational Therapy and Physical Dysfunction, Principles, Skills and Practice, fifth ed. Churchill Livingstone, Edinburgh.

Gan, C., Campbell, K., Snider, A., et al., 2008. Giving Youth a Voice (GYV): a measure of youths' perceptions of the client-centredness of rehabilitation services. Canadian Journal of Occupational Therapy 75 (2), 96–104.

Hobson, S., 1996. Being client centred when the client is cognitively impaired. Canadian Journal of Occupational Therapy 63 (2), 133–137.

Hong, C.S., Pearce, S., Withers, R.A., 2000. Occupational therapy assessments: how client centred can they be? British Journal of Occupational Therapy 63 (7), 316–319.

Jamieson, M., Krupa, T., O'Riordan, A., et al., 2006. Developing empathy as a foundation of client-centred practice: evaluation of a university curriculum initiative. Canadian Journal of Occupational Therapy 73 (2), 76–85.

Lane, L., 2000. Client centred practice: is it compatible with early discharge hospital at home policies? British Journal of Occupational Therapy 63 (7), 310–315.

Larrson-Lund, M., Tamm, M., Braenholm, I., 2001. Patients' perceptions of their participation in rehabilitation planning and professionals' view of their strategies to encourage it. Occupational Therapy International 8 (3), 151–167.

Law, M., Baptiste, S., McColl, M., et al., 1990. The Canadian Occupational Performance Measure: an outcome measure for occupational therapy. Canadian Journal of Occupational Therapy 57 (2), 81–87.

Law, M., Baptiste, S., Mills, J., 1995. Client-centred practice: what does it mean and does it make a difference? Canadian Journal of Occupational Therapy 62 (5), 250–257.

Law, M., Polatajko, H., Baptiste, S., et al., 1997. Core concepts of occupational therapy. In: Townsend, E. et al. (Eds.), Enabling Occupation: an Occupational Therapy Perspective. CAOT Publications ACE, Ottawa.

Law, M., Baum, C., Dunn, W., 2001. Measuring Occupational Performance. Slack, Thorofare, NJ.

Lewin, S.A., Skea, Z.C., Entwistle, V., et al., 2008. Interventions for providers to promote a patient-centred approach in clinical consultations (Review). Cochrane Collaboration, John Wiley.

Liu, K., Chan, C.C.H., Chan, F., 2005. Would discussion on patients' needs add value to the rehabilitation process? International Journal of Rehabilitation Research 28 (1), 1–7.

Maitra, K., Erway, F., 2006. Perception of client-centred practice in occupational therapists and their clients. American Journal of Occupational Therapy 60 (3), 298–310.

Mew, M., Fossey, E., 1996. Client-centred aspects of clinical reasoning during an initial assessment using the Canadian Occupational Performance Measure. Australian Occupational Therapy Journal 43, 155–166.

Moats, G., Doble, S., 2006. Discharge planning with older adults: towards a negotiated model of decision making. Canadian Journal of Occupational Therapy 73 (5), 303–311.

NHS Connecting for Health, 2004. Choose and Book: Patients' Choice of Hospital and Booked Appointment. HMSO, London.

Palmadottir, G., 2003. Client perspectives on occupational therapy in rehabilitation services. Scandinavian Journal of Occupational Therapy 10 (4), 157–166.

Parker, D.M., 1995. An Evaluation of the Canadian Occupational Performance Measure. Unpublished MSc thesis, University of Exeter.

Peloquin, S.M., 1997. Should we trade person-centred service for a consumer based model? American Journal of Occupational Therapy 51 (7), 612–615.

Polatajko, H.J., 1992. Naming and framing occupational therapy: a lecture dedicated to the life of Nancy B. Canadian Journal of Occupational Therapy 59 (4), 189–200.

Pollock, N., 1993. Client centered assessment. American Journal of Occupational Therapy 47 (4), 298–301.

Rebeiro, K.L., 2000a. Client perspectives of occupational therapy practice: are we truly client centred? Canadian Journal of Occupational Therapy 67 (2), 7–14.

Rebeiro, K., 2000b. Reconciling philosophy with daily practice: future challenges to occupational therapy's client centred practice. Occupational Therapy Now 2, 4–12.

Rogers, C.R., 1939. The Clinical Treatment of the Problem Child. George Allen and Unwin Ltd, London.

Rogers, C., 1951. Client Centred Therapy. Houghton Mifflin, New York.

Simon, C., Daub, M., 1993. Human development across the lifespan. In: Hopkins, H., Smith, H. (Eds.), Willard and Spackman's Occupational Therapy, eighth ed. JB Lippincott, Philadelphia.

Sumsion, T., 1993. Client centred practice: the true impact. Canadian Journal of Occupational Therapy 60 (1), 6–8.

Sumsion, T., 1997. Environmental challenges and opportunities of client-centred practice. British Journal of Occupational Therapy 60 (2), 53–56.

Sumsion, T., 1999. Client-Centred Practice in Occupational Therapy: A Guide to Implementation. Churchill Livingstone, Edinburgh.

Sumsion, T., 2000. A revised definition of client centred practice. British Journal of Occupational Therapy 63 (7), 304–310.

Sumsion, T., Smyth, G., 2000. Barriers to client-centredness and their resolution. Canadian Journal of Occupational Therapy 67 (1), 15–21.

Townsend, E., 1998. Occupational therapy language: matters of respect, accountability and leadership. Canadian Journal of Occupational Therapy 65 (1), 45–50.

Townsend, E., Stanton, S., Law, M., et al., 1999. Enabling Occupation: an Occupational Therapy Perspective. CAOT Publications ACE, Ottawa.

Turner, A., 2002. Theoretical frameworks. In: Turner, A. (Ed.), Occupational Therapy and Physical Dysfunction, Principles, Skills and Practice, fifth ed. Churchill Livingstone, Edinburgh.

Whalley Hammell, K., 2002. Informing client-centred practice through qualitative inquiry: evaluating the quality of qualitative research. British Journal of Occupational Therapy 65 (4), 175–185.

Wilkins, S., Pollock, N., Rochon, S., et al., 2001. Implementing client-centred practice: why is it so difficult to do? Canadian Journal of Occupational Therapy 68 (2), 70–79.

Wressle, E., Eeg-Olofsson, A., Marcusson, J., et al., 2002. Improved client participation in the rehabilitation process using a client centred goal formulation structure. Journal of Rehabilitation Medicine 34, 5–11.

The cognitive behavioural frame of reference

12

Edward A.S. Duncan

OVERVIEW

Cognitive behavioural therapy (CBT) is a popular and evidence-based psychotherapeutic approach. Whilst its guiding principles are associated with ancient Greek thought, current developments emanate from the modern theoretical frameworks of behavioural therapy and cognitive therapy. Contemporary CBT represents a broad church of theoretical developments, interventions and professional groupings (British Association for Behavioural and Cognitive Psychotherapies 2003).

This chapter outlines the development and general principles of CBT. It continues by examining CBT's theoretical framework and general characteristics. Having provided an overview of CBT in general, the chapter explores the various uses of a cognitive behavioural frame of reference in occupational therapy. In doing so, the criticisms that have been made of occupational therapists' use of CBT to date are acknowledged and proposals for ways in which the strengths of a cognitive behavioural frame of reference can be integrated within occupationally focused practice are offered.

Key points

This chapter:
- provides an accessible overview of the historical development of CBT
- outlines a cognitive behavioural frame of reference in occupational therapy
- presents criticisms of the use of CBT in occupational therapy

Key points—cont'd

- illustrates how a cognitive behavioural approach can be integrated within occupational therapy practice.

Introduction

'Cognitive Behavioural Therapy (CBT) is the term given to a specific psychological approach to conceptualizing and addressing clients' difficulties' (Duncan 2003a). Whilst CBT is frequently associated with the work of psychologists, it is more accurately described as a shared intervention by a variety of health professionals.

CBT's robust and developing evidence base has consistently drawn occupational therapists to use it in practice. However, in doing so, the potential to become a general mental health practitioner and not an occupational therapist has been noted. Considerable debate has taken place regarding the fact that occupational therapists may carry out CBT as a form of psychotherapy. The case for occupational therapists' use of their shared skills in this respect has been given elsewhere (Duncan 1999, 2003a,b, Harrison 2003, Stewart 2003) and will not be repeated here. Distancing from the occupational therapy role is, however, not essential in order for a clinician to use a CBT approach in practice. In fact, the incorporation of a cognitive behavioural frame of reference within occupational therapy is not only achievable but also highly desirable. Therefore, this chapter focuses on the use of a cognitive behavioural frame of reference within an occupational therapy context.

What is CBT?

Historical development

CBT is a dynamic body of knowledge that has developed since the 1950s. It is strongly influenced by the theoretical and therapeutic traditions of behavioural therapy and cognitive therapy. Behavioural therapy, in turn, has been significantly shaped by the evolutionary perspective of health. Its developmental roots stretch back to the beginning of the 20th century, when animal behaviour research was carried out and related to human beings (Hawton et al 1996). Cognitive therapy, whilst developing later than behavioural therapy, claims more historic roots. It cites the Roman emperor Epictetus, who wrote, 'Men are disturbed, not by things, but of the view they take of them', as an example of the early recognition of the power of thought on health (Beck et al 1979).

Behavioural therapy

Two principles of animal learning theory have affected the development of behavioural therapy: classical conditioning and operant conditioning (Bernstein 1996). Both classical and operant conditioning are briefly outlined below; however, readers are encouraged to refer to other texts for a more comprehensive overview of these important theories.

Classical conditioning

Ivan Pavlov, a Russian physiologist, developed the theory of classical conditioning at the turn of the 20th century. However, the original development of this theory could not have been further from its eventual applied role within behaviour therapy. Classical conditioning was discovered during an experiment into the digestive process of dogs, a study that would win Pavlov the Nobel Prize for Physiology/Medicine in 1904. In 1913, John Watson employed classical conditioning theory in the development of behaviourist theory. Watson's theory was popular, as it offered an objective and measurable basis for human behaviour, an approach that was in stark contrast to the other predominant psychological theories of the time (Hawton et al 1996, Duncan 2003a).

Operant conditioning

The second influential learning theory in the development of behavioural theory was operant conditioning.

This outlines 'the Law of Effect', whereby a behaviour that is rewarded will tend to be repeated, and behaviour that is punished will diminish (Hawton et al 1996).

Burrhus F. Skinner, an American psychologist, developed Pavlov's work by extending the principle of reinforcement. Previously, an action was considered to be reinforced if it increased or decreased behaviour. Skinner explored different types of reinforcers and consequences. It was observed that different types of reinforcers had different effects on behaviour, depending upon the nature of the action. Together, classical and operant conditioning provided the theoretical foundation for a variety of behaviour therapy interventions, mainly in mental health settings (Hawton et al 1996).

Whilst the benefits of behaviour therapy were widely recognized, the late 1960s and early 1970s witnessed a developing disillusionment with behaviour therapy as the theoretical shortcomings and practical failures associated with the approach came into focus. Such disillusionment, at least amongst some, supported the birth of another, related form of therapy known as cognitive therapy.

Cognitive therapy

The original attribution of a cognitive approach to therapy is given to Mechinbaum (1975). However, it is the work of Aaron T. Beck, an American psychiatrist, that has become synonymous with the term cognitive therapy.

'Aaron Beck (b. 1921) developed cognitive therapy though an examination of the links between the environment, the person and his/her emotion and motivation. Surprisingly, Beck, a medical doctor, did not come from a foundation in behaviorism. Instead, Beck's theoretical roots were found in the psychoanalytical perspective' (Duncan 2003a). Beck's career commenced in psychiatry, and he trained in psychoanalytical theory and practice. Despite initially questioning the nature of psychoanalytical theory, he embraced the approach, even undertaking research aimed at proving the efficacy of the approach in relation to depression. However, this study reignited his initial doubts about psychoanalytical theory and in doing so led to the development of cognitive therapy. Subsequently, Beck has published extensively on the theory and practice of cognitive therapy. For those who are interested in finding out more about Aaron Beck, a biography of his life and work has been published (Weishaar 1993).

Cognitive therapy and behaviour therapy, whilst taking significantly different views about the causal factors of a disorder (i.e. that it has a cognitive or behavioural root), have many commonalities. It was perhaps inevitable, therefore, that both theories became combined into the generally accepted framework of cognitive behavioural therapy.

Conditions in which CBT is commonly used

Owing to its strong evidence base in a variety of contexts (e.g. anxiety, depression and psychosis) (Department of Health 2001) and support in a range of clinical guidelines from both the National Institute of Health and Clinical Excellence (NICE) and the Scottish Intercollegiate Guidelines Network (SIGN), CBT has become an increasingly popular method of intervention and has swiftly developed over the last 20 years. As well as having a strong evidence base for practice in the forenamed conditions, CBT is often associated with interventions to address alcohol abuse (e.g. Longabaugh & Morgenstern 1999), personality disorders (e.g. Young 1999, Davidson et al 2006), family therapy (e.g. Epstein 2003) and drug abuse (e.g. Beck et al 1993, Waldron & Kaminer 2004). As well as conditions traditionally found within the mental health spectrum of interventions, CBT has also been positively associated with various other conditions, including chronic pain (Strong 1998, McCracken & Turk 2002, Vlaeyen & Morley 2005) and chronic fatigue syndrome (Prins et al 2001, Price et al 2008).

An introduction to the theoretical framework of CBT

CBT takes a problem-focused perspective of life difficulties and focuses on five aspects of life experience:

- thoughts
- behaviours
- emotion/mood
- physiological responses
- the environment (Greenberger & Padesky 1995).

Each aspect of life experience is influenced by the social and physical environment in which they are placed (Fig. 12.1). CBT suggests that changes in any factor can lead to an improvement or deterioration in the other factors. For example, if we exercise (behaviour), we feel better (mood); if we feel nervous (mood), we may experience an increased heart rate or sweat more (physiological reaction); if we find large social gatherings difficult (social environment), we may avoid them (behaviour).

The way in which CBT is delivered depends on the training of the therapist and the needs of the client. In practice, the majority of clinicians using these approaches draw from its richness of technique and theory. However, therapists' training and personal preferences can lead to a greater emphasis on a cognitive or behavioural approach:

- Cognitive therapy places an emphasis on rapid and automatic interpretations of events and the importance of underlying beliefs and values.

Fig. 12.1 • The influence of the social and physical environment on aspects of life experience. (Reproduced with the permission of Kathlyn L. Reed.)

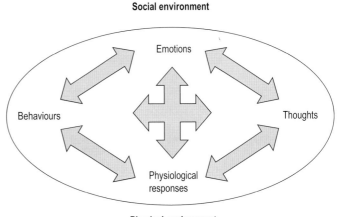

- Behaviour therapy emphasizes our automatic learned responses to stimuli and the way in which our behaviour is shaped by its consequences.

One of the key theoretical components to understanding the theoretical basis of CBT is its postulated levels of cognition.

Levels of cognition

Cognitions are the way in which we know, sense or perceive reality (Chambers 1994) (Box 12.1). Beck et al (1979), in their seminal text, *Cognitive Therapy of Depression*, outlined three levels of cognition that are amenable to therapeutic intervention. Key to this conceptualization is the idea that, unlike other psychotherapeutic approaches (e.g. psychodynamic psychotherapy), each of these levels is accessible by the client. The levels are hierarchical in nature, with automatic thoughts being the most frequently occurring and easily accessible, beliefs being more constant and core schema representing the building blocks of thought processes and being more challenging to shift.

Automatic thoughts

Automatic thoughts are habitual and plausible. They are the uninvited thoughts that pop into your head (e.g. 'I'll sound stupid if I ask a question in this class'). Everyone has automatic thoughts and it is likely that you will have some whilst reading this chapter (e.g. What am I having for tea? Is this going to help me with my assignment? When am I seeing my next client?). However, for clients, more often than not automatic thoughts will be negative in nature. Another characteristic of automatic thoughts is that they can be situation-specific — a client may be plagued by unhelpful automatic thoughts whilst in

a stressful work situation and find it difficult to cope, whilst appearing to function without difficulty when in the home environment.

It is useful to understand the automatic thoughts a client is having, as these can have a direct impact on their presentation in sessions and their ability to carry out day-to-day life activities. Several techniques can be used to elicit automatic thoughts.

- *Direct questioning.* What is (was) going through your mind just now?
- *Inductive questioning.* Use a series of open questions and reflexive statements to help a client recall an emotional situation (e.g. What happened next? What did you do?).
- *Re-enacting/recreating a situation.* Use imagery, role play and in vivo experiments.
- *Recording thoughts.* Use thought diaries and so on.

Where thoughts are recognized as being unhelpful, the therapist and clinician can work together to help the client to change the nature of their thinking — in the knowledge that this will help their behaviour. Importantly, changing thoughts is not the same as thinking more positively, which is unlikely in itself to lead to improved functioning (Greenberger & Padesky 1995). Challenging automatic thoughts is about gaining a sense of perspective on a situation, taking alternative perspectives and exploring new perspectives and solutions. Methods to challenge thoughts include:

- Looking at the evidence:
  - What do I know about this situation?
  - How well do my thoughts fit the facts?
  - Do I have experiences that suggest my thoughts are not completely true?
  - Would my thoughts be accepted as correct by other people?
- Looking at other possible interpretations:
  - Are there other interpretations that fit the facts just as well?
  - How might a friend think of this situation?
  - How will I think about this in 6 months or a year?
- Looking at the helpfulness of thinking this way:
  - If the facts are bleak, does my way of thinking help?
  - Is this type of thinking likely to make me feel worse?
  - Am I brooding over questions with no clear-cut answers?
  - Am I behaving in ways that may make the situation worse?

Box 12.1

Activity

Imagine you are asleep in bed … Suddenly you are awakened by a loud crashing sound from downstairs. How would you feel?

- How would you feel if you knew there had been a spate of violent burglaries in your neighbourhood?
- How would you feel if you had just bought a new kitten that has been knocking over everything in sight?

The nature of feelings is largely determined by the way we think.

Beliefs

These are conditional beliefs that we hold about ourselves. They may be unhelpful in nature (e.g. 'I always make a fool of myself when I meet my friends in the pub'). Whilst automatic thoughts are often easily accessible, beliefs tend to be slightly less obvious. They can sometimes be inferred from individuals' actions. If beliefs are to be put into words, then they often take the form of 'if . . . then . . .' sentences (e.g. *If* I cannot do my job to perfection, *then* everyone will think I am a failure') or of statements that contain 'should' (e.g. I *should* be the life and soul of a party) (Greenberger & Padesky 1995). Conditional beliefs lie beneath and shape the automatic thoughts that pop into our head; they can be viewed as guiding principles that affect our daily life experiences. All lives are governed by beliefs to a certain extent and these in turn govern our behaviour. Some people, however, develop unhelpful beliefs about a range of issues and these can often significantly affect the way in which they lead their lives.

Whilst unhelpful beliefs can be varied in nature, there are several categories in which the most common beliefs can be placed. It is often helpful to discuss these categories with clients to see if any of them resonate with their experience (Box 12.2).

Box 12.2

Typical forms of unhelpful beliefs
Overgeneralization
- Making sweeping judgements on the basis of single instances. *'Everything I do goes wrong.'*

Selective abstraction
- Attending only to negative aspects of experience. *'Not one good thing happened today.'*

Dichotomous reasoning
- Thinking in extremes, also known as black and white thinking. *'If I can't get it right, there's no point in doing it at all.'*

Personalization
- Taking responsibility for things that have little or nothing to do with oneself. *'I must have done something to offend him.'*

Arbitrary influence
- Jumping to conclusions without enough evidence. *'This course is rubbish'* (when you have only just started it!).

Core schemas

Schemas are the most stable of the three cognitive constructs. These are absolute core beliefs that we hold about ourselves. Schemas are formed during the early years of life and are influenced by childhood experiences and genetic composition. Often when working with clients with mental health difficulties, schemas are found to be unhelpful in nature, e.g. 'I am worthless' or 'I am bad'. A useful analogy to understand core schemas is to consider them as the building blocks of cognition. From the core schemas develop the beliefs, and from the beliefs come our automatic thoughts. Core schemas are not as immediately accessible as automatic thoughts or beliefs; however, through specialist CBT it is possible for a client to become aware of these processes (Young 1999). Changing a client's schemas is, however, very difficult, as these processes are deeply ingrained within each person. This is a specialist skill and should be left to individuals with specialist cognitive behavioural training. Interestingly, however, significant differences can be made to a person's life using cognitive and behavioural principles, without ever exploring the issue of core schemas.

General characteristics of CBT

CBT can be distinguished from other psychotherapeutic approaches by its general characteristics.

Present-focused

Whilst historic information (e.g. about a client's childhood and family relationships) can provide helpful information to give a context to a client's difficulties, this information is not the focus of traditional CBT. Therapists using CBT are much more interested in exploring what a client's current difficulties are and examining ways in which these can be directly addressed.

Time-limited

CBT is a time-limited procedure. The guiding principle here, however, is not predetermining the length of the intervention, but that an agreement is made between the therapist and client regarding the approximate length of intervention and agreed time-points for evaluation of therapy.

Collaborative

Beck et al (1979) describe the relationship between a therapist and a client as one of 'collaborative empiricism', in which both parties work together and develop a shared understanding of a client's problem.

Problem-focused

Cognitive behavioural therapists take a problem-focused approach. Frequently, the first form of collaboration between the therapist and client is the development of a 'problem list'. Together, the therapist and client then decide upon the priorities for intervention, and the focus of interventions is consequently developed.

Assessment and formulation

Assessment is an ongoing process within CBT. Initial assessment focuses on information-gathering and appraisal of a client's problems. This is achieved through a variety of methods including interviews, questionnaires, observational techniques and self-monitoring (Wells 1997). Information gathered from these assessments is then considered in the development of an individual case formulation. A case formulation is a conceptualization of the therapist's understanding of the client's problems. It takes into account the effects of the client's thinking, behaviour, physiological responses, emotions and environment, as well as other related information. This formulation is shared with the client by the therapist as a method of explaining their perspective of the client's problems. Crucially, the therapist should introduce the formulation and ask the client for their feedback on their perception of its accuracy. In doing so, the formulation becomes a collaborative effort to understand a client's difficulties. This document often becomes a key component of the intervention and can be referred to and refined throughout the course of therapy (Duncan 2003a).

Socialization

Socialization is the term given to the education of clients about the theoretical basis of CBT. This education enables clients to understand the rationale for therapy and empowers them as collaborators in the therapeutic process. Educating clients about the theoretical background to CBT can occur in a variety of manners, including verbal explanations and the provision of written or audiovisual material as well as providing examples and demonstrations of the links between cognition and behaviour and emotion.

Intervention

CBT interventions are very varied. Whilst cognitive behavioural therapists frequently engage clients in didactic (one-to-one) interaction, they are also found out of such settings *doing* therapy whilst engaged in specific *activities* (e.g. shopping, using public transport, etc.). Such an active engagement in therapy can bear close resemblance to occupational therapy and, again, gives an indication of why so many occupational therapists are attracted to this frame of reference.

Concluding therapy

One of a cognitive behavioural therapist's key objectives is to assist a client to become their own therapist. This is again an empowering process. It involves educating a client about the triggers that have initiated their problems and the development of effective strategies for dealing with them in the future. Through this process, known as 'relapse prevention', the chances of future difficulties are decreased.

Each of these characteristics resonates with the guiding principles of occupational therapy practice today. Indeed, many of the interventions even appear to be similar to occupational therapy in practice. Perhaps it is these factors, together with CBT's impressive evidence base, that attracts so many occupational therapists to embrace CBT in practice.

The cognitive behavioural frame of reference in occupational therapy

CBT describes a range of approaches developed under a shared theoretical umbrella. Indeed, CBT is so vast in its development and application that the professional body that represents CBT in the UK has asked, 'What is CBT?' (British Association for Behavioural and Cognitive Psychotherapies 2003).

Within occupational therapy, the practice of CBT is complicated. Occupational therapists can describe using cognitive behavioural theory or practice within an occupational therapy framework, but refer to it as CBT (Duncan 2003a). In order to avoid confusion, it is important to clarify terminology. It is proposed that all forms of primarily didactic psychotherapy that use a CBT approach are referred to as CBT, whilst the use of cognitive behavioural theory or practice within core skill occupational therapy is referred to as employing a cognitive behavioural frame of reference.

History of CBT and the cognitive behavioural frame of reference in occupational therapy

Cognitive behavioural interventions within occupational therapy can be traced back as far as 1969 (Braund & Moore 1969). Later, the basic concepts of behaviour therapy were summarized and their use in the practice of occupational therapy outlined. Behaviour therapy was viewed as 'particularly relevant to occupational therapists' work because it concentrates on the behavioural repertoire of the patient and his interaction with the environment rather than on his internal state' (Jodrell & Sanson-Fisher 1975).

Despite an apparent lack of integration of CBT into occupational therapy, it continued to be used in practice. Taylor (1988) rationalized the use of cognitive behavioural techniques in the following manner:

> To function in everyday life, a person must be able to perform skills that enable him or her to engage in a variety of adaptive behaviors. If anger regularly interferes with an individual's ability to perform adaptive behaviors, it is the responsibility of the occupational therapist to assist such a person in the management of anger.

Taylor (1998) also attempted to ground the cognitive behaviour approach within an occupational performance context and highlighted the benefits to occupational therapists as follows:

- The approach is based on theories already familiar to occupational therapists and readily incorporated into practice.
- The methods of assessment are also familiar to therapists.
- The flexibility of the approach is attractive to the client group with whom occupational therapists often work.
- The approach lends itself to scientific investigation.

Taylor (1998) justifies the use of CBT within occupational therapy by illustrating the impact that such interventions have on occupation. However, the nature of the therapy Taylor (1998) describes is essentially a CBT intervention, not occupational therapy. Several other publications support occupational therapists' embracement of CBT as a method of skill enhancement (O'Neil 1989, Gilbert & Strong 1994, Keable 1997, Prior 1998a,b).

Whilst some colleagues from other disciplines have expressed surprise at occupational therapists' use of CBT (Stewart 2003), occupational therapists' continued use of cognitive behavioural techniques, especially within mental health settings, appears to be generally well accepted. Meeson (1998) found that anxiety management and problem-solving techniques (both cognitive behavioural approaches) contributed towards 28% of intervention choices in a survey of British occupational therapists working in community mental health teams.

Recently, in an initial attempt to articulate a cognitive behavioural frame of reference within occupational therapy, Duncan (2003a) highlighted the shared areas of concern and practice of CBT and occupational therapy, illustrating the overlap that existed in several areas of practice (Fig. 12.2). This articulation of the potential role of a cognitive behavioural frame of reference in occupational therapy was in response to the growing criticism of its use. However, it was only a partial explanation of cognitive behavioural theory's relevance to occupational therapy.

Criticisms of the use of CBT in occupational therapy

Acceptance of CBT without a direct occupation focus has been criticized as leading to role blurring and dilution of therapeutic expertise (e.g. Kaur et al 1996, Forsyth and Kielhofner 2005 in Chapter 6, p.53). Another concern is that occupational therapists' use of CBT is a response to dissatisfaction about the perceived effectiveness of occupational therapy and a desire for enhanced professional respect (Mocellin 1996, Harrison 2003). These concerns appear to be supported by Harrison and Hill (2003), who outline 'personal interest' and the 'impact of the intervention' as decisive factors in the use of CBT by a group of occupational therapists in mental health.

Integrating a cognitive behavioural approach within occupational therapy

Using cognitive behavioural techniques in occupational therapy

One method in which occupational therapists can effectively use a cognitive behavioural frame of reference is to integrate cognitive behavioural

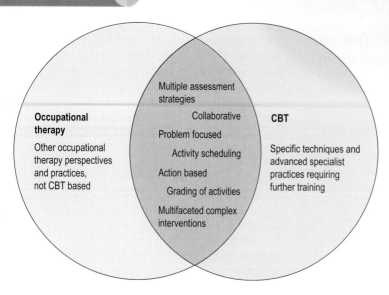

Fig. 12.2 • The relationship between CBT and occupational therapy. (From Everett, T., Donaghy, M., Fearver, S. (Eds), Interventions for Mental Health: an evidence based approach (2003) pulished by Butterworth Heinemann, reprinted with permission of Elsevier Ltd.)

techniques appropriately into their occupational therapy-focused interventions. Indeed, the use of cognitive behavioural techniques in occupational therapy has, at times, been deemed a research priority (Fowler Davis & Bannigan 2000). Such techniques include the use of anxiety management strategies (e.g. deep breathing exercises, relaxation, thought-challenging, diary-keeping, etc.) and techniques used for assisting people with phobias (e.g. systematic desensitization) or chronic fatigue (e.g. graded activity scheduling). An example of how cognitive behavioural techniques can be used appropriately within occupational therapy practice is outlined below.

CASE STUDY

John: the use of cognitive behavioural techniques in practice

John is a 21-year-old law student in his second year of university. He has recently moved back to his family's home from the city where he is studying, as he is having difficulty coping with living independently. After a successful first year of university (both academically and socially), John became unwell in the first semester of his second year. After several months, he was diagnosed with chronic fatigue syndrome. He has now missed several months of course work and the university is suggesting that he re-enter second year. John worries that even this may not be possible, as he continues to find it difficult to complete simple tasks at home.

John's GP referred him to an occupational therapist, who carried out an initial assessment in John's family home.

During the assessment, John informs the occupational therapist that he wishes to return to university, but cannot see how he will achieve this. Taking a goal-setting approach, the occupational therapist encourages John to view return to university as his aim and discusses with John what short-term goals they can develop to work towards this. The occupational therapist leaves John with an *activity diary* and requests that he complete this diary each day, describing each activity he undertakes, his level of fatigue following the activity and his enjoyment of the activity (both levels were rated by John using a 1–4 Likert scale).

The occupational therapist returned to see John the following week and together they reviewed the diary. Examining the diary, they agree that John appears to spend large parts of his days doing very little and then attempts a relatively large task (e.g. going to the supermarket), which results in him feeling exhausted and needing to rest for several hours/days. The occupational therapist proposes to John that a short-term goal, which may be useful for his recovery, would be to undertake smaller, more graded activities each day. Amongst other activities, John and the occupational therapist agreed a weekly programme of *graded activity scheduling*. In this way, John gradually builds up his strength and experiences satisfaction in the activities he carries out.

Activity diaries and *graded activity scheduling* are only two of the cognitive behavioural techniques that are used by occupational therapists in practice. There are numerous cognitive behavioural techniques and their appropriate use is outlined in a variety of specialist cognitive behavioural textbooks (e.g. Beck et al 1979, Greenberger & Padesky 1995, Hawton et al 1996, Burns 1999).

Cognitive behavioural techniques are undoubtedly useful tools for occupational therapists to have as part of their therapeutic repertoire. However, these should not be employed lightly, as they can appear to be deceptively simple. Careless employment of such techniques without consideration being given to the broader conceptualization of a client from a cognitive behavioural frame of reference can result in a therapist becoming 'gimmick orientated' (Beck et al 1979).

Theory of mind

A 'theory of mind' is an understanding of the inner psychological workings of a person (Wellman & Lagattuta 2004). There are numerous conceptualizations of how people understand each others' interactions, behaviours, relationships and lives in general. Daily, we form opinions about the rationale of other people's actions, a process that has become known as 'folk psychology' (Wellman & Lagattuta 2004). Some theories of mind are formalized (e.g. the psychodynamic frame of reference discussed in Chapter 13 and the cognitive behavioural frame of reference discussed in the current chapter). Rather than relying on idiosyncratic folk psychology to guide a clinician in their interactions and conceptualization of clients, I propose that clinicians should develop the ability to use an evidence-based theory of mind. The cognitive behavioural approach has undergone rigorous research to underpin its theoretical basis. I contend that the evidence base and pragmatic here-and-now philosophy of the cognitive behavioural frame of reference mean that it lends itself to being the theory of mind of choice for occupational therapists in practice. The benefit of using a cognitive behavioural frame of reference as a theory of mind is outlined in the case vignette below.

CASE VIGNETTE

Helen: using a cognitive behavioural theory of mind in occupational therapy practice

Helen works as an occupational therapist in a medium-secure forensic unit. She has been qualified for 8 months. One afternoon she enters a ward day room to gather together a group of clients due to attend their regular kitchen session. Two of the clients willingly get up and prepare for the group; however, the third (Jack) shouts from a distance saying that 'she can stuff her group!'. Helen approaches Jack and suggests that she is surprised that he does not want to attend, as he had appeared to be getting a lot of satisfaction from previous sessions. In response, Jack launches into a verbally aggressive discourse about his feelings about the unit and several of the staff. He concludes by stating that he wants nothing more to do with her, occupational therapy or any of the other staff. Clients and staff watch to see how Helen will react. Initially, she feels like walking away — after all, he has made his position very clear! However, taking a cognitive behavioural theory of mind, Helen is aware that the real issue for Jack may not be being verbalized at present and in fact his current behaviour is likely to be a consequence of other issues. Helen sits down near Jack (but mindful of her own safety). She acknowledges Jack's anger and states that she respects his right to make decisions about his care. Jack appears a little surprised at this and states, 'nobody cares about my side of things'. Helen recognizes this as a verbalization of an unhelpful automatic thought and asks Jack what he means. Jack continues by explaining (in an angry but less aggressive manner) that he has just found out that his request for an unescorted leave of absence from the unit has been rejected. Continuing to use the cognitive behavioural approach as her guiding theory of mind, Helen understands that Jack's outburst at her (emotion) and refusal to attend his occupational therapy session (behaviour) were a result of a recent decision by the clinical team (social environment). Helen acknowledges Jack's disappointment and asks if she can return later to chat to him some more. Jack replies that he still does not want to go to the group today, but would be happy for Helen to return later. He appears more settled now and is talking at an appropriate rate and in an appropriate tone. Helen leaves, having a greater understanding of Jack's problem and with an invitation from Jack to continue the conversation.

There can be many occasions when it is useful to use a theory of mind when engaging with clients. Had Helen not used a cognitive behavioural theory of mind, she may well have left the day room without engaging any further with Jack, or alternatively responded in a way that would not have been constructive. Conscious use of an evidence-based theory of mind enhances a clinician's ability to reason about clinical situations and lessens the potential for them to be influenced by their own biases and feelings.

The cognitive behavioural frame of reference and conceptual models of practice

The cognitive behavioural frame of reference does not enable an occupational therapist to have a detailed understanding of a client's occupational performance and identity needs. However, it can be readily employed in conjunction with a clinician's guiding occupation-focused conceptual model of practice. Conversely, occupation-focused conceptual models of practice provide excellent theories and tools upon which an occupational therapist can conceptualize the occupational challenges facing a client but do not contain all the theoretical basis required for an occupational therapist to practise effectively. Taking the Model of Human Occupation (see Chapter 6, p.65), 'occupational therapists using MOHO will also need to use other frameworks in order to understand and address performance capacity. A combination of frameworks can, therefore, be used to support a full understanding of the client's occupational engagement.'

The cognitive behavioural frame of reference is one such approach that assists the occupational therapist to understand the client more comprehensively and work collaboratively with them in order to address their occupational performance challenges. However, such use of a cognitive behavioural frame of reference is not as straightforward as cutting and pasting from CBT literature. It requires an explicit use of a cognitive behavioural frame of mind and judicious use of cognitive behavioural techniques in practice, in clear conjunction with the therapist's occupation-focused conceptual model of practice.

Summary

This chapter has explored the historical basis and theoretical framework of CBT. CBT's broad evidence base was acknowledged. The guiding principles of CBT (problem-focused, working in the here and now, collaborative and time-limited) were recognized as principles that resonated with occupational therapy theory and practice. It is suggested, therefore, that the principles of CBT should be integral to occupational therapy practice. This proposal would certainly resonate with Aaron Beck, who stated (cited in Salkovskis 1996):

> I hope in 10 years it no longer exists as a school of therapy ... what we call cognitive therapy ... will be taken

for granted as the basics of all good therapy, just as Carl Rogers's principles of warmth, empathy and genuine regard for patient were adopted as necessary basics for all therapy relationships.

Whilst the principles and characteristics of CBT appear congruent with occupational therapy, the method of their integration into practice has drawn criticism. Critics suggest that the use of CBT in occupational therapy practice has led to a loss of professional confidence and identity. In order to address these criticisms, this chapter has explored methods by which occupational therapists can effectively use a cognitive behavioural frame of reference in occupational therapy practice whilst remaining true to their professional role and identity. It is proposed that the cognitive behavioural frame of reference, when used in conjunction with an occupation-focused conceptual model of practice, enhances a clinician's therapeutic potential by increasing their understanding of a client and allowing appropriate and judicious use of cognitive behavioural techniques within an occupational context. Examples of how this can be achieved have been outlined.

Reflective learning

- Can you explain to a friend who is not a health professional what CBT is? Try to use everyday language, but give as in-depth a description as you can.
- What differentiates between an occupational therapist using CBT and an occupational therapist taking a cognitive behavioural frame of reference?
- Recall a practice setting in which you have had a placement or worked. How could a cognitive behavioural frame of reference been applied in this setting?
- What differentiates the cognitive behavioural frame of reference from other psychological frames of reference presented in this text?
- What are the similarities between the cognitive behavioural frame of reference with other psychological frames of reference presented in this text?

References

Beck, A.T., Rush, A.J., Shaw, B.F., et al., 1979. Cognitive Therapy of Depression. Guilford, New York.

Beck, A.T., Wright, F.D., Newman, C.F., et al., 1993. Cognitive Therapy of

Substance Abuse. Guilford, New York.

Bernstein, D., 1996. Psychology. Houghton Mifflin, Boston.

Braund, J.L., Moore, R.J., 1969. The use of behaviour therapy in occupational therapy with psychiatric patients. Australian Occupational Therapy Journal 16 (3), 27–32.

British Association for Behavioural and Cognitive Psychotherapies, 2003. BABCP away day. BABCP News 31 (1).

Burns, D., 1999. Feeling Good. The New Mood Therapy. Avon, New York.

Chambers, 1994. The Chambers Dictionary. Chambers, Edinburgh.

Davidson, K., Norrie, J., Tyrer, P., et al., 2006. The effectiveness of cognitive behavior therapy for borderline personality disorder: results from the Borderline Personality Disorder Study of Cognitive Therapy (BOSCOT) Trial. Journal of Personality Disorders 20 (5), 450–465.

Department of Health, 2001. Treatment Choice in Psychological Therapies and Counselling. DOH, London.

Duncan, E.A.S., 1999. Occupational therapy in mental health: it is time to recognise that it has come of age. British Journal of Occupational Therapy 62 (11), 521–522.

Duncan, E.A.S., 2003a. Cognitive-behavioural therapy in physiotherapy and occupational therapy. In: Everett, T., Donaghy, M., Feaver, S. (Eds.), Interventions for Mental Health: An Evidence Based Approach. Butterworth–Heinemann, Edinburgh.

Duncan, E.A.S., 2003b. Cognitive behaviour therapy: seeking a common understanding. British Journal of Occupational Therapy 66 (5), 231.

Epstein, N., 2003. Cognitive-behavioral therapies for couples and families. In: Hecker, L.L., Wetchler, J.L. (Eds.), An Introduction to Marriage and Family Therapy. Haworth Clinical Practice Press, Binghamton, NY.

Forsyth, K., Kielhofner, G., 2005. The model of human occupation: embracing the complexity of occupation by integrating theory into practice and practice into theory. In: Duncan, E.A.S. (Ed.), Hagedorn's Foundations for Practice, fifth ed. Churchill Livingstone, Edinburgh.

Fowler-Davis, S., Bannigan, K., 2000. Priorities in mental health research: the results of a live research project. British Journal of Occupational Therapy 63 (3), 98–104.

Gilbert, J., Strong, J., 1994. Dysfunctional attitudes in patients with depression: a study of patients admitted to a private psychiatric hospital. British Journal of Occupational Therapy 57 (1), 15–19.

Greenberger, D., Padesky, C.A., 1995. Mind Over Mood. Change How You Feel By Changing How You Think. Guilford, New York.

Harrison, D., 2003. The case for generic work in community mental health occupational therapy. British Journal of Occupational Therapy 66 (3), 110–112.

Harrison, D., Hill, S., 2003. Mental health occupational therapy and cognitive behaviour therapy. Mental Health Occupational Therapy 8 (3), 101–105.

Hawton, K., Salkovskis, P., Kirk, J. et al. (Eds.), 1996. Cognitive Behaviour Therapy for Psychiatric Problems: A Practical Guide. Oxford University Press, Oxford.

Jodrell, R.D., Sanson-Fisher, R., 1975. An experiment involving adolescent girls. American Journal of Occupational Therapy 29 (10), 620–624.

Kaur, D., Seager, M., Orrell, M., 1996. Occupation or therapy? The attitudes of mental health professionals. British Journal of Occupational Therapy 59 (7), 319–322.

Keable, D., 1997. The Management of Anxiety: A Guide for Therapists. Churchill Livingstone, Edinburgh.

Longabaugh, R., Morgenstern, J., 1999. Cognitive-behavioral coping-skills therapy for alcohol dependence: current status and future directions. Alcohol Research and Health 23 (2), 78–86.

McCracken, L., Turk, D., 2002. Behavioral and cognitive-behavioral treatment for chronic pain: outcome, predictors of outcome, and treatment process. Spine 27 (22), 2564–2573.

Meichenbaum, D., 1975. A self-instructional approach to stress management: A proposal for stress inoculation training. In: Spielberger, C., Sarason, I. (Eds.), Stress and anxiety in modern life. Winston, New York.

Meeson, B., 1998. Occupational therapy in community mental health, part 1: intervention choice. British Journal of Occupational Therapy 61 (1), 7–12.

Mocellin, G., 1996. Occupational therapy: a critical overview, part 2. British Journal of Occupational Therapy 59 (1), 11–16.

O'Neil, H., 1989. Managing Anger. Whurr, London.

Price, J.R., Mitchel, E., Tidy, E., et al., 2008. Cognitive behaviour therapy for chronic fatigue syndrome in adults. Cochrane Database of Systematic Reviews 16 (3) CD001027.

Prins, J.B., Bleijenberg, G., Bazelmans, E., et al., 2001. Cognitive behaviour therapy for chronic fatigue syndrome: a multicentre randomised controlled trial. Lancet 357, 841–847.

Prior, S., 1998a. Determining the effectiveness of a short term anxiety management course. British Journal of Occupational Therapy 61 (5), 207–213.

Prior, S., 1998b. Anxiety management: results of a follow up study. British Journal of Occupational Therapy 61 (6), 284–285.

Salkovskis, P.M. (Ed.), 1996. Frontiers of Cognitive Therapy. Guilford, New York.

Stewart, A., 2003. The case for generic working in mental health. British Journal of Occupational Therapy 66 (4), 180.

Strong, J., 1998. Incorporating cognitive-behavioural therapy with occupational therapy: a comparative study with patients with low back pain. Journal of Occupational Rehabilitation 8 (1), 61–71.

Taylor, E., 1988. Anger intervention. American Journal of Occupational Therapy 42 (3), 147–155.

Vlaeyen, J.W.S., Morley, S., 2005. Cognitive-behavioral treatments for chronic pain: what works for whom? Clinical Journal of Pain 21 (1), 1–8.

Waldron, H.B., Kaminer, Y., 2004. On the learning curve: the emerging evidence supporting cognitive-behavioral therapies for adolescent substance abuse. Addiction 99 (Suppl. 2), 93–105.

Weishaar, M., 1993. Aaron T. Beck. Sage, London.

Wellman, H.M., Lagattuta, K.H., 2004. Theory of mind for learning and teaching: the nature and role of explanation. Cognitive Development 19, 479–497.

Wells, A., 1997. Cognitive Therapy for Anxiety Disorders: A Practical Manual and Conceptual Guide. Wiley, Chichester.

Young, J.E., 1999. Cognitive Therapy for Personality Disorders: A Schema-Focused Approach (Practitioner's Resource Series). Professional Resource Exchange, Sarasota, FL.

An introduction to the psychodynamic frame of reference

13

Margaret A. Daniel   Sheena E.E. Blair

OVERVIEW

Everyone in the helping professions should have a psychotherapeutic attitude, be familiar with the simpler forms of psychotherapeutic methods, and be aware of the scope and availability of more specialised forms of psychotherapy.

(Bateman et al 2001, p.220)

This is the underlying premise from which this chapter will proceed. Both authors of the chapter have retained a fascination with this approach to understanding people, organizations and society for over 30 years. So, regardless of whether careers have progressed within the direction of education, management, research or consultancy, an awareness of dynamic factors concerning anxiety, conflict, the effects on development of early life experience and the vibrancy of our inner lives has been retained. This approach celebrates the complexity of our emotional lives, attempts to understand and deal with corresponding feelings, and, in partnership with the person, couple, family, team or organization, seeks to find workable and helpful routes towards managing issues that negatively complicate human relations. In relation to our core professional values, we have not personally experienced a conceptual or professional tension between an interest in this approach and the practice of occupational therapy. Rather, the relationship between 'doing' and 'feeling' has always seemed intrinsically connected. Consider the times when a person is at a transitional point in their life and the frequent tendency to exclaim 'What am I going to do!' Our contention is that the dynamic relationship between feeling, thinking, doing and becoming needs to be continually reflected upon and understood. We also consider that an understanding of dynamic

factors in human relations enables practitioners, managers and researchers to employ a unit of analysis which can facilitate change at a personal or a systems level.

Key points

This chapter:
- traces the evolution and current practice of psychodynamic thinking in occupational therapy
- analyses the relationship between occupational therapy and the psychodynamic approach
- considers the dynamics of doing and the occupational imperative
- explores group work within this approach
- explores the contribution to health and well-being.

Introduction

From its inception, the profession of occupational therapy took its identity from the notion of occupation and the therapeutic belief that this contributed towards health and well-being (Wilcock 1998). The psychodynamic approach has contributed to our conceptual foundations alongside others now commonly described as 'related-knowledge' models of practice. Occupational therapy has striven to establish a corpus of knowledge specifically related to the understanding of occupational performance and how to comprehend the occupational nature of human beings. The historical development of this phenomenon has, according to some sources, been characterized by certain epistemological crises, particularly in the 1950s and 1970s. The concern was that related models did not focus on occupation clearly or specifically enough as the potential change mechanism for people who used the services of occupational therapy.

A renaissance of interest in occupation was stimulated by the development of discipline-specific models of practice such as the Model of Human Occupation (Kielhofner 2002). Related models of practice are multidisciplinary in nature. As such, this requires practitioners to employ a specific professional lens or 'occupational filter', a term that was coined by Forsyth and Mallinson (personal communication 2000). This ensures that the primary concern of occupational therapists is how — in the case of the psychodynamic approach — complicating feelings and issues in both internal and external worlds affected occupational lives.

This chapter intends to engage the reader in a wish to understand and evaluate critically this intriguing area within contemporary practice rather than offer a definitive account. Our contention is that, regardless of whether occupational therapists use a psychodynamic approach in their daily practice, a psychodynamic attitude as outlined by Bateman et al (2001) is an asset to their professional repertoire and enhances clinical reasoning and reflective practice.

Introduction to key ideas from psychodynamic practice

Any writer on the subject of psychodynamic practice would acknowledge the work of Sigmund Freud (1856–1939). He was a unique thinker and prolific writer whose ideas have continued to attract both admiration and derision. Two characteristic issues underpin Freudian thinking. They are the role of the unconscious and the impact of instincts. Freud used the contemporary cultural ideas of the late 19th century to evolve his concept of psychoanalysis. Just as a film projector transports an image on to a blank screen, Freud believed the inner working of the mind (psyche) could also influence our outer vision by expanding and creating additional layers to what is experienced, influenced by earlier past events. These representations, he believed, were contained in the unconscious and not fully in the control of the whole person (Gomez 1997). However,

Freud's biological training as a doctor and neurologist made him aware that his ideas would not be well received, as they were introspective and retrospective, influenced by personal insights that resulted in his continual reviewing and reshaping of his concepts. From the start, science and feelings were in conflict (Hughes 1999).

The central tenets of psychoanalysis are that symptoms are produced by conflicting unacceptable ideas about oneself or another. The emotions are translated into anxiety or psychic pain, and are defended against by actively locking them away in the unconscious (repression), enabling incompatible views to exist together. Defence mechanisms (Box 13.1) have a protective function that serve to deny, suppress or disown what we do not want to tolerate, and can be both helpful and harmful. Unacceptable feelings surface as motivational instincts, more commonly known as drives (Bateman et al 2001). They emerge from the unconscious as slips of the tongue, jokes, symptoms, or by the most direct route through our dreams. An example of this occurred when, after a talk about occupational therapy and psychodynamic work to undergraduate nurses, they seemed singularly unimpressed and the ensuing questions verged on confrontation. However, at the end of the allotted time, the tutor thanked the presenter profusely for coming, and she in turn tried to regain her composure and replied by thanking them for their 'hostility' instead of their 'hospitality'! This inner experience won out over rational responses, everyone laughed and it served to illustrate a point about defence mechanisms, which everyone in the room recognized!

Psychoanalysis is seen as a way of retrieving these censored memories, but it has been considerably modified since Freud's time. This is an issue that is often overlooked in criticisms of this approach. As an intervention today, it offers a less intense and briefer form of therapy called psychodynamic psychotherapy, which seeks to give personal meaning to a person's symptoms through understanding the relevance of the past to their present difficulties. It focuses on listening to the person's story, with attention paid to how their early childhood experiences can be projected on to present relationships, inducing others to take up familiar roles from their past. Within the therapeutic relationship, the therapist can be on the receiving end of these feelings (transference), which can evoke the therapist's feelings (counter-transference) and be used as a tool to deepen understanding (Bateman et al 2001).

Box 13.1

Defence mechanisms used to protect against anxiety

Repression

- The unconscious creates memory lapses that prevent painful, conflicting or difficult thoughts

Denial

- Complete avoidance of unpleasant reality that can induce anxiety

Projection

- Unacceptable feelings/impulses are attributed to others

Reaction formation

- Exaggerated behaviour, which is the opposite of the actual feelings experienced

Intellectualization

- Deliberately removing emotion from the issue by dealing only with logic

Rationalization

- Extreme attempts to justify behaviour or thoughts by giving numerous reasons

Suppression

- Carrying on without avoiding the reality of the difficulty

Regression

- Behaving in ways characteristic of a much younger age

Sublimation

- Substituting something in place of a desired experience

Compensation

- Seeking to excel in something to reduce feelings of failure in another area

Splitting

- A primitive way in which reality is separated and distorted into polarized extremes, e.g. good/bad; right/wrong

Structuring the mind

Freud outlined three structural models of the mind, which neuroscience is beginning to map out on to the emerging contours in the psychoanalytic landscape, revealing, perhaps, what Freud was striving to attain (Balbernie 2001). His earliest theory believed that actions are affected by unconscious thoughts and feelings, creating symptom formation due to the dynamic tensions between conflicting conscious and unconscious thoughts and wishes. This became the basis of the first topographical theory, and was divided into three spatial levels: the conscious, preconscious and unconscious. The second structural model (Box 13.2) focused on drives in which the mind attempts to have its wishes satisfied. This new version was composed of the id, the ego and the superego. Berne (1961) subsequently adapted this concept to transactional analysis, using parent (superego), adult (ego) and child (id) to represent his psychic construction. Freud's final model is the developmental theory, which suggested that early life proceeds in stages modifying adult activity.

Influenced by Charles Darwin, Freud based his ideas on the continuation of the species, which he believed had to be sexually driven. For example, a baby's pleasure is sought through body sensations, and moves from oral activity around the first year of life, through interest in anal activity in the second and third years, and finally to the genital phase around 3–5 years of age. These stages shape later life, and if the baby experiences trauma of either too little or too much stimulation at any of these stages it can

Box 13.2

Freud's structural theory of the mind

Id

- This area is unconscious, and creates an overwhelming urge that takes over the individual with no thought for others. It is linked to the need to satisfy the drives of sex and aggression

Ego

- This more thoughtful and mainly conscious part of the mind can rationalize and consider others' needs as well as those of the individual

Superego

- This area stems from the parental and authority influences that have been internalized and become the conscience that can be supportive or critical. It is part conscious and part unconscious hinder development and create problems later in life (Symington 1986). Erikson's (1980) interest in child development emphasized the conscious and unconscious progression through eight life stages, resulting in a strengthened synthesis of thoughts and feelings. Freud's longstanding friend and colleague, Sandor Ferenczi, continued to work with the environmental concept of trauma, realizing that, like children, his adult patients with neurosis longed to have what was passively beyond their grasp (Ferenczi 1949). For this to happen, trust had to be established, so that the shift into active engagement could take place. The later object–relations theorists, Winnicott (1971), Bion (1961) and Bowlby (1988), took up Ferenczi's belief in a form of maternal love (Ferenczi 1984) to counterbalance what had been lost. This was provided through attentive listening, sensitivity and piecing together of the trauma without overstepping boundaries. Object relations theory departed from the exclusive focus on the self by exploring the individual's relationship with the environment and the urge to form relationships in the pursuit of well-being and the effective achievement of goals (Sutherland 1969). The intention of object relations is to attach meaning to relationships, artefacts or abstract concepts. Those were the ideas that caught the imagination of Fidler and Fidler (1963), whose communication process in occupational therapy revolved around activity, communication and the relationship with objects. Likewise, Mosey (1970) was interested in how symbolism and object relations were evident within clients' engagement with activities. In Scotland, Batchelor (1970), while still an undergraduate, sought to differentiate occupational therapy from mainstream psychotherapy by the presence of objects that were ready-made, offered or created.

Donald Winnicott's attention to the mother–infant relationship (Winnicott 1971) overlaps with the idea of object relations, and gives a sense of reciprocity that can lead to the first sense of unfolding identity. Winnicott, like Bion, saw the start of the infant's inner emotional and intellectual life as being separate from, yet able to relate to, the outer world. He considered that, from the onset, the infant is part of a couple, and the intensity of this relationship gives the child the illusion that they exist as a single entity. Winnicott's (1971) 'holding environment' allows the infant the possibility of tolerating their surroundings, not unlike the therapeutic relationship. To assist an infant in coping with the gains and losses of separating, an object, such as a cloth or toy, is utilized to help

make the alteration. Winnicott called this substitute used to replace the wanted object a 'transitional object', and it forms the first symbol of language. The absence of the object allows space for play, which, with 'good enough mothering', extends into adult life through culture and creative activity. In the occupational therapy literature, this idea has been embraced by Fidler and Velde (1999) in exploring the meanings that are inherent in activities, and more recently Blair (2000) has entertained the notion that certain occupations can be understood as protective during times of stressful transition. From a research base, the Swedish occupational therapist Eklund (2000) emphasizes the need for an integrative approach to gain a broader understanding of human activity performance. She uses the cultural work of Harry Sullivan and Donald Winnicott to argue that an object relations perspective is comparable with Kielhofner's (1997) requirements for a conceptual model of occupational therapy practice.

What can be deduced from this brief overview of underpinning theories, all of which focus on the notion of successful change occurring in the mind of the individual, is the way that complex ideas have emerged and been adapted over the years. The therapeutic relationship, as Jenkins (1999) suggests, is seen as pivotal within occupational therapy. This frame of reference underpins specific work in child and family work, palliative care, substance abuse and certain areas of mental health. Apart from occupational therapy, the ideas have substantially influenced the practice of art therapy, mental health nursing, social work, education, organizational studies and, more recently, mental health promotion.

Over the last decade there have been a number of therapeutic developments (Box 13.3) that have striven to address the perceived imbalance or restrictions of the classical psychoanalytical therapy. These include a concern over the length of time that psychodynamic therapy takes, its cost and the lack of empirical research. Dialogic methods have become more widespread, and often depart from insight-oriented pursuits to those more linked to action, which is synonymous with an occupational therapy approach to adaptation and change.

The psychodynamic frame of reference has stood the test of time despite concerns from Barris et al (1983) that it had little to offer the contemporary practice of occupational therapy and that it had actively contributed to a crisis of identity within the profession. Perhaps success can be gauged by the extent to which Freud's work has stimulated

Box 13.3

Contemporary developments

Solution-oriented brief therapy

- The accent is on solutions rather than problems, and people are set problem-oriented goals that are mutually explored using techniques such as the miracle question, scaling questions and joint discussion of future possibilities

Interpersonal psychotherapy

- A time-limited therapy that focuses on present-day problematic relationships, elevating mood level through active involvement with others. The focus is less on transference, and relies on a joint approach to improve well-being

Conversational model of psychodynamic–interpersonal therapy

- A collaborative and interpersonal approach incorporating psychodynamic aspects with humanistic and interpersonal components. It aims to achieve sensitive attunement to the feelings aroused in the session, and deepen understanding of how these emotions affect past and present relationships. It is a bridge between interpersonal psychotherapy and traditional psychotherapy

Cognitive behavioural therapy

- A pragmatic approach initially used for depression by altering unhelpful thinking processes evident in symptom formation. Recent trends are beginning to re-examine the role of the unconscious. The therapist takes an active informative role, encouraging the client to monitor patterns of automatic thinking on a daily basis. The focus is on recognizing unhelpful thoughts and feelings, so that new strategies can be incorporated to alter the patterning

Cognitive analytic therapy

- An integrative form of therapy, using past recollections and information acquired from the transference and counter-transference arising in the session. It also uses the cognitive choices a person makes by focusing on the effect this has on present relationships

---

controversy, how it was one of the first theories to have a specific mode of practice, how it remains a crucial theme in the arts, and how it has acted as the springboard for subsequent therapies. Indeed, the original psychoanalytical ideas, which acted as both a theory and a form of treatment, became broadened into a diverse collection of neo-Freudian theories/models such as child psychotherapy, milieu therapy, family and marital therapy and group therapy, all of which retained a legacy to the ideas of Freud. This is not to deny that the approach is above legitimate criticism, as feminist writers have articulately documented (Appignanesi & Forrester 2000).

Psychodynamic thinking in all of those approaches and in current practice refers to the interchange between intrapersonal and interpersonal issues. This accentuates the process of therapy and the relationships that foster change, regardless of whether they are didactic or within a group setting.

The relationship between occupational therapy and the psychodynamic approach

It is interesting to reflect upon the way that psychodynamic ideas and ideas that acknowledged the value of occupation for mental health ran in parallel.

At the turn of the 20th century, a new approach to the management of mental health was being developed across the Western world; it was called 'mental hygiene'. The core belief was that mental ill health could be prevented by understanding the cause of mental illness. In doing this, people could achieve insight into their problems and surmount them by engaging in therapy. This was the crucial Freudian premise. Simultaneously, in the USA, a Swiss physician called Adolf Meyer was interested in transforming mental illness through occupation as a way to 'normalize', adapt and give meaning to peoples' lives, both socially and environmentally (Winters 1951). There is every likelihood that the profession of occupational therapy owes some of its originating ideas to a psychobiological approach that attempted to synthesize neuroscience with psychoanalytical ideas.

Meyer spent time in the UK, and a network of like-minded clinicians was created within Scottish psychiatry. The eminent physician, David Henderson, actually delayed taking up a post in Glasgow to continue working for Meyer after his training in New York was complete. He subsequently returned to Gartnavel Royal Hospital in Glasgow in 1915, bringing with him Meyer's clinical vision of occupation as a therapeutic resource. Meyer believed in a process of providing opportunities for people with mental health problems rather than the ubiquitous provision of medicines. His ideas of balance between activities and the use of meaningful daily occupations that reflected physical, psychological, social, emotional and spiritual components of our lives constituted a powerful blending of ideas. It was a vision that nurtured the origins of occupational therapy, and has been one which has sustained it through various ontological and epistemological crises.

In the 1950s, in the USA, an analytical approach was advocated by the work of Azima and Azima (1959), who outlined a theory of occupational therapy based on object relations theory, and it was in this article that the first mention of projective group therapy arose. This work substantially influenced that of Fidler and Fidler (1963), who wrote the seminal text for this approach alongside the work of Mosey (1970). The original text by the Fidlers remains the most innovative approach to analysis of activity in this frame of reference, despite changing contexts of practice and social change. Other authors in diverse parts of the world who have attempted to summarize work in the psychodynamic tradition all acknowledge the debt to those writers.

Within a Scottish context, the late 1960s and 1970s were a time when therapists were experimenting with explorative ways of using the creative arts range of activity primarily within a group context. This range of activities, which included art, music, poetry, pottery and drama, were used as ego-explorative activities, and were interspersed within treatment programmes with ego-supportive activities, which allowed insights and increased self-awareness to be put into practice. The choice of those activities was based upon a careful activity analysis of their properties, and a balance was always considered necessary between activities that sought to explore and those that were more supportive in nature. This was an integral part of an interdisciplinary psychodynamic approach to practice, which recognized that not all clients could find solace in purely verbal forms of psychotherapy. Batchelor (1970) was one of the first occupational therapists to publish on this topic, and was followed by Drost (1971), who discussed occupational therapy in groups; later, Affleck (1977) sought to introduce projective work within a unit for the treatment of alcohol problems. Blair (1974) worked primarily on the topic of occupational therapy and group work, while her colleague, Malcolm (1975), wrote about the versatility of painting within a psychodynamic approach.

Occupational therapists working within mental health across various countries became interested in projective techniques, which were defined by Remocker and Storch (1982, p.157) as 'methods used to discover an individual's attitudes, motivations, defensive manoeuvres and characteristic ways of responding through analysis of their responses to unstructured, ambiguous stimuli'. Their work is concentrated upon action techniques within a group setting, and is similar to the action-oriented methods used for organizational and human relations work. The work of Brown (1990), by contrast, focused upon drama, and used Moreno's (1948) principles of 'show me' rather than 'tell me' within an analytical psychotherapy day unit in Glasgow. Amongst her ideas about this medium was a belief that occupational therapists were particularly suited to working with psychodrama because it was about the 'psyche in action'.

Levens (1986) sought to outline the dynamics of activity, which in many ways echoed the earlier work of the Fidlers, and this served to sustain the interest of therapists in this area of practice into the 1980s. Robertson (1984) took a 'broad-brush' approach to the topic, and outlined the role of the occupational therapist within a psychotherapeutic setting, while Stockwell (1984) commenced the shift to the notion of creative therapies. In the 1990s, as Perez-Franco (1998) has highlighted, few articles appeared within the professional literature; nevertheless, there was a steady interest in specific areas such as group work within a unit for alcohol problems based upon Yalom's (1970) work by Ogilvie et al (1995), a psychodynamic perspective on work with older people by Banks and Blair (1997), and the use of poetry for health and well-being (Jensen & Blair 1998). Findlay (1997) produced two texts, one on psychosocial occupational therapy and one on group work, which have acted as key texts since their creation.

The interest in creative therapies was developed by Stockwell (1984), nurtured by others such as Steward (1996), and culminated in an excellent text by Atkinson and Wells (2000), which they call a 'psychodynamic approach within occupational therapy'. This is noteworthy for a number of reasons. Firstly, it is a clear exposition of theory and the links between psychodynamic practice and occupational therapy, and secondly it continually notes the relationship between ideas and creative therapy. The turn of the 21st century did not go unmarked by work in this area, and the links between a psychodynamic attitude and supervision within occupational therapy were outlined by Daniel and Blair (2002).

Table 13.1 Occupational therapists who have written about psychodynamic work and occupational therapy

1950	1960	1970	1980	1990	2000
Azima & Azima (1959)	Fidler & Fidler (1963)	Batchelor (1970)	Remocker & Storch (1982)	Brown (1990)	Atkinson & Wells (2000)
		Mosey (1970)	Robertson (1984)	Ogilvie et al (1995)	Eklund (2000)
		Drost (1971)	Stockwell (1984)	Piergrossi & Gilbertoni (1995)	Ingram (2001)
		Blair (1974)	Levens (1986)	Telford & Ainscough (1995)	Bruce & Borg (2002)
		Reilly (1974)	Bruce & Borg (1987)	Steward (1996)	Daniel & Blair (2002)
		Malcolm (1975)		Banks & Blair (1997)	Finlay (2002)
		Affleck (1977)		Jenson & Blair (1998)	Nicholls (2003)
				Perez-Franco (1998)	MacKenzie & Beecraft (2004)
				Thompson & Blair (1998)	Jackson (2005)
					Hyde (2006)
					Munro (2008)
					Nicholls (2008)

Ingram (2001), along with Telford and Ainscough (1995), discussed the role of psychotherapeutic work within child and family psychiatry, and Nicholls (2003, 2008) has, through postgraduate study and further publication, sustained the profile of psychodynamic work in relation to occupational therapy. Nicholls is interested in the synthesis of work by Menzies Lyth (1988, 1990) in relation to how occupational therapists tolerate the pain of the clients with whom they work. MacKenzie and Beecraft (2004) use an observational perspective to acknowledge the emotional impact of unconscious processes on staff working with older people. Jackson (2005) endorses their paper, seeing containment as the core to reflective practice, which Munro (2008) illustrates in her personal account of being seconded to a psychotherapy department, in which she emphasizes the need to have space to think. Extending the psychodynamic gaze further, Hyde's (2006) organizational observations encourage staff to reflect on and develop an understanding of the unconscious to help them talk about their work.

The key issue about this type of work is that it is multidisciplinary in nature, and the occupational therapy process operates within this frame of reference using core skills in relation to psychodynamic principles. Shared concerns within the team are the therapeutic relationship, the process of therapy, support for the client throughout the process, reporting and recording, and evaluation. All of the aforementioned aspects are dealt with in a multidisciplinary forum. In addition, a supervision system (whether individual- or group-oriented) is always

part of the process, and attention to team skills is a necessary concern. Within occupational therapy, attention to the way that a client's occupational life has been compromised by emotional difficulties is part of the assessment process. This is explored through dialogue rather than formal testing, and is always shared with the team. Planning for intervention involves an appraisal of the balance between ego-supportive and ego-explorative activities, combination of techniques, times for review and length of intervention. This usually involves creative activities, either in groups or individually, and the focus of the occupational therapist is always on how occupational behaviour and performance is changing as a result of psychotherapeutic interventions. Table 13.1 demonstrates the sustained interest in this work from a variety of areas of practice.

The dynamics of doing and the occupational imperative

Occupational lives are dynamic and complex. Attempts to harness this complexity by occupational therapists have led to the subdivision of occupational behaviour into self-care, work and leisure as domains of concern. However, therapists have become increasingly interested in the meaning of what we do, how we do it and why we do it, for example (Krupa 2003). Spirituality became the core of the Canadian Occupational Performance Measure (COPM) from the late 1990s, and represents a movement away from a focus on the observable.

There is a link here with ideas from psychodynamic practice, where inner turmoil and issues are not immediately obvious but projected on to or through actions and reactions. Curiously, while ideas from psychodynamic practice are still treated with suspicion by some occupational therapists, aspects connected with a notion of spirituality are embraced. For the therapist who is interested in a synthesis between psychodynamic thinking and the use of occupation for therapeutic ends, certain questions arise:

- What is the link between emotion and action?
- What constitutes defensive doing?
- What actions are prompted by unconscious motivation?
- Can involvement in occupation act as a container for anxiety?
- What are the dynamics between the therapist, the person and the act of occupation?
- How can occupation hinder or facilitate emotional growth?

It is important to stress that these dynamic issues are no less relevant for the therapist or team to reflect upon than for whoever is the recipient of such services. Our belief is that, in the spirit of critical reflection, practice can be enhanced by attention to intrapsychic and interpersonal factors within the context of doing.

As the development of discipline-specific models of practice gathered speed over the last 20 years, particularly in the USA, Canada and Australia, this has had an impact upon research, practice and education. A renaissance of interest in Meyer's original ideas and the work of Mary Reilly (1974) caught the imagination of therapists, and a new professional identity and confidence seemed to emerge. With the emergence of occupational science in 1989 at the University of Southern California, a new language began to develop, and occupational discourse emerged. Correspondingly, curricula within universities altered over time to reflect those changes, with the study of occupation featuring as the core topic. Social and biological science was still perceived as valuable to the profession of occupational therapy, but the selection of material from those areas was severely reduced.

In such a climate of innovation and optimism, it may have seemed heretical to consider that the phenomenon of occupation may require analysis of its counterproductive features. To those interested in both psychodynamic ideas and indeed critical social theory, questions concerning this omission would be raised. One of the few writers to offer such a critique is Nicholls (2003, 2008), who explores the perpetually optimistic discourse that underlies practice. In a brief but poignant opinion piece, she considers that this may be a form of 'manic defence' against the difficulties that clients endure. Using the work of Menzies Lyth (1988, 1990), her argument is that occupational therapists may deal with attendant anxiety by repressing and denying dependence, pain and exclusion and focusing wholeheartedly upon action. Ultimately, this can cause professional weariness and burnout, whereby the therapeutic zeal diminishes and therapists can be left bewildered and disenchanted.

The role of insight is commonly thought to be important within psychodynamic practice. Heightened self-awareness can indeed pave the way for emotional change, and this frequently includes reflecting on the reasons for certain occupational involvement. This is part of the occupational therapy process, and is not a luxury or side issue. We may work too hard, spend too much time at the gym or in the bar, become obsessively interested in our weight or use our hobbies as the main source of pleasure in our lives. This may be considered as occupational imbalance within our professional discourse, and there may be a recognition that change is necessary, but the reasons for such behaviour may be seen to be outside the remit of occupational therapy. From a psychodynamic perspective, attempts would be made to engage the person in some mutual understanding of the behaviour and the underlying reasons for it. This does not mean that the therapist relinquishes an occupational perspective but rather seeks to incorporate the emotional connotations within it.

Involvement in chosen activities is meaningful not only in an obvious way: for example, to develop a skill or make something grow. Extrinsic motivation is not the only spur to action. Our unconscious links us with the artefacts, activities and objects of our past. Our inner lives may be given voice through symbol, metaphor and recurrent patterns of actions and interactions. This was recognized by Fidler and Fidler (1963), and also by Levens (1986) in her overview of the psychodynamics of activity. Interestingly, it is also a theme of continuity in the work by Fidler and Velde (1999, p.13), who celebrate the 'affective richness of inner life', and maintain that this enhances a 'fuller understanding of how human activities at one level influence processes at another'.

If we need to use occupation as a defence against anxiety, we almost certainly need to use it as a safe deposit for emotions that are in transition or flux. People need bridges between one way of being and another, and engagement in occupation provides this intersection. The notion of the 'therapeutic space' is used by creative arts therapists more than occupational therapists to represent the working through of an issue, but it is our contention that this may be a missed opportunity. Ultimately, the greatest controversy seems to reside in what actually promotes therapeutic change — understanding or action. It is not a negation of the value of occupation to recognize that dynamic factors reside within the process.

CASE STUDY

Cara: a case story from supervision

The occupational therapist wanted to discuss in supervision a difficulty he was having with one of his clients. Each week for a few months he had been seeing Cara, a mother in her thirties, who had a diagnosis of borderline personality disorder.

The therapist had noticed that, although he had a sense of being in control when he collected Cara from the ward, he felt his professional role leave him as they entered the occupational therapy department. Now feeling helpless, he was unable to function without experiencing an intense anxiety that made it difficult for him to think clearly.

At the start of the session Cara chose to work on a collage and the therapist gradually found himself caught up in doing more of the work, encouraged by Cara to add torn pieces from magazines to the collage.

Discussion of these dynamics in supervision helped the therapist to see that he was caught up in an experience in which he felt as if he was one of Cara's children. This new understanding about *why* he had felt so helpless in the session resulted in the therapist gradually becoming less anxious and deskilled as Cara's therapy progressed. His professional role returned and Cara became able to work in a more collaborative way.

At points, however, the feeling of being deskilled would return but the therapist now noticed that this happened when Cara felt anxious or defensive. In response, he became less reactive, holding back slightly. No longer feeling that he had to make things better, he reached Cara simply by listening. This enabled her to talk about her emotions, which, like the torn pieces of paper in her collage, resembled the emotional tears within her marriage.

In being able to take a less defensive stance, the therapist was able to remain curious about what was happening in the therapeutic process, which in turn assisted Cara to explore her pain around issues of not being in control.

Group work within a psychodynamic frame of reference

Consider all the groups you have been involved with, your family, an evening out with friends, a team meeting at work or a discussion after a lecture. These groups can be 'natural' or 'created', and are influenced by cultural surroundings (Douglas 1983). A group is a complex dynamic entity, not unlike an individual, continuously evolving and influenced by relationships with others. Although people have unique individual worlds, they seek sameness, by forming social groups within a variety of time spans. The 'known' is always preferable to the 'not known', which can engender fear, shaped by transgenerational and transpersonal experiences from the past.

Sigmund Freud was curious about what constituted a group, its influencing power and its ability to modify psychic change (Freud 1921). Moreno (1948) was also developing an interest in action instead of words, and developed psychodrama as a way to demonstrate problematic areas expressively through the spectators' involvement as the principal players. The Second World War contributed to the shaping of group approaches through the influential work of Bion and Foulkes. They worked with servicemen who had been psychologically traumatized, and both believed that a group is a whole unit and more than just an assemblage of individuals. Their work took them on divergent paths, leading Foulkes (1964), influenced by gestalt therapy and Kurt Lewin's 'field theory', towards an more analytic concept and interest in the 'group matrix', the intermeshed tangle of group communications and relationships. Lewin (1947) closely linked his ideas to psychoanalytic thinking, coining the term 'group dynamics' from the unseen psychological forces that influence people. The family group itself arises out of creativity in the form of new life.

Bridger (1990) integrated paths taken by Bion and Foulkes, by emphasizing reflection on activity, which became the foundations of the therapeutic community, and Main's (1977) dualistic approach of psychoanalytic psychotherapy was complemented by activity groups. Bion (1961) described a group as a function of interrelated individuals joined in a collective task. Two types metaphorically co-exist, influenced by unconscious phantasies: the 'work group' and the 'basic assumption group'. The 'work group' relates to the real piece of work (primary task) that the group is required to achieve. This sophisticated group requires the skills, knowledge and motivation to complete the task, and will review and learn from their actions (Rioch 1975).

Group work and occupational therapy

Group work is a substantial part of occupational therapy practice in mental health, where emphasis is on the therapeutic relationship and the group process. To facilitate change, a bounded process that Milner (1950) calls the 'frame' is required, so that trust can be established to explore and think symbolically about emotions, fears and the deeper relationship of the group. Bruce and Borg (1987, 2002) emphasize that, within this containing environment, openness allows for negative as well as positive expression. Groups can vary in intensity from practical activity groups to explorative insight-oriented groups with specific individual as well as group aims. Finlay (2002) conceptualizes a continuum of activity of 'task–social–communication psychotherapy', which can all be present in any one group depending on the nature of the activity and the members' reactions. Groups can be directive, task-oriented and non-explorative; non-directive, allowing the unconscious to emerge with interpretation of the group process; or theme-centred — all of which vary in complexity and purpose. Theme-centred groups offer a structure arising out of the group's interactions or from collaborative discussion. From this, group or individual activities can emerge within contained boundaries where suitable themes stimulate the group into a creative process. Like Yalom's (1970) concept of universality, this can bond a group, working at different levels without the group feeling fragmented.

Occupational therapy focuses mainly on the dual areas of task and individual needs; however, seeing the group as a whole also includes the less than popular aspect of the management of the group through the therapeutic process. Attention is given to what is going on in the here and now, between and among the group members, and this highlights the importance of process. Through the use of creative and projective techniques such as art, music, poetry, drama, writing and dance, emotions can be expressed with or without words to gain a deeper insight through interpretation and the exploration of underlying meaning. This relies on the therapist using themselves as a tool within the therapeutic context, so that new learning can occur in what Robertson (1984) describes as the 'working through' process. One distinctive occupational therapy approach to group work is that advanced by Howe and Schwartzberg (2001), and is described as a functional approach based upon five areas: group dynamics, effectance, needs hierarchy, purposeful activity and adaptation. This account acknowledges the historical development of group work in the USA, and describes the functional group work model as the 'first comprehensive model of the profession's group practice' (Howe & Schwartzberg 2001, p.104).

Groups are composed of individuals, and therefore also use social defences that form and distort the characteristics of the organization. A feature of group process, especially within the UK National Health Service and community care, is the need to shield against the disturbance or dis-ease that the nature of the work can engender. This is resolved by projecting intolerable feelings into other groups, creating feelings of helplessness, inadequacy and confusion that can be experienced across the boundary between the practitioner and the client/patient. To manage this phenomenon, the feelings can go underground and resurface in more distant groups of staff or agencies, e.g. management. The original group's anxieties are bypassed, relieving them of their distress. Especially, heightened tensions occur around change, distorting perceptions and hindering communication, creating what Klein (1946) called splitting: relief gained by placing the problem in the other, which in turn creates upset, conflict and distrust. These projections can leave groups feeling excluded, driving a professional wedge between intra-agencies that is seldom addressed, yet needs to be acknowledged to support the staff and reduce tensions.

Unconscious uncontrolled effects are produced, and this begs the question as to where the demotivation goes in the optimistic image of occupational therapy? Klein described the depressive position as the point where the oppositional forces can be understood; for this to happen, space to think is essential so that patterns are not re-enacted (projective identification) and can be understood through support and maintaining communication. Hence the need for supervision, time to consider how the team is functioning and human relations training. As Savage (1983) suggests, there is a need to create, not impoverish, the transitional space for human growth and development. Our contention is that engagement in occupation facilitates this.

Contribution to health and well-being

The combination of this related knowledge and occupational therapy can contribute to health and well-being for clients, staff and organizations.

Basic tenets of this are:

- an opportunity to increase self-awareness and understand the dynamics of doing
- working with an emotional language — expressing feelings in mutually respectful ways
- learning to work with others and appreciate intrapersonal and interpersonal dynamics
- provision of a therapeutic space from which to practise and learn
- the need to operationalize insight through occupation and be able to reflect upon this
- to reach an understanding that there are different levels of meaning and to recognize which is helpful to pursue at any one time
- to have a place to reflect upon 'doing and being' while remaining curious.

Our occupational lives frequently reflect our emotional lives. We strive, we work too hard, we ventilate our emotions through different pursuits, we try to get thin, get fit, perfect our living spaces or seek out new ones. All have a sense of meaning and a set of activities associated with them. The activities often act as the barometer for how our lives are going and how contented or otherwise we are. Certainly, there is the possibility for negative doing as well as positive doing. For clients, an overview of their occupational lives acts as our means of assessment and understanding of their occupational behaviour and performance — we ask people what they do and how satisfied they are, and how they want things to be in the future. The language that is often used by people to describe their current state of health is interesting — 'How are you doing?', 'Doing away', 'I'm done for', all of which registers the unconscious links between feelings and what people do. It is a powerful means of access to inner life.

A psychodynamic attitude is a helpful component in the professional repertoire of all people who work within teams. It can help explain professional rivalry, professional distance, the lack of cohesion in a team or why change is experienced as a threat. Most importantly, it allows individuals to locate themselves within the network. This is not a luxury within our busy and hectic working lives; reflection is actively encouraged as part of continuing professional development. Clearly, the establishment of trust is the pivot around which this can work, and it can take some considerable time to build a relationship of trust with either an individual or a group. And so it should — there is no automatic right to this, but it is something that should be worked at and acknowledged openly as part of the learning process.

People who seem to be attracted to the synthesis of psychodynamic work with occupational therapy often tend to be interested in process rather than merely measurable outcomes. There is a belief in the possibility of learning from the dynamics that occur within the experience of a group, within an individual interaction or from the way an organization operates. Active reflection, mutual problem-posing and 'trying on for size' certain interpretative possibilities facilitate this phenomenon. However, those issues are not easily measured, and reflect emotional reactions and interactions, which can help or hinder the process of constructive change. One of the central tenets is the possibility of knowing yourself better or of achieving some insight into why similar patterns in relationships or events recur in your life. Although the 'working-through' process is part of the therapeutic activity, one of the main criticisms of this is that at a verbal level it remains a cerebral activity rather than a practical change. The first process does not automatically incur the other.

Our mental health requires us to have a reasonably balanced view of ourselves. We need to be aware of our impact on other people and be capable of ameliorating that if necessary. For example, a tendency to work long hours and always be available for advice sets up expectations, which may rebound on other people within an organization. Psychodynamic thinking to aid the development of human relations within organizations has been used for over 50 years. Trist (1989) notes Bridger's unpublished work in this area, relating to the management of change. For successful transition within organizations, he considered the need to 'tune in, work through and design' — a conscious way to select what is relevant, while tolerating the emotional disruption of letting go of the old routines, to provide room for the potential of creative play (design). It is only once individuals have internalized the change that the organization can begin to alter. This is the dual task of reflection and review through a transitional learning space.

Occupational therapy offers a number of possibilities to enhance the psychodynamic encounter. Firstly, it can provide a place to explore troubling feelings and ideas through the use of creative activities. Not everyone can verbalize their emotions, or indeed possesses the emotional language with which to explain their feelings. Also, the possibility actively to operationalize changes, which have been discussed within a psychodynamic setting, is the remit of occupational therapy. This also has a reciprocal effect in providing the experiential material for reflection in the next individual or group session. It can enhance the quality of the interaction and give live examples of where conflicts, defences or anxieties still reign. The idea of a 'therapeutic space', such as the engagement in meaningful occupations, is shared with other creative therapies such as art therapy. However, occupational therapy is considered to be involved in real life narratives — that is, it ultimately inhabits the realm of the commonplace daily round of activities rather than the esoteric discussions about exploration of conflict and where it originated. Feelings, however, permeate out of the daily round of activities; they are not conveniently stored until the time is right for ventilation, and this is the beauty of combining an insight into psychodynamic thinking with the analysis of occupational performance. Piergrossi and Gilbertoni (1995) emphasize the inner significance of activity, essential in contributing towards a sense of wellness and its considerable practical utility.

Summary

This chapter began by highlighting that a psychotherapeutic attitude towards health and well-being is a helpful attribute in our professional repertoire, with the importance of this frame of reference being summed up by the following points:

- There is a rich history and heritage of writing.
- It continues to stimulate contemporary thinkers across many disciplines.
- It is intimately concerned with process — the study of how things occur, change and progress.
- It helps people and organizations understand and deal with feelings, meanings and an emotional language.
- It acknowledges that people and organizations are gloriously complicated.
- It deals with introspection, reflection and how to follow this through into emotional and practical change.
- It offers insights across the lifespan.

The profession takes its identity and its means of change from ideas that link occupation with health and well-being. Professional confidence about this important construct is evident from the proliferation of texts concerning human occupation over the last decade. Many changes within health and social care have been negotiated, but curiously occupational therapy has never been considered as an alternative or complementary therapy despite its philosophical departure from medicine. So it has remained associated with mainstream health provision but with a somewhat ambivalent relationship to medicine. The literature over the last decade reveals that the profession can tolerate a shift to the inclusion of spirituality, creative therapies, the meaning of everyday occupation and narrative approaches to systematic inquiry. Occupational lives can be compromised by unconscious forces. Ideas from the psychodynamic tradition offer one perspective to illuminate why this may happen and how it impacts upon occupational behaviour.

Therapeutic occupation in this tradition offers the opportunity to explore meanings, to adjust to the consequences of those meanings and to work towards manageable occupational solutions. There is evidence of a steady and sustained interest in the links between psychodynamic ideas and the contemporary practice of occupational therapy. Perhaps the current interest in meaning, and recognition of the experience of occupation for both the therapist and clients, is the 'therapeutic space' by any other name.

Reflective learning

- In the spirit of reflexivity, explore and analyse how your own emotional state influences your practice.
- Anxiety affects us all. Consider ways in which you try to defend yourself through possible defence mechanisms.
- Can you explain how emotional health impacts on all other aspects of health and well-being?
- Does our 'doing' reveal our emotional state and how do we use that to engage with our clients?
- Is there a relationship between the therapeutic space and the notion of an occupational space?

References

Affleck, I.S., 1977. Poetry as medium in a unit for the treatment of alcoholism. British Journal of Occupational Therapy 40 (11), 277.

Appignanesi, L., Forrester, J., 2000. Freud's Women. Penguin, London.

Atkinson, K., Wells, C., 2000. Creative Therapies: a Psychodynamic Approach Within Occupational Therapy. Stanley Thornes, Cheltenham.

Azima, G., Azima, J., 1959. Outline of a dynamic theory of occupational therapy. American Journal of Occupational Therapy 13, 5.

Balbernie, R., 2001. Circuits and circumstances: the neurobiological consequences of early relationship experiences and how they shape later behaviour. Journal of Child Psychotherapy 27 (3), 237–255.

Banks, E.T., Blair, S.E.E., 1997. The contribution of occupational therapy within the context of the psychodynamic approach for older clients who have mental health problems. Health Care in Later Life 2 (2), 85–95.

Barris, R., Kielhofner, G., Watts, J., 1983. Psychosocial Occupational Therapy Practice in a Pluralistic Arena. Ramsco, Laurel.

Batchelor, L.J., 1970. The occupational therapist as a therapeutic medium. Scottish Journal of Occupational Therapy 83, 16–28.

Bateman, A., Brown, D., Pedder, J., 2001. Introduction to Psychotherapy: an Outline of Psychodynamic Principles and Practice, third ed. Routledge, London.

Berne, E., 1961. Games People Play. Penguin, Harmondsworth.

Bion, W.R., 1961. Experiences in Groups, and Other Papers. Tavistock, London.

Blair, S.E.E., 1974. Projective techniques. Scottish Journal of Occupational Therapy 96, 16–19.

Blair, S.E.E., 2000. The centrality of occupation during life transition. British Journal of Occupational Therapy 63 (5), 231–237.

Bowlby, J., 1988. A Secure Base: Clinical Applications of Attachment Theory. Routledge, London.

Bridger, H., 1990. The discovery of the therapeutic community: the Northfield experiments. In: Trist, E., Murray, H. (Eds.), The Social Engagement of Social Science, vol. 1. The Socio-Psychological Perspective. Free Association, London, pp. 68–87.

Brown, T., 1990. Drama and occupational therapy. In: Creek, J. (Ed.), Occupational Therapy and Mental Health. Churchill Livingston, Edinburgh, pp. 211–227.

Bruce, M.A., Borg, B., 1987. Object relations frame of reference. In: Bruce, M.A., Borg, B. (Eds.), Psychosocial Occupational Therapy: Frames of Reference for Intervention. Slack, Thorofare, NJ, pp. 39–83.

Bruce, M.A., Borg, B., 2002. Psychodynamic frame of reference — person, perspective and meaning. In: Bruce, M.A., Borg, B. (Eds.), Psychosocial Frames of Reference: Core for Occupation-Based Practice, third ed. Slack, Thorofare, NJ, pp. 69–119.

Daniel, M.A., Blair, S.E.E., 2002. A psychodynamic approach to clinical supervision: 1. British Journal of Therapy and Rehabilitation 9 (6), 237–240.

Douglas, T., 1983. Groups: Understanding People Gathered Together. Tavistock, London.

Drost, H., 1971. Occupational therapy in groups. Scottish Journal of Occupational Therapy 3 (86), 27–39.

Eklund, M., 2000. Applying object relations theory to psychosocial occupational therapy: empirical and theoretical considerations. Occupational Therapy in Mental Health 15 (1), 1–26.

Erikson, 1980. Identity and the Life Cycle. WW Norton, New York.

Ferenczi, S., 1949. Notes and fragments 1930–32. International Journal of Psycho-analysis 30 (4), 231–244.

Ferenczi, S., 1984. Confusion of tongues. In: Masson, J.M. (Ed.), The Assault on Truth: Freud's Suppression of the Seduction Theory. Penguin, Harmondsworth, pp. 145–188.

Fidler, G.S., Fidler, J.W., 1963. Occupational Therapy: a Communication Process in Psychiatry. MacMillan, New York.

Fidler, G.S., Velde, B.P., 1999. Activities Reality and Symbol. Slack, Thorofare, NJ.

Finlay, L., 1997. The Practice of Psychosocial Occupational Therapy. Stanley Thornes, Cheltenham.

Finlay, L., 2002. Groupwork. In: Creek, J. (Ed.), Occupational Therapy in Mental Health. Churchill Livingstone, Edinburgh, pp. 245–264.

Foulkes, S.H., 1964. Therapeutic Group Analysis. Maresfield Reprints, London.

Freud, S., 1921. Group psychology and the analysis of the ego. In: Strachey, J. (Ed.), Standard Edition of the Complete Psychological Work of Sigmund Freud, vol. XVIII. Hogarth, London, pp. 67–143.

Gomez, L., 1997. An Introduction to Object Relations. Free Association, London.

Howe, M.C., Schwartzberg, S.L., 2001. A Functional Approach to Group Work in Occupational Therapy. Lippincott Williams & Wilkins, Philadelphia.

Hughes, P., 1999. Dynamic Psychotherapy Explained. Radcliffe Medical, London.

Hyde, P., 2006. A case study of unconscious processes in an organisation. In: Ballinger, C., Finlay, L. (Eds.), Qualitative Research for Allied Health Professionals: Challenging Choices. John Willey, Chichester, pp. 218–231.

Ingram, G., 2001. Psychodynamic theories. In: Lougher, L. (Ed.), Occupational Therapy for Child and Adolescent Mental Health. Churchill Livingstone, Edinburgh, pp. 97–110.

Jackson, S., 2005. The use of psychodynamic observation [letter]. British Journal of Occupational Therapy 68 (1), 48–99.

Jenkins, M., 1999. Shifting ground or sifting sand? In: Creek, J. (Ed.), Occupational Therapy: New Perspectives. Whurr, London, pp. 29–46.

Jensen, C.M., Blair, S.E.E., 1998. Rhyme and Reason: the relationship between creative writing and mental well-being. British Journal of Occupational Therapy 60 (12), 525–530.

Kielhofner, G., 1997. Conceptual Foundations for Occupational Therapy. FA Davies, Philadelphia.

Kielhofner, G., 2002. Model of Human Occupation, third ed. Lippincott Williams & Wilkins, Baltimore.

Klein, M., 1946. Notes on some schizoid mechanisms. International Journal of Psycho-analysis 33, 433–438.

Krupa, T., 2003. The psychological–emotional determinants of occupation. In: McColl, M., Law, M., Stewart, D. (Eds.), Theoretical Basis of Occupational Therapy, second ed. Slack, Thorofare, NJ, pp. 94–116.

Levens, M., 1986. The psychodynamics of activity. British Journal of Occupational Therapy 49 (3), 87–89.

Lewin, K., 1947. Frontiers in group dynamics. Human Relations 1 (1), 5–41.

MacKenzie, A., Beecraft, S., 2004. The use of psychodynamic observation as a tool for learning and reflective practice when working with older adults. British Journal of Occupational Therapy 67 (12), 533–539.

Main, T., 1977. The concept of the therapeutic community: variations and vicissitudes. Group Analysis 10 (2), 1–16.

Malcolm, M., 1975. Occupational therapy techniques. British Journal of Occupational Therapy 40 (10), 147–148.

Menzies Lyth, I., 1988. Staff support systems: task and anti-task in adolescent institutions. In: Menzies Lyth, I. (Ed.), Containing Anxiety in Institutions. Free Associations, New York, pp. 197–207.

Menzies Lyth, I., 1990. Social systems as a defence against anxiety. In: Trist, E., Murray, H. (Eds.), The Social Engagement of Social Science. Free Associations, New York, pp. 463–475.

Milner, M., 1950. On Not Being Able to Paint. Heinemann, London.

Moreno, J.L., 1948. Psychodrama 1. Beacon House, New York.

Mosey, A., 1970. Three Frames of Reference in Mental Health. Slack, Thorofare, NJ.

Munro, K., 2008. The psychological therapies. Occupational Therapy News (Feb), 28–29.

Nicholls, L., 2003. Occupational therapy on the couch. Therapy Weekly 10 July, 5.

Nicholls, L., 2008. A psychoanalytic discourse in occupational therapy. In: Creek, J., Lawson-Porter, A. (Eds.), Contemporary Issues in Occupational Therapy: Reasoning and Reflecting, second ed. John Willey, Chichester, pp. 55–84.

Ogilvie, S.S., Blair, S.E.E., Paul, L.A., 1995. Survey of patients on an alcohol in-patient unit in relation to group therapeutic factors. Occupational Therapy International 2 (4), 257–277.

Perez-Franco, A., 1998. The Use of a Psychodynamic Approach in Mental Health and its Value for Occupational Therapy. BSc(Hons) dissertation. Oxford Brookes University, Oxford.

Piergrossi, J.C., Gilbertoni, C., 1995. The importance of inner transformation in the activity process. Occupational Therapy International 2, 36–47.

Reilly, M., 1974. Play as Exploratory Learning: Studies of Curiosity Behavior. Sage, Beverly Hills.

Remocker, J., Storch, E.T., 1982. Actions Speak Louder: a Handbook of Non-verbal Group Techniques. Churchill Livingstone, Edinburgh.

Rioch, M., 1975. The work of Wilfred Bion on groups. In: Colman, A.D., Bexton, W.H. (Eds.), Group Relations Reader 1. AK Rice Institute, Jupiter, pp. 21–31.

Robertson, E., 1984. The role of occupational therapy in a psychotherapeutic setting. British Journal of Occupational Therapy 47 (4), 106–110.

Savage, J., 1983. The role and training of a creative therapist: some reflections. In: Jennings, S. (Ed.), Creative Therapy. Dramatherapy Consultants/Kemble, Banbury, pp. 199–227.

Steward, B., 1996. Creative therapies. In: Willson, M. (Ed.), Occupational Therapy in Short Term Psychiatry, third ed. Churchill Livingstone, Edinburgh, pp. 173–194.

Stockwell, R., 1984. Creative therapies. In: Willson, M. (Ed.), Occupational Therapy in Short Term Psychiatry. Churchill Livingstone, Edinburgh, pp. 182–204.

Sutherland, 1969. Psychoanalysis in the post-industrial society. International Journal of Psycho-analysis 50, 637–682.

Symington, N., 1986. The Analytic Experience: Lectures from the Tavistock. Free Association, London.

Telford, R., Ainscough, K., 1995. Non-directive play therapy and psychodynamic theory: never the twain shall meet? British Journal of Occupational Therapy 58 (5), 201–203.

Thompson, M., Blair, S.E.E., 1998. Creative arts in occupational therapy: Ancient history in contemporary practice? Occupational Therapy International, 5(1), 48–64.

Trist, E., 1989. Psychoanalytic issues in organisational research and consultation. In: Klein, L. (Ed.), Working with Organisations: Papers to Celebrate the 80th Birthday of Harold Bridger. Kestral, Loxwood, pp. 50–58.

Wilcock, A., 1998. An Occupational Perspective of Health. Slack, Thorofare, NJ.

Winnicott, D.W., 1971. Playing and Reality. Tavistock, London.

Winters, E.E. (Ed.), 1951. The Collected Papers of Adolf Meyers, vol. II. Psychiatry. Johns Hopkins, Baltimore.

Yalom, I.D., 1970. The Theory and Practice of Group Psychotherapy. Basic, New York.

The biomechanical frame of reference in occupational therapy

14

Ian R. McMillan

OVERVIEW

This chapter explains why studying a biomechanical frame of reference within occupational therapy is relevant in today's practice. The profession continues to have a contract with society to provide a service that focuses on human occupation. Occupational therapists are concerned with the relationship between people's occupations and their health, and assess people's disengagement from their occupations, provide ways for them to re-engage in their occupations, or suggest alternatives so that people's quality of life may improve. Core values and beliefs about the importance of occupation to humans constitute a paradigm of occupation. In daily practice, occupational role issues that individuals may experience can be appreciated by referring to conceptual models of practice using a 'top-down' approach. Examples of such models of practice are the Canadian Model of Occupational Performance (CMOP) (see Chapter 7 for further information) and the Model of Human Occupation (MOHO) (see Chapter 6 for further information). Such models provide the knowledge, skills and attitudes necessary to understand how we can analyse, intervene and evaluate individuals in relation to their roles and efficacy of occupational performances, e.g. in self-care, work and leisure. However, in order to understand the individual's specific occupational performance problems, it is also necessary to analyse and understand their 'performance capacities' in more detail. Performance capacities refer to cognition, behaviour, neural development, personal interactions and, most importantly for this chapter, movement. The biomechanical frame of reference deals exclusively with the capacity for *motion*, whilst other frames of reference deal with other capacities, e.g. the cognitive behavioural frame of reference deals with cognition and behaviour. A biomechanical frame of reference may be useful in assessment, intervention and evaluation with people who have occupational performance problems, created primarily by some disease, injury or event that impinges on their voluntary movement, muscle strength, endurance or usually a combination of all three. The loss of one or more of these capacities will interfere to some degree with an individual's ability to perform their occupations to their satisfaction. The biomechanical frame of reference assists in understanding the assessment, intervention and evaluation strategies associated with changing physical performance capacities in order to help individuals re-engage in their occupations.

Key points

- This chapter explores the evolution and use of a biomechanical frame of reference in occupational therapy.
- The biomechanical frame of reference can be located within a 'top-down' and a 'bottom-up' approach to occupational therapy.
- The biomechanical frame of reference deals with a person's problems related to their capacity for movement in daily occupations.
- The biomechanical frame of reference can be used to shape assessment, intervention and evaluation strategies, in order to help individuals re-engage in their occupations.

Introduction

The 'biomechanical frame of reference', in its original form, was not necessarily compiled by occupational therapists for occupational therapy practice today and therefore some translation of the original frame of reference (from a professional perspective) is necessary in order to ensure a 'fit' with the philosophy of occupational therapy. Therefore, this chapter describes and articulates a biomechanical frame of reference from an occupational therapist's perspective.

The biomechanical frame of reference used in occupational therapy has a long tradition and at different points in history has been termed Baldwin's reconstruction approach 1919, Taylor's orthopaedic approach 1934, and Licht's kinetic approach 1957 (Turner et al 2002). This frame of reference continues to be widely used today and different occupational therapists are continuing to present this frame of reference in different ways (for example, Trombly appears to have incorporated a biomechanical frame of reference into the Occupational Functioning Model; Trombly & Radomski 2002).

Reflecting on this biomechanical frame of reference (which encompasses a variety of knowledge, skills and attitudes) broadens a professional's knowledge base and provides more insight into fieldwork experiences and therefore an understanding of how practice can inform theory-building and vice versa.

Conceptual models of practice

Occupation (Kielhofner 1997, Canadian Association of Occupational Therapists 2002), within the context of occupational therapy, is part of the human condition, is necessary to society and culture, is required for physical and psychological well-being, entails underlying performance components and is a determinant and product of human development. Further, the intrinsic values of occupational therapy as a practice grounded in humanism affirm the dignity and worth of individuals, the participation in occupation, self-determination, freedom and independence, latent capacity, caring and the interpersonal elements of therapy, human uniqueness and subjectivity, and mutual cooperation in the therapeutic process. Occupation and occupational performance are usually expressed in terms of self-care/daily living tasks, work/productivity and leisure/play (Kielhofner 1997, Canadian Association of Occupational Therapists 2002).

This infers that studying and considering human occupation has to be paramount and is the core business of being an occupational therapist. When necessary, occupation can be analysed (e.g. the biological, psychosocial, environmental, etc.) regarding its content and meaning for the individual, to determine 'dysfunctional elements' that may occur because of disease and injury. Occupational therapists who can expertly analyse occupations are then able to perceive the meaning for that person and to assist them in regaining the necessary skills (or compensate for their permanent loss) through the medium of occupation and/or by modifying the environment or the attitudes of others in society and so on.

If an individual has temporarily or permanently lost an occupational role because of occupational performance problems primarily concerning movement, then the biomechanical frame of reference is likely to inform the therapist and assist the overall therapeutic process.

Ultimately, the majority of clients seen by an occupational therapist will have problems of 'body and mind' (irrespective of diagnostic labels), which can only be discerned within the context of that individual's environment, perspectives and value systems. This requires adopting a top-down approach to practice (Kramer et al 2003) by using an occupational therapy conceptual model of practice to appreciate the significance of an individual's occupational performance problems and then using the biomechanical frame of reference and others to appreciate the performance capacity issues.

Top-down approach to practice

The values and beliefs inherent in an occupation paradigm imply that occupational therapists need to view their clients as occupational beings. We therefore need to choose conceptual models of practice that focus on describing the occupational nature of the client. There are a number of unique occupational therapy models of practice available to choose from, such as the Model of Human Occupation (MOHO) (Kielhofner 2007), the Canadian Model of Occupational Performance (CMOP) (Law et al 2005) and the Person–Environment–Occupation Model (Law et al 1996, Strong et al 1999). Practice can then be further supported with other frames of reference when required (e.g. the biomechanical frame of reference), so that

Fig. 14.1 • The 'top-down' approach. Reproduced with permission from Forsyth and McMillan, personal communication, (2001).

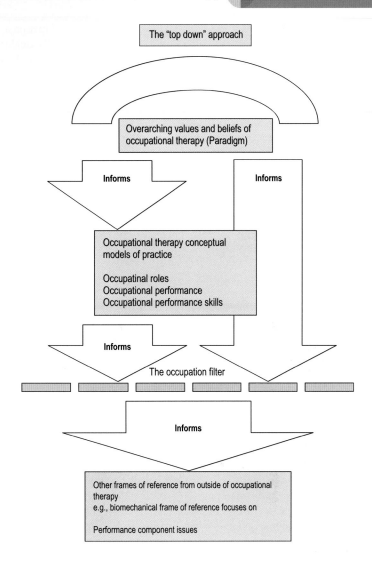

occupational performance issues relative to motion in occupations can be more specifically analysed and managed.

Figure 14.1 implies that the occupation paradigm influences every aspect of an occupational therapist's practice. The use of knowledge located in a biomechanical frame of reference needs to be filtered (occupation filter) by values that an occupational therapist embodies, which are located within the occupation paradigm. This ensures that the focus of interventions remains occupational in nature. The focus of the biomechanical frame of reference is the musculoskeletal capacity to create movement (range of motion), strength and endurance in order to carry out meaningful occupations. Movement,

strength and endurance can then be assessed within the context of a person completing their occupations and using occupations to restore/maintain/compensate for lack of movement, strength and endurance.

Occupation filter

The following criteria constitute the occupation filter and occupational therapists ought to reflect on these statements when using the technology of the biomechanical frame of reference to enrich practice (Mallinson & Forsyth, personal communication 2000):

- *Person's occupational performance.* The primary concern here is understanding how the phenomena from the biomechanical frame of reference (movement, strength and endurance) influence the person's performance of their occupational roles.
- *Assess through occupation.* Analyse and assess the phenomena from the biomechanical frame of reference (movement, strength and endurance) within the context of the person's performance of their occupational roles.
- *Occupation restores/maintains.* This reinforces the person's performance of occupational roles during the restoration and/or maintenance and/or compensation of movement, strength and endurance.
- *The outcome of occupational therapy is satisfying/meaningful performance in occupations.* Occupational therapists ought to view the satisfying, meaningful performance of occupation as the primary outcome of therapy (Mallinson & Forsyth, personal communication 2000).

Using the top-down approach above implies that a biomechanical frame of reference used by an occupational therapist will be different from a biomechanical frame of reference used by other health professionals.

Occupation and occupational performance that incorporate movement and its potential restoration are the key to understanding the use of this frame of reference in our professional practice. Movement for the sake of movement is more likely to be the aim of other professionals, reflecting a bottom-up approach (Kramer et al 2003).

Details of the biomechanical frame of reference

The biomechanical frame of reference in occupational therapy is primarily concerned with an individual's motion during occupations. Motion in this context can be understood in more detail as the capacity for movement, muscle strength and endurance (the ability to resist fatigue).

An individual's quality of motion may be compromised as they carry out their occupations due to the effects of disease or injury. These effects may compromise specific body systems and structures (e.g. bones and joints) that help create motion seen during occupational performance. Additionally, an individual's quality of movement has to be viewed in the context of the environment that may facilitate or inhibit their occupations.

Aim and objectives

The biomechanical frame of reference aims to address the quality of movement in occupations. Specific objectives are to:

- prevent deterioration and maintain existing movement for occupational performance
- restore movement for occupational performance, if possible
- compensate/adapt for loss of movement in occupational performance.

Compensation and adaptation are terms that have often been associated with 'rehabilitation' or the 'rehabilitative model'. Some practitioners believe the biomechanical frame of reference deals comprehensively with the topic of compensation and some believe that a rehabilitation model deals with compensation. This author believes that rehabilitation may be viewed as an 'aim' and that compensation is more comprehensively addressed within the biomechanical frame of reference.

Who would you use the biomechanical frame of reference with?

This frame of reference is principally used with individuals who experience the following problems in their daily occupations.

Limitations in movement during occupations

This describes the capacity of the person to use their muscles in conjunction with bones and joints to move freely when engaging in occupations. This is usually due to one or more of the following problems:

- shortening (contracture) of soft tissues, i.e. muscle tissue, muscle connective tissues, tendons, ligaments, fibrous capsules and skin
- the presence of inflammation, oedema or haematoma

- localized destruction of bone (e.g. rheumatoid arthritis, osteoarthrosis)
- amputation
- congenital abnormalities
- acute and chronic pain
- maladaptive environmental conditions.

Inadequate muscle strength for use in occupations

This describes the capacity of the person to initiate and maintain muscle strength during their occupations (e.g. using the forearm muscle groups to facilitate gripping an object effectively in the hand). Inability to do this may be due to one or more of the following problems:

- limitations in movement
- disuse or atrophy of muscle (e.g. post-fracture immobilization)
- primary muscle pathology (e.g. muscular dystrophy)
- anterior horn cell pathology (e.g. motor neurone disease)
- peripheral neuropathy (e.g. diabetes)
- peripheral nerve damage (e.g. mononeuropathy of the median nerve)
- acute and chronic pain
- maladaptive environmental conditions.

Loss of endurance in occupations

This describes the ability of the person to resist subjective fatigue and therefore sustain their occupations over time and distance to their satisfaction. Issues in this area are usually due to one or more of the following problems:

- limitations in movement
- inadequate muscle strength
- compromised cardiovascular and/or respiratory function
- acute and chronic pain
- maladaptive environmental factors.

Biomedical conditions

People who experience limitations in movement, inadequate muscle strength and loss of endurance whilst engaging in their occupations may have a diagnosis of one or more of the following biomedical conditions:

- rheumatoid arthritis, osteoarthrosis or a combination of the two, or the individual may have experienced surgical arthroplasty
- amputations, burns and other soft-tissue damage frequently seen in hand and limb injuries
- fractures and various orthopaedic conditions
- Guillain–Barré syndrome, muscular dystrophy, motor neurone disease and the long-term effects of poliomyelitis (post-polio syndrome)
- peripheral neuropathy, mononeuropathy, brachial plexus lesions
- cardiac problems in the form of ischaemic heart disease (angina, myocardial infarction), cardiac failure or the effects of bypass surgery
- respiratory problems in the form of various obstructive airways diseases
- chronic pain due to occupational overuse syndrome (OOS), back injuries, neck injuries or pain associated with any of the conditions outlined above.

To appreciate the application of the biomechanical frame of reference fully implies an understanding not only of the biomedical conditions outlined above but also of the anatomical and physiological details of certain body systems and structures, which are outlined below:

- the musculoskeletal system, which comprises muscles, tendons, ligaments, bone and related tissues, and synovial joints (fibrous capsules, synovial tissues)
- the peripheral nervous system, comprising neural and connective tissues
- the integumentary system, comprising the epidermis, dermis, blood vessels, hair follicles, sebaceous glands and sweat glands
- the cardiorespiratory system, comprising the heart, blood vessels and lungs.

It should also be understood that, because the biomechanical frame of reference principally concerns the capacity to execute purposeful movement in everyday occupations, it is important to understand other factors that underpin this concept.

Other factors

It is helpful to have an understanding of the following factors. Understanding the biomechanical basis of movement includes knowing the locomotor system (how bones and joints perform together, especially in relation to the appendicular skeleton), active and passive joint range of movement (a.ROM and p.ROM), the function of skeletal muscle, types of muscle work (concentric and eccentric, isotonic and isometric contraction), muscle architecture and role, the peripheral nervous system (motor, sensory and autonomic) and the relationship between the peripheral nervous system (synaptic transmission and innervation) and muscles (sliding filament theory).

In addition, the biomechanical basis of movement includes understanding concepts of force, gravity, friction, resistance, leverage, stability and equilibrium, and how these elements interact to affect the nature of motion in human beings (Spaulding 2005).

The relationship between occupational performance and the biomechanical frame of reference requires understanding locomotion and the stance and swing phases of the gait cycle, prehension and the prehensile patterns of hand grips (power and precision), skeletal muscle and cardiovascular endurance, and the effects of fatigue on human occupations, all of which have to be considered for the execution of purposeful motion. Tyldesley and Grieve (2002) provide a detailed explanation of all of the above and this text is recommended as further reading to understand these factors in greater detail.

In summary, the capacity for movement (and occupational performance) is a synthesis of forces (the capabilities of the musculoskeletal system and the nervous system coordinating the work of groups of muscles to produce movement and stabilize joints) acting on the body. Endurance (the ability to sustain occupational performance) is predominantly a function of muscle physiology and the ability of the body systems to transport the required material towards, and waste materials away from, the muscle tissues.

Individuals' problems that can be addressed through the biomechanical frame of reference *should* have an intact, fully matured central nervous system. In other words, no evidence of biomedical conditions or pathology that might affect the following body systems should be evident:

- motor control systems (cortex/basal ganglia/cerebellum)
- sensory discrimination (cortex/thalamus/cerebellum)
- perceptual qualities (association areas of the cortex and parietal lobe functions)
- cognition (localization of function)
- behaviour (localization of function).

This is because the individual with movement problems described in the biomechanical frame of reference still has the capacity in their central nervous system to initiate the production of smooth, controlled isolated movements (Dutton 1998). This is in sharp contrast to individuals with central nervous system (CNS) damage who would have different types of motor problem and therefore a different frame of reference would have to be considered, i.e. the theoretical approaches to motor control and cognitive function (see Chapter 15 for further information). However, it is also apparent that occupational therapists do use the technology of the biomechanical frame of reference at certain times with selected individuals who *do have* CNS damage in the form of stroke, multiple sclerosis and so on. This is because, inevitably, some individuals do sustain *permanent* loss of the control of movement in various parts of their body, and in the long term *compensating* for this loss of motion in occupational performance is required.

The next part of this chapter concentrates on the assessment of movement seen in occupational performance.

Principles of assessment and measurement

Rationale for assessment

Occupational therapists ought to be concerned with the principles of assessment and measurement in their practice to facilitate collaborative goals, build intervention plans and document measures of outcomes. This process of assessment can be undertaken through client-driven assessment, therapist observation and the use of standardized and non-standardized instruments.

Assessment facilitates the collection of quantitative and qualitative data, which, when analysed, permit the interpretation of the effectiveness of an intervention by both the client and the therapist. This interpretative process, in relation to hard and soft data, assists in monitoring and implementing change, helps in building goals, facilitates decision-making and produces evidence that is readily understood, for the benefit of clients and of health professional and managerial colleagues.

General aims of assessment

The aims of occupational therapy assessment are generally agreed to:

- decide whether occupational therapy is appropriate or necessary
- establish abilities, disabilities and the effects of the environment on an individual's occupations
- formulate a package of information (data collection) to plan future goals
- formulate a baseline to compare progress and regress
- assist decision-making regarding the modification of intervention plans
- involve, inform, educate and motivate the individual (client)
- establish the efficacy (and evidence base) of occupational therapy intervention
- assist resource decision-making regarding demands on service provision
- produce tangible outcomes/evidence for the benefit of the individual and of healthcare and management colleagues.

Methods of assessment

In the context of the biomechanical frame of reference these may consist of:

- observation of occupational performances
- interviews (informal/unstructured through to formal/structured)
- questionnaires (open and closed questions)
- checklists (paper and pencil, computer)
- rating scales (paper and pencil, computer)
- performance evaluations (specific tasks, electrical, mechanical and computer equipment).

Framework for assessment and occupation

Assessments frequently reflect the theoretical perspectives of certain conceptual models of practice or frames of reference. It is important to reflect on which theoretical perspectives have informed the construction of assessments administered in practice. Although occupational therapists utilize a wide range of assessments, Mathiowetz (1993), Kielhofner (2007) and Fisher (1998), all occupational therapists, assert that in concert with the values and philosophy of the profession, assessment ought to be focused on occupation,

with a view to re-engaging the person in their occupations, and be as comprehensive as possible within the constraints of time. Because assessments have arisen from conceptual models of practice and frames of references, it is important to understand the difference between assessments constructed by occupational therapists and assessments constructed by others. These differences reflect varying professional philosophies and need to be understood, so that it is clear when to use multiple assessments appropriately.

Mathiowetz (1993) and more recently Molineux (2004) believe that a hierarchical order should be imposed on assessment, with occupational role and occupational performance being more important than the assessment of performance components. Mathiowetz (1993) advocated this approach (reflecting Kramer et al's (2003) 'top-down' view) because he believed occupational therapists ought to be primarily concerned with the daily effects of loss of occupational performance, thus reflecting the importance of the link between individuals and occupations. Specific assessments, e.g. the Worker Role Interview (Braveman et al 2005) and the Canadian Occupational Performance Measure (COPM) (Law et al 2005), would capture occupational performance as described above. However, Wilby (2007) also believes that performance components ought to be recognized in occupational therapy practice and that specific assessments *are* required in specialist areas of practice that are drawn from other frames of reference. This would help inform therapists about specific performance component issues that are the building blocks of occupational performance; that is, an occupational therapist would assess loss of movement, which influences occupational performances. This approach could be described as a 'bottom-up' approach (see Kramer et al 2003 for a detailed explanation of this terminology).

In summary, assessments are drawn from occupational therapy models first and then more detailed data about movement, strength and endurance (performance components) could also be collected using specific instruments to provide a comprehensive picture of the individual. Figure 14.2 reflects this approach.

Assessment of performance components for occupation

As previously mentioned, an area of expertise within the biomechanical frame of reference is to collect data from individuals, which provides greater

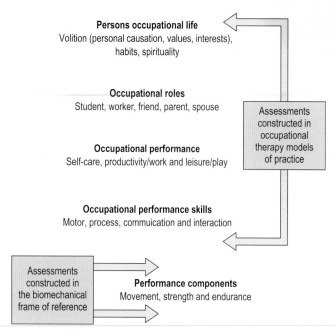

Persons occupational life
Volition (personal causation, values, interests),
habits, spirituality

Occupational roles
Student, worker, friend, parent, spouse

Assessments
constructed in
occupational
therapy models
of practice

Occupational performance
Self-care, productivity/work and leisure/play

Occupational performance skills
Motor, process, commuication and interaction

Assessments
constructed in
the biomechanical
frame of reference

Performance components
Movement, strength and endurance

Fig 14.2 • Assessment and occupation. Reproduced with permission from McMillan and Forsyth (2001).

detailed evidence to understand an individual's specific occupational performance problems. Because of the nature of the biomechanical frame of reference, assessments mostly relate to movement. There are various methods (mostly quantitative) available to assess occupational performance components in terms of movement, strength and endurance. The majority of these are readily available and can be easily applied with some practice. During the last few years there has been an increase in electronic and computer technology to assist the assessment process. Table 14.1 identifies specific testing procedures and sources of reference related to assessing the capacity for movement, strength and endurance. This table also details other factors, such as sensation (including pain) and other tests of function, which may fall within the remit of the biomechanical frame of reference.

Assessment of specific performance components

Occupational therapists frequently use tests of 'function'. These tests tend to examine performance components related to the upper limb and especially power and precision grips of the hand. Examples of these include (Turner et al 2002):

- Bennett Hand Tool Test
- Jebsen–Taylor Hand Function Test
- Moberg Pick Up Test
- Valpar Work Samples.

Principles of intervention

The principles of intervention located in a biomechanical frame of reference should reflect the philosophy and values of our profession. This implies filtering the knowledge associated with the biomechanical frame of reference through the occupation paradigm. Therefore, the philosophy and values of occupation provide the rationale for coherent principles, skills and techniques that are applied to meet the needs of individuals, with regard to movement and occupational performance problems.

Occupation in therapeutic intervention

Occupational therapy intervention varies considerably in terms of contact time with individuals. This may range from performing an assessment and discharge planning service (1 day) to constructing programmes where the individual may be seen by you for longer periods of time (especially on an outpatient basis). This helps distinguish, to some

Table 14.1 Tests of function

Test	Reference
Movement	
Range of motion (ROM) in joints	
Observation	Pedretti & Early (2001)
Goniometry	Neistadt & Crepeau (1998)
Odstock method	Roberts (1989)
Strength	
Muscle power	
Oxford Rating Scale	Trombly & Radomski (2002)
Other scales	Neistadt & Crepeau (1998)
Grip strength in the hand	
Dynamometer	Trombly & Radomski (2002)
	Pedretti & Early (2001)
Pinch strength in the fingers	
Pinch meter	Trombly & Radomski (2002)
Muscle bulk	
Observation	Trombly & Radomski (2002)
Tape measure	Trombly & Radomski (2002)
Presence of swelling in limbs	
Observation	Turner et al (2002)
Tape measure	Neistadt & Crepeau (1998)
Volumeter	Pedretti & Early (2001)
Endurance	
Observation	Neistadt & Crepeau (1998)
Cardiorespiratory	Neistadt & Crepeau (1998)
Functional	Neistadt & Crepeau (1998)
Sensation	
Light touch and pressure	Trombly & Radomski (2002)
Weinstein monofilament	Trombly & Radomski (2002)
Thermal sensation	Trombly & Radomski (2002)
Pain*	Trombly & Radomski (2002)

*The management of pain as part of the biomechanical frame of reference is a contentious issue. Pain is a *perception* (not merely a sensation) formulated in the cerebrum and is therefore within the remit of a different frame of reference; however, pain can be apparent in a multitude of conditions that fall within the remit of the biomechanical frame of reference and affect the occupational performance of individuals.

extent, practice that attempts to restore, maintain or compensate for 'lost' (temporarily or permanently) occupational performance. The use of meaningful occupation energizes intervention and defines the unique philosophy of occupational therapy (Trombly 1995, Ferguson & Trombly 1997, Fisher 1998, Perrin 2001). In summary, principles related to the quality of movement, intervention techniques and meaningful occupation are blended together to manage the problems that the individual experiences. This usually relates to restoring (or compensating) an individual's physical performance in terms of movement, strength and endurance in order to carry out tasks in self-care, work and leisure in different contexts of practice.

Practice settings

Occupational therapists tend to be employed in different practice settings, and usually these are denoted by specialized areas of expertise. The application of techniques associated with the biomechanical frame of reference is usually experienced within the following areas of practice:

- amputation and amputee problems
- assistive technology (wheelchairs, orthotics and other devices for home and personal use)
- burns and plastic surgery
- cardiac rehabilitation

- general medical problems
- hand therapy
- housing (ergonomic) modifications in the community
- older people (usually problems with falls, stability and mobility)
- orthopaedics
- orthotics and prosthetics
- pain management
- spinal cord injury
- work rehabilitation
- worksite modification.

All of the above may take place in hospital or community settings.

In order to link the theory described in this chapter clearly with practice, the next part of this chapter will illustrate the use of the biomechanical frame of reference with a hypothetical case study of a person who has difficulties in her daily life with some occupational performances.

CASE STUDY

Ms A

Ms A is a 40-year-old woman who currently lives independently in her own apartment, with a very supportive partner. She has a 5-year history of rheumatoid arthritis (RA) and reports that the main effects of her condition on her occupational lifestyle are fatigue at work and some experience of pain.

Ms A is employed full-time in an office as a clerical assistant, mainly using a computer for multiple tasks in her worker role.

She still pursues leisure interests in terms of socializing with friends, reading and listening to music, but has given up skiing, cycling and generally keeping fit.

Ms A appears to manage (in her own words) her occupational roles; however, she does report having some minor difficulties during an initial interview with the occupational therapist.

ASSESSMENT

The occupational therapist could utilize various rigorous assessments drawn from MOHO (Kielhofner 2007) or use the COPM (Law et al 2005) to collect self-report data regarding occupations. Assessments related to movement, strength and endurance are then administered to collect objective data on specific performance components. Based on the client's perceived problems (from the selected occupational therapy conceptual model of practice assessments) and objective assessments from the biomechanical frame of reference, the following is apparent:

- *Occupational roles*. No major concerns expressed at this time in terms of fulfilling her role expectations of being a partner, daughter, worker and friend.

- *Occupational performance*. No self-care problems evident except in relation to heavy housework (lack of endurance). Work and productivity (especially using a computer keyboard) provoke more anxiety in terms of future capability. Leisure is not reported as being problematic.
- *Occupational performance skills*. Problems at times in terms of mobility, reaching, bending, manipulating and endurance in her occupations.
- *Occupational performance components*. Objective findings related to loss of muscle bulk, strength, hand grip and overall endurance.
- *Environment*. Problems with work environment, attitudes towards her productivity and minor problems in her home environment.

INTERVENTION

The aim of the biomechanical frame of reference in this case study is to address the quality of movement in Ms A's occupations. General objectives relative to Ms A are to:

1. prevent deterioration and maintain existing movement for occupational performance (computer usage at work, joint protection techniques and acknowledging/managing pain)
2. restore movement for occupational performance, if possible (improving muscle strength)
3. compensate/adapt for loss of motion in occupational performance (energy conservation techniques and using assistive technology).

It should be noted that, whilst individual objectives are documented above, all three objectives are probably being addressed simultaneously when Ms A engages in any occupation in a therapeutic manner.

Using computers at work

Ms A uses a computer at her work every day and therefore the topic of ergonomics is relevant to her situation. Ergonomics is the application of scientific information concerning human beings to the design of objects, systems and environments for human use (Pheasant 1991).

This subject is principally associated with the design of everyday objects in the environment, and, in this case, analysing the computer at the point of interaction with Ms A, to prevent OOS, postural deformity, excessive fatigue and pain, whilst also ensuring safety.

In relation to occupational performance in its widest context, occupational therapists should be concerned with biological efficiency, health and safety in the home and workplace, and the comfort and ease of use of objects (Nicholson 1999, Hignett 2000). The College of Occupational Therapists has produced a vocational rehabilitation strategy (2008) and this document would provide more information on this important role for an occupational therapist intervening with Ms A.

OOS is defined as those disorders that are caused, precipitated or aggravated by repeated exertions or movements of the human body. It involves a number of similar conditions arising from overuse of soft tissues (tendons, muscles, nerves, vascular structures), usually of the upper limb, and is due to repeated 'micro trauma' rather than sudden instant injury (McNaughton 1997). Ms A may be at risk of developing OOS because of repetitive or prolonged keyboard use, awkward postures due to poorly designed chairs, localized contact stress on her forearms and hands due to the table edge and poorly designed work stations in general. Ms A may complain of stiffness, discomfort, pain, alteration in sensation and clumsiness because of OOS, in addition to the problems associated with rheumatoid arthritis. In response, intervention may be delivered in terms of altering the ergonomics of her computer work station and reinforcing the following elements.

Chair

Ensure that Ms A uses the correct chair, which should have a five-spoked base with castors and an adjustable backrest. The backrest angle should be adjusted to 110%, and ought to support her lumbar region up to the inferior aspect of her scapulae. Adjust her chair for height; when her fingers are placed on the keyboard, her forearms ought to be roughly parallel with the floor. Ensure that her feet are firmly placed on the floor with her knee angle at roughly 90–110%. If her feet are not touching the floor, use a footrest (a strong ringbinder would suffice if cost is an issue for her employer). Some space between the top of the thighs and the underside of the desk ought to exist.

Work station

Adjust the position of Ms A's monitor by ensuring that her feet are flat on the floor and her head is in the midline; when she is looking straight ahead, the top of the screen should be at or just below eye level height. The monitor should be at least 18–30 inches from her eyes (arm's length). The posture of her hands on the keyboard is important. Preferably, the hands and wrists should be neutral relative to the forearm (no excessive flexion, extension, or radial or ulnar deviation). Instruct her to hold the mouse loosely and to avoid resting the forearm or wrist on the edge of the desk. Discourage hyperextending the little finger and advise her to use a light touch when clicking the mouse. Use work-station devices, e.g. a copy stand or document holder, a gel wrist rest, a gel mouse mat, a lumbar roll if necessary, and a footrest and telephone headset if appropriate. Check her arc of reach on the desk when seated and place important objects to hand to prevent overstretch (Jacobs & Bettencourt 1995).

Lighting

Try to reduce glare on the computer screen by placing the monitor at right angles to a window (light source), if possible, using blinds on windows if these are fitted. Tilt the monitor slightly so that overhead lighting does not create screen glare. Use the brightness, colour and contrast controls on the monitor to compensate for glare.

Posture

Encourage Ms A to take frequent breaks from keyboarding, by varying her routines and walking about to perform other tasks, e.g. a 30-second break every 10 minutes.

The same advice would be applied to Ms A if she also uses a computer at home for work or leisure. You should consult Holmes (2007) for further information on vocational rehabilitation.

Joint protection and occupational performance

Joint protection is principally an educational and training programme used in conjunction with connective tissue diseases, and has historically been utilized in the management of rheumatoid disease in the upper limb. The principles are designed to teach Ms A about the inflammatory process and potential deformities seen in rheumatoid arthritis (Hammond 1997, Hammond & Lincoln 1999). Instruction in joint protection techniques addresses the following points:

- reducing joint stress
- decreasing pain
- preserving joint structure
- maximizing occupational performance and conserving energy.

Ms A will require careful instruction, so that joint protection techniques can be consistently employed in all of her occupations to maintain maximal capacity for motion and to prevent damage and long-term deformity.

Seven principles of joint protection are outlined below in title only, and further research is recommended in order to understand fully the detail required for implementing each of these principles before instructing Ms A in their application. The detail regarding these principles can be found in most occupational therapy textbooks related to physical dysfunction (e.g. Pedretti & Early 2001):

- Respect pain at all times.
- Maintain muscle strength and joint range of movement.
- Avoid positions of deformity and deforming stress.
- Use each joint in its most stable, anatomical and functional position.
- Use the strongest joints available for the activity.
- Avoid using muscles or holding joints in one position for any undue length of time.
- Never begin an activity that cannot be stopped immediately.

The success of these techniques with Ms A depends on the need for education in terms of teaching her about preventing deterioration or maintaining her present occupational performance. Occupational therapists are constantly required to reinforce existing knowledge or impart new skills, which may alter habits in some way to facilitate change. In relation to Ms A, the key to learning (and teaching) involves using the techniques in conjunction with her occupational performances in self-care, work and leisure that she has identified as problematic. Effective learning methods also imply planning ahead, imparting information at the correct level, providing clear instructions, eliciting feedback, evaluating learning, promoting the highest level of learning and using different methods to impart new information (French et al 1994, Neistadt & Crepeau 1998).

Ms A may also have a problem with chronic pain. Although it is beyond the remit of this chapter to deal with the extensive information about the management of chronic pain, attention to computer usage, joint protection techniques and pacing during occupations may help to change the perception of chronic pain. Tyldesley and Grieve (2002) give further information regarding the occupational therapist's role in the management of pain and also present a related case study.

Improving muscle strength

Muscle strength is the amount of force that can be exerted by a single muscle or groups of muscles in a voluntary contraction. Muscle strength can be seen in isometric and isotonic activity, both of which are required for occupational performance. There is a relationship between the recruitment of motor units and the production of maximum muscle tension in response to external loads on muscle groups. Periods of muscular inactivity due to disease or trauma may lead to muscle atrophy (decreased strength), the inability to sustain performance and a loss of co-ordination during occupational performances. In order to increase muscle strength, stress (demand) has to be applied to a muscle through the use of occupational performances in order that all the motor units are recruited

to maintain and restore the muscle. This activity will ensure maximum (or near-maximum) contraction of the muscle, thus hypertrophying muscle fibres by influencing changes in the amount of contractile proteins. An increase in the amount of proteins and cross-bridges improves muscle cross-sectional size and therefore strength (Jackson et al 2002).

Hypothetically, muscle tension needs to reach 50–67% of the maximum potential capability of that muscle or group of muscles, and an increase in strength will result. This implies that, as the muscle increases in strength, the amount of stress placed upon it should also be increased over time, to increase strength further. This is termed the 'overload principle' and requires grading of stress through occupations, placed on the client's affected muscle groups over time. Overloading is a positive stressor and will improve adaptation to the demands placed on Ms A when carrying out her self-care, work and leisure performances. Trombly & Radomski (2002) argue that *occupation as a means* of therapeutic change and *occupation as an end result* have to be apparent to the individual.

Muscle strengthening (through overloading) involves the analysis and grading of occupation and is dependent on the following factors:

- type of occupation (self-care, work/productivity and leisure)
- intensity (resistance of muscles against the performance)
- duration (time taken to complete the occupation)
- speed (of the limbs and so on during the occupation)
- frequency (how often the occupation is undertaken).

Occupations should be motivating and have meaning for Ms A in relation to her occupational performances. The most important factor other than the occupation itself is the intensity, which concerns the muscle groups being resisted whilst attempting to produce motion for occupation. Resistance can be altered by changing the position of Ms A relative to the occupation, changing the length of lever arms, changing the materials used, increasing the difficulty of the occupation, using different tools, and changing the weight of any objects used for the occupation.

Engaging in occupational performance is usually aimed at restoring muscle strength and improving motion in one area of the body: for example, the upper limbs. However, in order to carry out her desired occupations in a sustained fashion, Ms A's muscular (whole-body) endurance also has to be improved. For example, this could be attained by looking at the weight of the clothes that she loads into her washing machine and gradually increasing that load over time. The 'reserve' of the cardiorespiratory system in resisting fatigue is then considered as part of the occupation. Pedretti (1996) provides further detail on increasing cardiorespiratory reserve.

Energy conservation

Energy conservation techniques are generally used in the management of chronic pathological conditions in which strength and particularly endurance are compromised. This implies compensation on a temporary or permanent basis. The aims of the techniques are to eliminate wasted body motion in order to preserve physical and psychological energy resources. This is especially the case when Ms A perceives a relapse in the clinical course of her condition of rheumatoid arthritis.

Ms A could be instructed to reduce energy expenditure (physical and psychological) by planning ahead, organizing storage in the home and at work, sitting to perform kitchen work instead of standing where possible, reducing the weight of briefcases, bags of shopping and so on, and ensuring good working conditions with respect to lighting, ventilation and heating.

She could also utilize alternative sources of energy (human resources and assistive technology devices) by asking her partner, immediate family and relatives to undertake certain tasks for her at times (shopping, laundry, vacuuming). In the longer term, if her condition did deteriorate, then volunteer and 'home help' services (ironing, laundry, etc.) would be worth considering.

Assistive technology and occupational performance

This section describes technology that can help an individual maintain, restore or compensate for loss of occupational performance.

Assistive technology can be utilized over short or long periods of time, depending on the client's potential for restoration or compensation. Assistive technology in its simplest form includes personal and domestic devices: for example, adapted cutlery, plates, easy chairs, dressing devices, communication devices, bath boards, kitchen devices and manual wheelchairs. Some of these simpler devices may be appropriate for Ms A at certain times. On a more complex level, static and dynamic orthoses, prostheses, burn pressure garments, electric wheelchairs, stair lifts, adapted vehicles and environmental control systems can also be viewed as assistive technology (Van Schaik 2000, Weilandt & Strong 2000).

One aspect of assistive technology that may assist Ms A temporarily is the use of a wrist–hand orthosis or splint. Orthotics (or splinting) involves the design, manufacture and application of thermoplastic material to manage individuals' biomechanical problems. Although thermoplastic orthoses can potentially be applied to any area of the body, occupational therapists most often apply orthoses to the prehensile structures, i.e. the hand and upper limb, and locomotor structures, i.e. the foot and lower limb.

In general, orthoses are biomechanical in design and are used to manage problems associated with limitations resulting from problems of the musculoskeletal system, peripheral nervous system and integumentary system. Despite the different designs (static and dynamic orthoses) and materials, orthoses are generally used to meet the following aims, dependent on the individual's problems:

- to achieve an optimal anatomical position and physiological state, therefore maximizing functional ability
- to provide pain relief
- to facilitate correct anatomical healing
- to prevent and correct soft-tissue deformity
- to maintain the function of unaffected parts
- to maintain the improvements achieved by other forms of treatment
- to restore or maintain joint alignment and stabilization
- to assist the function of weak muscles and prevent overstretch
- to provide a substitution for absent muscle power
- to protect vulnerable anatomical structures.

In addition to the skill of manufacture and application, comprehensive assessment procedures and specific knowledge regarding the musculoskeletal structures necessary for motion are necessary. Effective management of problems by the application of orthoses depends as much on efficient manufacture as the clients' attitudes to wearing the device. Individuals like Ms A have to understand why wearing the orthosis is important, this being accomplished through educational principles, which are the key to successful management and treatment. See Coppard and Lohman (2001) for further information about orthoses.

SUMMARY

Some occupational therapists have argued that a biomechanical frame of reference is essentially reductionist and narrow in its focus, because it is based on a biomedical view of the world (Turner et al 2002). However, this stance reflects a 'bottom-up' approach to practice, and occupational therapists who attempt to use the technology of the biomechanical frame of reference *in isolation* from occupational therapy conceptual models of practice will certainly find its usage frustrating.

In isolation, the biomechanical frame of reference is not universally applicable to every individual, even those with movement problems; however, the management of any individual (e.g. Ms A) will always require a blend of conceptual models of practice and frames of reference. For example, the successful management of Ms A will require knowledge about occupational therapy conceptual models of practice, the biomechanical frame of reference and probably the cognitive behavioural frame of reference (see Chapter 12 for further information) in order to address problems of occupational performance created by conditions that affect *mind and body together*.

Ultimately, it is not necessarily the theoretical base of a specific frame of reference that makes it narrow in application, but one's view of the world as an occupational therapist and how different conceptual models of practice/frames of reference are used to address the multiple needs of an individual like Ms A.

Areas for future research

Kielhofner (2009, p.76) documents the following areas of current interest in the application of a biomechanical frame of reference in occupational therapy:

- the relationship between musculoskeletal capacity and success in occupations
- muscle action and movement patterns used in different task conditions
- how the purpose and meaning of activities affect therapy compliance, effort, fatigue and improvement in movement capacity.

Summary

Kielhofner (2009, p.79) concludes that the biomechanical model is a unique model of practice in occupational therapy and states:

> Given the centrality of movement problems in occupational therapy clients and the long history of this approach in occupational therapy practice, there is no

doubt that the [biomechanical] model will continue to be a vital part of occupational therapy science and practice.

Reflective learning

- What features make a biomechanical frame of reference different from other frames of reference in this book?
- Which areas of human performance does a biomechanical frame of reference help you understand as an occupational therapy student?
- In what ways could a biomechanical frame of reference inform you how to assess and intervene with people who have issues in their daily occupations?
- What would be the consequences of assuming that a biomechanical frame of reference could be applied in isolation from models and other frames of reference in occupational therapy?
- Reflect on your most recent practice experiences. In what ways could you have enriched the interventions that you undertook with individuals with movement problems in their daily occupations?

References

Braveman, B., Robson, M., Velozo, C., et al., 2005. Worker Role Interview (WRI). MOHO Clearing House, Chicago.

Canadian Association of Occupational Therapists, 2002. Enabling Occupation: An Occupational Therapy Perspective. Canadian Association of Occupational Therapists, Ottawa.

College of Occupational Therapists, 2008. Vocational Rehabilitation Strategy. College of Occupational Therapists, London.

Coppard, B.M., Lohman, H., 2001. Introduction to Splinting: A Critical Thinking and Problem Solving Approach, second ed. Mosby, St Louis.

Dutton, R., 1998. Biomechanical frame of reference. In: Neistadt, M.E., Crepeau, E.B. (Eds.), Willard and Spackman's Occupational Therapy. ninth ed. Lippincott, Philadelphia.

Ferguson, J.M., Trombly, C.A., 1997. The effect of added-purpose and meaningful occupation on motor learning. American Journal of

Occupational Therapy 51 (7), 508–515.

Fisher, A.G., 1998. Uniting practice and theory in an occupational framework. British Journal of Occupational Therapy 52 (7), 509–521.

French, S., Neville, S., Laing, J., 1994. Teaching and Learning: A Guide for Therapists. Butterworth–Heinemann, Oxford.

Hammond, A., 1997. Joint protection education: what are we doing? British Journal of Occupational Therapy 60 (9), 401–406.

Hammond, A., Lincoln, N., 1999. The Joint Protection Knowledge Assessment (JPKA): knowledge and reliability. British Journal of Occupational Therapy 62 (3), 117–122.

Hignett, S., 2000. Occupational therapy and ergonomics: two professions exploring their identities. British Journal of Occupational Therapy 63 (3), 137–139.

Holmes, J., 2007. Vocational Rehabilitation. Blackwell, Oxford.

Jackson, J., Gray, J.M., Zemke, R., 2002. Optimizing abilities and capacities: range of motion, strength and endurance. In: Trombly, C.A., Radomski, M.V. (Eds.), Occupational Therapy for Physical Dysfunction, fifth ed. Lippincott Williams & Wilkins, Philadelphia.

Jacobs, K., Bettencourt, C.M., 1995. Ergonomics for Therapists. Butterworth–Heinemann, Boston.

Kielhofner, G., 1997. Conceptual Foundations of Occupational Therapy, second ed. FA Davis, Philadelphia.

Kielhofner, G., 2007. Model of Human Occupation: Theory and Application, fourth ed. Lippincott Williams & Wilkins, Philadelphia.

Kielhofner, G., 2009. Conceptual Foundations of Occupational Therapy, fourth ed. FA Davis, Philadelphia.

Kramer, P., Hinojosa, J., Royeen, C.B., 2003. Perspectives in Human Occupation: Participation in Life. Lippincott Williams & Wilkins, Philadelphia.

Law, M., Cooper, B., Strong, S., et al., 1996. The Person–Environment–Occupation Model: a transactive approach to occupational performance. Canadian Journal of Occupational Therapy 63 (1), 9–23.

Law, M., Baptiste, S., Carswell-Opzoomer, A., et al., 2005. Canadian Occupational Performance Measure, fourth ed. Canadian Association of Occupational Therapists, Toronto.

Law, M., Baptiste, S., Carswell, A., et al., 2005. Canadian Occupational Performance Measure. CAOT Publications ACE, Toronto.

Mathiowetz, V., 1993. Role of physical performance component evaluations in occupational therapy functional assessments. British Journal of Occupational Therapy 47 (3), 225–230.

McNaughton, A., 1997. Occupational overuse syndrome/repetitive strain injury: the occupational therapist's role. British Journal of Occupational Therapy 60 (2), 69–72.

Molineux, M., 2004. Occupation for Occupational Therapists. Blackwell, Oxford.

Neistadt, M.E., Crepeau, E.B., 1998. Willard and Spackman's Occupational Therapy, ninth ed. Lippincott, Philadelphia.

Nicholson, J., 1999. Management strategies for musculoskeletal stress in the parents of children with restricted mobility. British Journal of Therapy and Rehabilitation 62 (5), 206–212.

Pedretti, L.W., 1996. Occupational Therapy: Practice Skills for Physical Dysfunction, fourth ed. Mosby, St Louis.

Pedretti, L.W., Early, M.B., 2001. Occupational Therapy: Practice Skills for Physical Dysfunction, fifth ed. Mosby, St Louis.

Perrin, T., 2001. Don't despise the fluffy bunny: a reflection from practice. British Journal of Occupational Therapy 64 (3), 129–134.

Pheasant, S., 1991. Ergonomics, Work and Health. MacMillan, London.

Roberts, C., 1989. The Odstock Hand Assessment. British Journal of Occupational Therapy 52 (7), 256–261.

Spaulding, S.J., 2005. Meaningful Motion: Biomechanics for Occupational Therapists. Churchill Livingstone, Edinburgh.

Strong, S., Rigby, P., Stewart, D., et al., 1999. Application of the Person–Environment–Occupation Model: a practical tool. Canadian Journal of Occupational Therapy 66 (3), 122–133.

Trombly, C.A., 1995. Occupation: purposefulness and meaningfulness as therapeutic mechanisms. British Journal of Occupational Therapy 49 (11), 960–972.

Trombly, C.A., Radomski, M.V., 2002. Occupational Therapy for Physical Dysfunction, fifth ed. Lippincott Williams & Wilkins, Philadelphia.

Turner, A., Foster, M., Johnson, S.E., 2002. Occupational Therapy and Physical Dysfunction: Principles, Skills and Practice, fifth ed. Churchill Livingstone, Edinburgh.

Tyldesley, B., Grieve, J.I., 2002. Muscles, Nerves and Movement in Human Occupation, third ed. Blackwell Science, Oxford.

Van Schaik, P., 2000. Adapted technology for people with special needs: the case of smart cards and terminals. British Journal of Occupational Therapy 63 (3), 111–114.

Wielandt, T., Strong, J., 2000. Compliance with prescribed adaptive equipment. British Journal of Occupational Therapy 63 (2), 65–75.

Wilby, H.J., 2007. The importance of maintaining a focus on performance components in occupational therapy practice. British Journal of Occupational Therapy 70 (3), 129–132.

Theoretical approaches to motor control and cognitive–perceptual function

15

Sally Feaver   Leisle Ezekiel

OVERVIEW

Stroke is a major cause of disability and often results in significant occupational dysfunction. The stroke survivors' ability to engage in their occupations may be affected by motor, cognitive or perceptual dysfunction. Consequently, occupational therapists have an important part to play in stroke rehabilitation.

Occupational therapists use a variety of approaches to aid their planning of interventions for people with stroke and often aim to maximize the recovery that occurs following stroke. This chapter focuses on some of the main approaches used to address motor dysfunction and cognitive–perceptual dysfunction in adults.

Firstly, the motor control frame of reference is explored. This frame of reference includes both the normal movement (neurodevelopmental) and the task-orientated approach. Secondly, the adaptive approach and the remedial approach for cognitive and perceptual dysfunction are introduced. The theory, practice and evidence base for all of these approaches are considered and case scenarios provide clear examples of how each affects occupational therapy intervention.

The chapter concludes with a comment about the need for standardization of practice using these approaches, as the lack of protocols and guidelines for specific assessments and implementation of approaches makes conducting evidence-based practice difficult.

Key points

- Developments in neuroscience and movement science have influenced our understanding of motor control and its organization within the central nervous system.

Key points—cont'd

- Normal movement and motor relearning are two widely used approaches in occupational therapy for the treatment of motor problems following stroke.
- Both approaches reflect current theories of motor control and reacquisition of motor skill but have a limited evidence base to support their efficacy.
- Approaches used to design interventions for cognitive and perceptual dysfunction are not as cohesively supported by a set of theories as the motor control frame of reference.
- There is considerable evidence to support the use of the adaptive approach for cognitive and perceptual dysfunction and some evidence to support specific interventions that might fall under the remedial approach.

Introduction

Stroke is the second most common cause of death and one of the leading causes of disability, in both the UK and the rest of the world (Murray & Lopez 1997, World Health Organization 2002). In 2001, it was estimated that stroke caused almost 10% of all deaths worldwide (World Health Organization 2002) and over two-thirds of these occurred in developing countries (Truelsen 2006). Within Europe, there are currently 6 million people who have survived a stroke and this figure is set to rise over the next 20 years (Truelsen 2006). It is difficult to give a global picture of the overall cost of stroke in terms of health, social care and loss of earnings but a recent study conducted for the National Audit Office calculated the cost of stroke in the UK to be £7 billion a year (Saka et al 2006).

It is vital, therefore, that effective initiatives are developed both to prevent stroke and to reduce the levels of disability experienced following stroke. On a micro scale, this provides occupational therapists with the imperative to offer effective rehabilitation interventions and to maximize the individual's occupational performance and occupational engagement in their recovery from stroke.

Stroke care and rehabilitation is an area of practice that is rapidly changing. The introduction of the National Service Framework established standards of care, the national stroke clinical guidelines identified best practice for clinicians (Intercollegiate stroke working party 2008) and there is an increasing evidence base to support interventions (Saka et al 2006). Key healthcare individuals work together, learn together, and draw on common publications and practice guidelines.

Approximately 40% of people who experience stroke are left with a substantial level of disability; this may be as a consequence of hemiplegia, cognitive difficulties or perceptual problems (Kwan 2001). The often complex nature of stroke and its sequelae has a profound impact on the person's occupational engagement. Occupational therapists often aim to remediate some of these problems in the acute phase of recovery or use compensatory approaches as a focus for their interventions (Walker et al 2000). However, there is no consensus on which is the best approach to use or on the exact nature of occupational therapy practice for this group of people (Walker et al 2000).

Consequently, this chapter aims to explore the main approaches currently used to plan occupational therapy interventions for people experiencing stroke (motor dysfunction and cognitive–perceptual dysfunction), as well as their theoretical basis and available evidence.

The motor control frame of reference

Traditionally, in occupational therapy practice, several intervention approaches have been used to enable people with neurological dysfunction to achieve optimal occupational performance. Following theorists from the 1960s, these approaches have been based on assumptions about the hierarchical nature of motor control (Shumway-Cook & Woollacott 2007). In recent years, these traditional approaches have been challenged, as the understanding of neuroanatomy and neuroplasticity has advanced.

One specific example of this, with clinical application for occupational therapy, is the previously held assumption about the way in which damage to the central nervous system in adults could be remediated. Using assumed knowledge of the hierarchical nature of neurodevelopment, the mastery of gross motor tasks was a necessary precursor to developing fine motor movement.

As our knowledge has advanced, some of the assumptions upon which the approaches were based have been disproved. A systems approach is now a major influence in our understanding of motor control and describes motor control as distributed across several interconnected subsystems of the central nervous system that act in parallel (Gentile 1998). Current practice has taken account of this new understanding, embracing a more contextual approach or systems approach to motor functioning.

The following approaches all come under the broad heading of 'motor control'. They require an understanding of motor control and of how the central nervous system processes sensory and perceptual information and coordinates muscles and joints to produce controlled movement. Motor control, however, is about action and purposeful movement as part of an activity or task (Shumway-Cook & Woollacott 2007).

The implications of this are that a person's movements are affected by the environment in which they are performed and the demands of the task. For example, a standing person reaching for a bottle of water and taking a drink elicits different movements from those of a person sitting and drinking from a cup. The task of reaching, grasping and taking a drink is altered by the person's position and the size and weight of the object being held. Motor control intervention approaches must therefore consider both the activity being conducted and the environments in which it is performed, when looking at a person's recovery and improvement in motor performance (Mathiowetz 2004).

The main assumptions of the motor control approaches are that:

- Motor learning results in reorganization of the cortex (Teasel et al 2008).
- Motor control is a prerequisite for precise or skilled movement.
- Musculoskeletal and neurological systems need to work together to produce skilled movement.
- Sensory feedback and feedback from the environment are key in the development of skilled movement.

- There is an element of hierarchy in movement control.
- Skills practised over time form patterns of skilled movement (Shumway-Cook & Woollacott 2007).

The Bobath/normal movement/neurodevelopmental approach and the movement science/task-orientated approaches are now described in more detail. All of these approaches are considered to be remedial, as they focus on changing the primary pathology.

Bobath/normal movement/neurodevelopmental approach

Berta and Karel Bobath first developed the Bobath concept in 1940. They evolved this approach with the expectation that it might help improve motor performance. The two main principles of treatment were based on the inhibition of abnormal movements and the facilitation of more normal movement patterns. Sessions were traditionally 'hands-on', with the focus being on reducing tone and the facilitation of both active and passive movement (Bobath 1990).

Since then, the Bobath concept has evolved in light of new understanding about motor control and motor learning (Howle 2003). However, this evolution has proven problematic both because of the oral tradition of passing down skills and beliefs in this approach, and because of the slow development of its theoretical underpinning (Lennon & Ashburn 2000). Despite this uncertainty, the Bobath concept continues to be a dominant approach in the recovery of motor control following stroke, in both the UK and the USA (Walker et al 2000, Natarajan et al 2008).

The main aim of the normal movement approach is to facilitate the recovery of movement resulting from neuroplasticity and physiological changes following stroke. The more general aims of intervention are to achieve functional patterns of movement through addressing underlying problems such as abnormal tone, poor postural control and the use of sensory and proprioceptive control to facilitate movement (IBITA 2008). The following is a description of the basic principles and theoretical assumptions of this approach, as used with adults with hemiplegia.

- Recovery of function is based on neuroplasticity (namely, the ability of the adult central nervous system to change following damage).
- Recovery of function is influenced by the person's positioning and how they attempt to move (IBITA 2008).

- A systems model of motor control of the central nervous system.
- Neuroplasticity is shaped by manipulation of sensory inputs, mainly proprioceptive (Lennon & Ashburn 2000).
- The relearning of normal movement occurs through experience and with the active participation of the person (Lennon & Ashburn 2000).
- The development of postural control is an essential part of skill development.
- Postural control uses feedback and feedforward mechanisms (i.e. it is anticipatory).
- Postural control activity is initiated at the base of support (Connelly & Montgomery 2002).
- Problems with strength are secondary (Lennon & Ashburn 2000).
- Facilitating the components of normal movement will lead to improvement in functional tasks.

Principles of intervention

The main components of normal movement include the central postural control mechanism (i.e. balance reactions, tone, reciprocal innovation and sensory–motor feedback).

Interventions include the use of proximal and distal key points, postural sets, facilitation and inhibition. Whilst the postural alignment of key areas of motor control, use of inhibitory or facilitatory techniques to influence tone, and the facilitation of normal movement patterns remain key features, there is now greater emphasis on the integration of postural control with task-specific movement (IBITA 2008).

The essential focus of intervention is the facilitation of movement on the affected side, trying to achieve symmetry of both body and movement. Initially, the therapist uses handling techniques to guide movements until the client is able to maintain some control. Some essential principles for intervention include orientation towards the affected side, facilitation of normal movement and the development of coordinated use of both hands. Positioning to achieve weight-bearing over the affected side and placing affected limbs in the field of vision are also important (Levit 2008).

Evidence base

The Bobath approach is widely used in Europe, although evidence continues to suggest that Bobath is not superior to approaches based on movement science (Luke et al 2004, Van Vliet et al 2005). There are elements of the Bobath approach that may, however, be in conflict with current evidence and recommended practice. For example, the use of manual guiding of movement is not indicated by our knowledge of motor learning; the Bobath approach traditionally does not incorporate the necessary emphasis on practice of tasks and task-focused movements, and therapists may limit the use of visual and verbal feedback, thereby affecting the person's motor performance (Lennon & Ashburn 2000).

The UK National Clinical Guidelines for Stroke (Intercollegiate Stroke Working Party 2008) advise that multiprofessional teams adopt the same approach towards rehabilitation of motor dysfunction, as consistency is important. It is also recommended that, whichever approach is used, the person with stroke is given as much opportunity as possible to practise movements and tasks in all the environments where these tasks are likely to be performed.

It is worth noting that research into the effectiveness of different therapeutic approaches predominantly considers physiotherapy and more research is needed to establish the efficacy of specific treatment approaches and techniques used by occupational therapists (Legg et al 2007).

In summary, there is no conclusive evidence that completely supports or refutes the use of the Bobath approach for people with stroke, and some traditional elements of the intervention may be in conflict with recommended practice. It is clear, however, that the Bobath concept needs to be defined and standardized so as to aid development of practice guidelines (Paci 2003).

Clinical application

An example of intervention following the normal movement/neurodevelopmental approach is given in the following case study.

CASE STUDY

Joe

Joe has difficulty dressing his upper body. He is able to sit independently and symmetrically. He finds he is unable to put his right arm into the sleeve of a jumper and pull the jumper over his head. He also struggles to put on his coat. He used to put his right arm in first and then pull the coat around to put his right arm in. However, he finds his shoulder movements are limited and describes his arm as 'feeling heavy'. He is able to grasp and release objects in his right hand and can oppose his thumb to each finger.

NEURODEVELOPMENTAL APPROACH

The occupational therapist observed Joe's attempts to put on his coat, and noted that he was limited in his range of movement, particularly shoulder flexion, extension and external rotation. He tended to compensate for his limited movements by flexing his trunk to his left side and abducting his shoulder in order to raise his right hand.

The occupational therapist further assessed Joe for his sense of proprioception in his upper limb, passive range of movement in his upper limb and shoulder girdle (particularly concerning his shoulder movements and considering any subluxation), postural tone in both his trunk and his upper limb, and alignment of key points.

After liaising with Joe's physiotherapist, the occupational therapist identified the fact that Joe's difficulties arose from the low tone and weakness he experienced in his shoulder and shoulder girdle. He also had limited movement in his scapula, which was having an impact on his shoulder movement and his ability to place his hand successfully and effortlessly.

In preparation for Joe practising a dressing task successfully, the occupational therapist considered the environment in which the task would be performed. The therapist identified how the environment might be used, and graded the task to facilitate both Joe's motor control and his successful completion of the task. The therapist decided to start the intervention with Joe seated on a plinth, thus providing a firm base for him to sit on (a lesser base of support than a chair would give, for example) and facilitating a general increase in his postural tone. The therapist then facilitated Joe into an aligned and upright sitting posture, and mobilized his shoulder and scapula so that his scapula was protracted, ensuring that Joe had sufficient muscle length to achieve the movement.

Joe then engaged with the task of dressing, with the therapist continually monitoring his position, movement and tone, using 'hand-over-hand' guiding when Joe attempted more difficult movements. The therapist recognized the importance of preventing Joe from adopting abnormal movement patterns during the task.

Once Joe began to demonstrate increased motor skill within this task, the therapist increased the difficulty of the task and changed the context in which it was practised. For example, Joe began to dress whilst sitting on the side of his bed, and also practised putting his coat on whilst standing.

Task-orientated approach

The task-orientated approach is based on a systems theory of motor control and includes movement science-based approaches such as motor relearning (Shumway-Cook & Woollacott 2007). Motor learning is concerned with the acquisition or modification of movement through practice or experience, which then leads to changes in the person's ability to produce skilled actions (Shumway-Cook & Woollacott 2007). Two key principles of motor learning are the interaction between the person, task and environment, and the importance of sensory and cognitive processes in the development of skilled movements. Motor learning and recovery cannot be considered outside of the context of functional tasks and the environments in which a person performs these tasks.

This approach is informed by theories arising from neuroscience and movement science about the organization of motor control, and the role of feedback in skills acquisition and learning processes. The following is a description of the theoretical assumptions and basic principles of the task-orientated approach:

- A distributed control model, i.e. the neural organization of motor control, is dependent on the task and is not reliant on the hierarchical position of the cortex (Connelly & Montgomery 2002).
- The existence of open-loop feedback mechanisms and closed-loop feedback mechanisms highlights the significance of feedback when learning a new motor skill (Connelly & Montgomery 2002).
- Acquisition of a motor skill involves developing the basic crude pattern of movement, which is then refined by experiencing the subtle interplay of passive and active components. Passive components consist of environmental factors (i.e. weight of cup, effect of gravity, air resistance); active components are the dynamic interactions between muscle contraction and joint movement (Gentile 1998). This is described as parallel learning processes: explicit learning (learning that occurs around the development of the crude pattern of movement and is therefore conscious) and implicit learning (i.e. learning that occurs from experiencing the interplay of active and passive components and is unconscious).

Principles of intervention

- The task orientated approach directs the therapist to understand the nature of a persons motor behaviour by considering the context in which the task is being performed, the strategies used to accomplish the task, the underlying sensory, motor, cognitive and perceptual difficulties experienced and how these interact to affect a persons functioning (Shumway-Cook & Woollacott 2007).
- The therapist needs to be aware of the role of information-processing and memory in skill acquisition because cognitive impairments may have an impact on the acquisition of a new skill/task.

- The therapist may use different interventions to facilitate explicit or implicit learning: for example, the use of verbal instruction, changes in environment and demonstration of task access explicit learning processes.
- Repetition of the movement task with as much variation as possible accesses implicit learning processes.
- Movement needs to be functional and goal-focused. The therapist supports problem-solving and memory through the use of prompts.
- Passive handling techniques interfere with the learning process, as the therapist becomes part of the environmental forces and the person does not develop the necessary mapping. The therapist recognizes that initially movements may be inefficient and uncoordinated; therefore, quality of movement is not considered at this stage.
- Extended practice is needed for the person to improve the quality of the movement (Gentile 1998).

Evidence base

The task orientated approach is a relatively new approach and has limited research to support the approach as a whole. However, this approach is based on current theories about motor control and motor relearning (Shumway-Cook & Woollacott 2007). There is also evidence to support specific aspects of the approach, for example, the role of feedback during the acquisition of skilled movement (Wulf, Shea & Lethwaite 2010).

Motor relearning approach

Carr and Shepherd developed the motor relearning approach in the 1980s (Carr & Shepherd 1987) as a result of what they saw as deficiencies in practice. The main assumption in this approach is that the principles of learning a motor skill are the same as relearning the skill (Connelly & Montgomery 2002).

The basic principles of motor relearning are as follows (Carr & Shepherd 2003):

- Motor control is essential to every aspect of performance.
- Regaining ability to perform motor tasks requires a learning process.
- Learning requires a specific goal, practice and feedback.

- The central nervous system uses anticipatory processes to make postural adjustments in preparation for movement to occur.
- Sensory input modulates performance of task.

The approach describes six sections, which represent essential functions of everyday life. These are the upper limb, oro-facial function, sitting up from supine, standing up, standing and walking.

Principles of intervention

Intervention involves the therapist observing the person with stroke whilst attempting identified tasks (such as reaching for an object). The therapist then analyses the movement and identifies which elements of the movement are missing or unsuccessful. Once this assessment is complete, the therapist devises a programme of exercises that enable the person with stroke to practise the missing movement components. During practice, the therapist offers instruction and feedback, as well as explaining the purpose of the exercises and identifying the movement goals. The aim is for the client to master the missing components of movement and practise the entire task. The person with stroke is then encouraged and supported in practising the task in different contexts and environments, to facilitate transference of learning.

Feedback is an essential part of the intervention. The therapist uses demonstration and verbal and visual feedback to support the motor relearning. As soon as some movement control is demonstrated, the person progresses to more complex activities. Reducing spasticity is not central to this approach (Carr & Shepherd 2003).

Movements that have previously been considered as abnormal movement patterns are now thought to be the person's attempts at adapting to the constraints placed by their impairments on their motor control (Carr & Shepherd 1998).

Evidence base

The evidence to support or refute the effectiveness of movement science-based approaches in their entirety remains inconclusive when considering the impact on upper limb function, movement and occupations. There is some evidence that motor relearning may result in shorter hospital stays (Van Peppen et al 2004) and small improvements in activities of daily living. However, in studies where movement science-based approaches resulted in short-term gains when compared with other approaches, those gains were not maintained in the longer term (French et al 2007).

There is evidence to support elements of movement science approaches. For example, the use of verbal feedback during motor skill acquisition, as well as visual and proprioceptive feedback, has been shown to affect motor relearning positively (Cirstea et al 2006).

Although Bobath continues to be a significant influence on occupational therapy practice, both in the UK and internationally (Walker et al 2000, Latham et al 2006, Natarajan et al 2008), there has been a shift towards the application of motor control and motor relearning approaches within functional tasks (Latham et al 2006). Defining the therapeutic content of occupational therapy remains problematic and this lack of standardization clearly raises issues for researchers when attempting to assess the effectiveness of one intervention compared with another (DeJong et al 2005).

Clinical application

An example of intervention following the movement science approach is given in the following case study.

CASE STUDY

Joe: motor relearning approach

As with the neurodevelopmental approach, the therapist observed Joe's movements whilst he dressed himself and noted which movements were difficult. The therapist jointly assessed Joe with the physiotherapist and completed three subsections of the Motor Assessment Scale (focusing on upper arm function, hand movements and advanced hand activities) (Carr et al 1985). This enabled the therapist to identify which aspects of movement Joe was missing when using his affected arm, and provided a baseline for measuring change. The assessment clarified that Joe had difficulty with shoulder flexion, protraction of his scapula and external rotation of his humerus.

Using the principles of motor relearning, the therapist devised a programme of tasks that focused on these separate movement components (Carr & Shepherd 2000). For example, to address difficulties with flexion of the shoulder, Joe completed a series of graded tasks. Firstly, he sat at a table and was asked to push cards across the table to the end of his arm's length. The therapist provided verbal guidance and feedback, and corrected any compensatory movements. Once Joe had mastered this task, he moved on to the next task, which involved a greater degree of shoulder flexion. (He was asked to pick up small objects and put them in a cup placed at the extent of his reach. Thus Joe had to reach and lift his arm without the support of the table.) This process continued until Joe was able to flex his shoulder to 90 degrees. He also practised the other missing components of movement, and was able to complete the exercises daily outside of the therapy sessions. Joe was also advised on how to rehearse mentally (visualize) the movements (Carr & Shepherd 2000).

Once Joe had mastered the movements of shoulder flexion, scapula protraction and external rotation of the humerus, he brought all three aspects of movement together within the task of dressing. He practised dressing in different environments and when sitting and standing, using a range of clothes (both lightweight and heavier ones). Such practice recognizes that the requirements of the task and the characteristics of the items being held and moved affect the types of movement, the amount of strength and the number of manipulations required (Carr & Shepherd 2003).

Finally, the therapist used the Motor Assessment Scale (Carr et al 1985) to re-assess Joe's arm and hand function.

Approaches to intervention for cognitive and perceptual dysfunction

Perceptual and cognitive problems are frequent consequences of stroke and may result in significant occupational dysfunction. Additionally, the presence of cognitive and perceptual problems affects the person's ability to engage with and benefit from occupational therapy intervention.

Occupational therapists use a variety of theoretical perspectives in addressing these issues. However, these perspectives fail to provide a cohesive theoretical framework that would justify the terminology of a frame of reference. They do, however, fall under two broad headings: adaptive approach and remedial approach.

Evidence from therapists surveyed in the UK suggested that both remedial and adaptive approaches were used. Walker et al (2003) found that 98% of therapists used adaptive approaches and 60% used remedial approaches in more than half of their case loads.

The adaptive approach

The adaptive approach focuses on a person's residual skills and abilities, aiming to maximize their occupational performance. It includes adaptation of environment, task/activity, functional task training (sometimes referred to as the functional or neuro-functional approach) and compensatory techniques (Toglia et al 2008). It may also be described as a top-down approach, as it focuses on the mastery of functional tasks rather than on improving specific cognitive or perceptual deficits (Unsworth 1999).

The main assumptions of the adaptive approach are that:

- The adult brain has limited potential to repair and reorganize itself after injury.

- The person with stroke can use their residual skills to reduce the impact of their cognitive or perceptual deficits on their daily life (Lee et al 2001).

- Training in specific, essential activities of daily living tasks is necessary because adults with brain injury have difficulty generalizing learning (Lee et al 2001).

- Functional activities require both perceptual and cognitive skills.

The main aim of this approach is to enable the person to engage successfully in their chosen occupations through application of compensatory strategies, environmental adaptation and learning of new skills (Toglia et al 2008).

Principles of intervention

- Application of the principles of occupational therapy, such as grading and adapting of tasks.

- Using demonstration, cueing, prompts, imitation or gesture to facilitate the person during activities (Edmans et al 2000).

- Repetition and practice of functional tasks.

- Teaching compensatory techniques: for example, the therapist teaches the person with visual neglect to turn their head towards their affected side during an activity.

- Trying to establish set patterns and routines for carrying out each activity.

- Adaptation of the environment.

- Teaching strategies such as use of self-talk to aid attention to a task.

- Teaching the person to use their meta-cognitive skills, such as organizational skills or increased self-awareness, to compensate for cognitive deficits.

- Use of external aids, such as notebooks, diaries and electronic devices (personal digital assistants, computers and pagers).

Evidence base

There is now considerable evidence to support the range of interventions considered under the adaptive approach. Examples of these are the use of strategy training to compensate for attention deficits during functional tasks, use of compensatory strategies and external aids for memory deficits (Cappa et al 2005, Cicerone et al 2005). The National Clinical Guidelines for Stroke (Intercollegiate Stroke Working Party 2008) recommend the practice of everyday tasks, use of compensatory strategies and external aids, and education regarding the impact of cognitive–perceptual deficits as the main evidence-based interventions to be used in rehabilitation.

Clinical application

An example of intervention following the adaptive approach is given in the case study at the end of the section on the remedial approach.

Remedial approach

The remedial approach (also known as the transfer of training approach) assumes that practice at a particular perceptual task will improve the underlying perceptual and cognitive skills (Toglia et al 2008). It can therefore be described as a bottom-up approach because it focuses on changing the underlying deficits (Unsworth 1999). The remedial approach assumes transference of improvement in perceptual and cognitive exercises to everyday functional tasks (Lee et al 2001). For example, a person with poor figure–ground discrimination would practise paper and pen exercises differentiating foreground objects from the background in the expectation that this would enable them to find utensils in a kitchen drawer. However, there is insufficient evidence to support transference of improvements in cognitive or perceptual performance to the performance of everyday activities (Lincoln et al 2000).

The remedial approach assumes that the way the brain repairs itself can be influenced by therapeutic interventions and lead to re-establishing synaptic connections or mapping new pathways (Toglia 2009).

The main disadvantage with the remedial approach is that people may object to abstract training (particularly perceptual exercises) and find it difficult to relate to their immediate problems (Edmans et al 2000). The approach also becomes problematic when considering people with complex cognitive and perceptual dysfunction, as there may be too many underlying deficits to address them on an individual basis. Indeed, Cicerone et al (2005) suggest that a more holistic and comprehensive rehabilitation programme addressing cognitive, functional and social impairments is most effective when working with people who have moderate to severe brain injury.

The main assumptions of the remedial approach are:

- The adult brain can repair and reorganize itself after injury.

- This repair and reorganization may be influenced by the process of retraining (i.e. the person takes part in perceptual and cognitive exercises focusing on specific cognitive and perceptual skills) (Lee et al 2001).
- Remedial training in perceptual skills will be generalized across all activities requiring those perceptual skills — thereby improving functional performance (Lee et al 2001).

The main aim of using the remedial approach is to increase and improve clients' cognitive and perceptual skills in order for people to engage in their everyday occupations.

Principles of intervention

- Use of specific exercises to address cognitive/perceptual deficits: e.g. visual scanning training to reduce visual neglect (Cicerone et al 2005).
- Use of pen and paper exercises to address problem-solving and perceptual skills (Toglia et al 2008).
- Practice of tasks designed to develop identified perceptual skills: e.g. use of face and body puzzles to develop body scheme skills, constructing two-dimensional and three-dimensional objects to address constructional apraxia (Quintana 2008).

Evidence base

There is little evidence to support the exclusive use of a remedial approach for treatment of cognitive deficits. Cicerone et al (2005) suggest in their recommendations for clinical practice that the main focus of interventions for cognitive deficits should be compensatory. However, it is worth noting that the current evidence does not explicitly address the overall impact of these approaches on occupational performance or levels of disability. Neither does it consider the long-term effects of intervention.

Cicerone et al (2005) also recommend systematic training of visuo-spatial skills for people with right hemisphere stroke (without neglect) as part of their overall rehabilitation. The evidence is not conclusive but suggests that interventions that specifically address visuo-spatial skills have better outcomes than conventional therapy alone.

In summary, whilst there is evidence to support a range of interventions for cognitive and perceptual deficits, the research is currently unable to differentiate between the clinical effectiveness of specific approaches (Cicerone et al 2005). However, interventions that are specifically designed to address cognitive and perceptual deficits are more effective than conventional occupational therapy, such as activities of daily living (Cicerone et al 2005). Lee et al (2001) suggest that occupational therapists use both approaches in a targeted and systematic way, which is defined by the stage of recovery of the person with stroke. This suggests that remedial approaches are used in the initial stages of recovery, with a progression towards adaptive approaches and focus on occupational performance as the person returns home.

Clinical application

An example of intervention following the remedial approach is given in the following case study.

CASE STUDY

Shamsun

Shamsun has been experiencing difficulties with her self-care activities following a right hemisphere stroke. She seems to have difficulty finding her clothes in the wardrobe and often puts them on inside out or back to front.

REMEDIAL AND ADAPTIVE APPROACH

As part of her initial assessment of Shamsun's abilities, the occupational therapist administered the Rivermead Perceptual Assessment Battery. The results indicated that Shamsun had visual perception problems, such as figure–ground discrimination, form constancy and depth perception. She explained the results of the assessments to Shamsun and described how these problems were affecting her in her daily activities.

Shamsun identified that she wanted to be able to wash and dress herself independently, as well as to continue to cook the family meals.

Initially, the occupational therapist engaged Shamsun with remedial tasks such as foreground/background discrimination exercises, and object recognition exercises using pen and paper tasks, as well as practising with everyday items.

As Shamsun became more proficient at these exercises, therapy sessions started to focus on practising washing and dressing, and making simple snacks and drinks in the occupational therapy kitchen. The therapist continued to encourage Shamsun to practise her skills but now started to include an adaptive approach. The therapist structured the environment to increase the contrast between the foreground and background, simplified the ways items were stored and organized, and taught Shamsun how to organize a task so as to reduce clutter and reduce the requirements on her perceptual skills. As Shamsun understood and became aware of her perceptual difficulties, she was able to develop her own compensatory techniques. The therapist continually provided cues and prompts throughout the therapy sessions.

In preparation for Shamsun returning home, the occupational therapist assessed Shamsun's abilities to complete self-care and food preparation successfully at home. She advised on adaptions to the home environment, as well as enabling Shamsun to apply the strategies learnt whilst an inpatient, in her home setting. As Shamsun became more successful with these activities, the therapist increased the complexity and continued to give Shamsun positive encouragement and feedback on her performance. Shamsun's husband was invited to participate in therapy sessions at home so that he also understood the nature of his wife's difficulties and how they affected her on a daily basis. He learned how to enable Shamsun, rather than simply taking over the task for her when she experienced difficulties.

Summary

There is evidence to support the effectiveness of occupational therapy for people who have experienced stroke but little that identifies which elements of intervention are effective (Legg et al 2007). Therapists need to adopt a range of approaches, as well as offering conventional occupational therapy.

Although there is limited published evidence of the benefits of using most of these approaches, it should be remembered that this does not signify that the interventions are ineffective. Instead, it highlights the lack of research evidence for the majority of rehabilitation approaches used by occupational therapists. Although evidence-based practice is a goal (Straus et al 2006) and the best evidence would be from randomized controlled trials, occupational therapists currently need to make standardization of practice a priority. Without working to standard guidelines and while following different approaches, eliciting concrete evidence to support best practice will remain elusive.

However, if there is no published randomized control trial evidence available, less rigorous levels of evidence can be used to guide good practice. An example of this is the levels of recommendations used in the National Clinical Guidelines for Stroke (Intercollegiate Stroke Working Party 2008).

From the evidence available, intervention following any of the approaches described in this chapter may be of benefit to clients. Occupational therapists need to be aware of the different approaches available, to enable them to make an informed choice and to decide which approach to use with each individual client. Intervention should be guided by goal-setting with each individual and the chosen occupations to be addressed. The occupational therapist should explain to the client how the intervention applies to the particular occupation, whichever approach is used.

Occupational therapy is evolving and responding to the changing environments in which practice is based. Within the UK, resources are increasingly being moved away from the acute hospital sector to primary care in the community. Occupational therapists need to adapt to these changing practice contexts. Additionally, occupational therapy is increasingly occupation-focused, and less emphasis is being placed on impairment-focused interventions. This is a timely change, fully congruent with the new International Classification of Functioning, where the focus is on activity (occupation) and participation (World Health Organization 2001).

These changes may accelerate the shift towards the more 'top-down' approaches discussed within this chapter, as they naturally cite the home environment as the optimum one, and focus on enabling individuals to achieve occupations required for quality of life.

Whatever the approach taken by therapists, the need for increasing the body and quality of evidence is clear. The poverty of conclusive, available evidence arises from the lack of standardization of practice; once therapists are able to reach a consensus on how these approaches are applied, research may be able to give the professional some definitive outcomes of effectiveness.

Reflective learning

- What are the main problems that occupational therapists encounter when attempting to establish an evidence base for their work?
- How strong would you consider the evidence base is for intervention in stroke rehabilitation, in comparison with other areas of practice?
- What are some of the strategies that help you develop an evidence base for your work?
- How can you break down an approach into its different parts: basic concepts, assessments, and intervention techniques and tools?
- How can this breakdown help you develop an evidence base for an intervention?

References

Bobath, B., 1990. Adult Hemiplegia Evaluation and Treatment. Heinemann Medical, Oxford.

Cappa, S.F., Benke, T., Clarke, S., et al., 2005. EFNS guidelines on cognitive rehabilitation: a report of an EFNS task force. European Journal of Neurology 12, 665–680.

Carr, J., Shepherd, R., Nordholme, L., et al., 1985. Investigations of a new motor assessment scale for stroke patients. Physical Therapy 65 (2), 175–180.

Carr, J.H., Shepherd, R.B., 1987. A motor relearning programme for stroke, 2nd edn. Heineman, London.

Carr, J., Shepherd, R., 1998. Neurological Rehabilitation - optimizing motor performance. Butterworth-Heinemann, Oxford.

Carr, J., Shepherd, R., 2000. Neurological Rehabilitation: Optimising Motor Performance, second ed. Butterworth–Heinemann, Oxford.

Carr, J.H., Shepherd, R.B., 2003. Stroke Rehabilitation: Guidelines for Exercises and Training to Optimize Motor Skill, third ed. Butterworth–Heinemann, Oxford.

Cicerone, K.D., Dahlberg, C., Malec, J.F., et al., 2005. Evidence-based cognitive rehabilitation: updated review of the literature from 1998 through 2002. Archives of Physical Medicine and Rehabilitation 86, 1681–1692.

Cirstea, C.M., Ptito, A., Levin, M.F., 2006. Feedback and cognition in arm motor skill reacquisition after stroke. Stroke 37 (5), 1237–1242.

Connelly, B.H., Montgomery, B.C., 2002. A framework for examination, evaluation and intervention. In: Connelly, B.H., Montgomery, B.C. (Eds.), Clinical Applications for Motor Control. Slack, Thorofare, NJ, pp. 1–24.

DeJong, G., Horn, S.D., Conroy, B., 2005. Opening the black box of stroke rehabilitation: stroke rehabilitations patients, processes and outcomes. Archives of Physical Medicine and Rehabilitation 82 (Suppl. 2), S1–S7.

Edmans, J.A., Webster, J., Lincoln, N.B., 2000. A comparison of two approaches in the treatment of perceptual problems after stroke. Clinical Rehabilitation 14, 230–243.

French, B., Thomas, L.H., Leathley, M.J., et al., 2007. Repetitive task training for improving functional ability after stroke (Review). Cochrane Database of Systematic Reviews (4). Available at: http://www.cochrane.org/reviews/en/ab006073.html (accessed 19.12.08.).

Gentile, A.M., 1998. Implicit and explicit processes during acquisition of functional skills. Scandinavian Journal of Occupational Therapy 5, 7–16.

Howle, J., 2003. Neuro-developmental Treatment Approach: Theoretical Foundations and Principles of Clinical Practice. Neurodevelopmental Treatment Association, Laguna Beach.

IBITA, 2008. Theoretical Assumptions and Clinical Practice. Available at: http://www.ibita.org/pdf/

assumptions-EN.pdf (accessed 19.12.08.).

Intercollegiate Stroke Working Party, 2008. National Clinical Guidelines for Stroke, third ed. Royal College of Physicians, London. Available at: http://www.rcplondon.ac.uk/pubs/brochure.aspx?e=254 (accessed 19.12.08.).

Kwan, J., 2001. Clinical epidemiology of stroke: continuing medical education. Journal of Geriatric Medicine 3 (3), 94–98.

Latham, N.K., Jette, D.U., Coster, W., Richards, L., Smout, R.J., James, R.A., Gassaway, J., & Horn, S.D., 2006. Occupational therapy activities and intervention techniques for clients with stroke in six rehabilitation hospitals. American Journal of Occupational Therapy 60, 369–378.

Lee, S.S., Powell, N.J., Esdaile, E., 2001. A functional model of occupational therapy. Canadian Journal of Occupational Therapy 68 (1), 41–50.

Legg, L., Drummond, A.E., Leonardi-Bee, J., et al., 2007. Occupational therapy for patients with problems in activities of daily living after stroke: systematic review of randomised trials. British Medical Journal 335, 922.

Lennon, S., Ashburn, A., 2000. The Bobath concept in stroke rehabilitation: a focus group study of the experienced physiotherapist's perspective. Disability and Rehabilitation 22 (15), 665–674.

Levit, K., 2008. Optimizing motor behaviour using the Bobath approach. In: Rodomski, M.V., Trombly, C.A. (Eds.), Occupational Therapy in Physical Dysfunction. sixth ed. Lippincott Williams & Wilkins, Philadelphia, pp. 643–666.

Lincoln, N., Majid, M., Weyman, N., 2000. Cognitive rehabilitation for attention deficits following stroke. Cochrane Database of Systematic Reviews (4).

Luke, C., Dodd, K.J., Brock, K., 2004. Outcomes of the Bobath concept on upper limb recovery following stroke. Clinical Rehabilitation 18 (8), 888–898.

Mathiowetz, V., 2004. Task-orientated approach to stroke rehabilitation. In: Gillen, G., Burkhardt, A. (Eds.),

Stroke Rehabilitation: A Functional Approach, second ed. Mosby, St Louis, pp. 59–74.

Murray, C.J.L., Lopez, A.D., 1997. Global mortality, disability and the contribution of risk factors. Global burden of the disease study. Lancet 349, 1436–1442.

Natarajan, P., Oelschlager, A., Agah, A., et al., 2008. Current clinical practices in stroke rehabilitation: regional pilot survey. Journal of Rehabilitation Research and Development 45 (6), 841–850.

Paci, M., 2003. Physiotherapy based on the Bobath concept for adults with post-stroke hemiplegia: a review of effectiveness studies. Journal of Rehabilitation Medicine 35, 2–7.

Quintana, S., 2008. Optimising vision, visual perception and praxis abilities. In: Rodomski, M.V., Trombly, C.A. (Eds.), Occupational Therapy in Physical Dysfunction, sixth ed. Lippincott, Williams & Wilkins, Philadelphia, pp. 728–747.

Saka, O., MacGuire, A., Wolfe, C.D.A., 2006. Economic Burden of Stroke in England. National Audit Office. Available at: http://www.nao.org.uk/system_pages/search.aspx?&terms=stroke+care (accessed 17.12.08.).

Shumway-Cook, A., Woollacott, M.H., 2007. Motor Control: Translating Research into Clinical Practice, third ed. Lippincott Williams & Wilkins, Philadelphia.

Straus, S.E., Richardson, W.S., Glasziou, P., Haynes, B.E.I., 2006. Evidence-based Medicine: How to Practise and Teach EBM. Churchill Livingstone, Edinburgh.

Teasel, R., Bayona, N., Bitensky, J., 2008. Background Concepts in Stroke Rehabilitation. Evidence Based Review of Stroke Rehabilitation. Available at: http://www.ebrsr.com/reviews_details.php?Background-Concepts-in-Stroke-Rehabilitation-12 (accessed 17.12.08.).

Toglia, J.P., Golisz, K.M., Goverover, J., 2008. Evaluation and intervention for cognitive–perceptual impairments. In: Crepeau, E.B., Cohn, E.S., Boyt Schell, B.A. (Eds.), Willard and Spackman's Occupational Therapy, eleventh ed. Lippincott Williams & Wilkins, Philadelphia, pp. 739–776.

Toglia, J.P., Goliz, K.M., Goverover, Y., 2009. Evaluation and Intervention for cognitive perceptual impairments. In: Elizabeth Blessedel Crepeau, Ellen. S. Cohn, Barbara A Boyt Schell (Eds.), Willard & Spackmans Occupational Therapy. Lippincott Williams & Wilkins, Philadelphia, pp. 739–776.

Truelsen, T., Begg, S., Mathers, C., 2006. The Global Burden of Cerebrovascular Disease. World Health Organization. Available at: http://www.who.int/healthinfo/statistics/bod_cerebrovasculardiseasestroke.pdf (accessed 20.04.10.).

Unsworth, C., 1999. Cognitive and Perceptual Dysfunction: A Clinical Reasoning Approach to Evaluation and Intervention. FA Davis, Philadelphia.

Van Peppen, R.D., Kwakkel, G., Wood-Dauphenee, S., et al., 2004. The impact of physical therapy on functional outcomes after stroke: what is the evidence? Clinical Rehabilitation 18, 833–862.

Van Vliet, P.M., Lincoln, N.B., Foxall, A., 2005. Comparison of Bobath based and movement science based treatment for stroke: a randomized controlled trial. Journal of Neurology, Neurosurgery, and Psychiatry 76, 503–508.

Walker, M.F., Drummond, A.E.R., Gatt, J., et al., 2000. Occupational therapy for stroke patients: a survey of current practice. British Journal of Occupational Therapy 63 (8), 367–372.

Walker, C., Walker, M., Sunderland, A., 2003. Dressing after a stroke: a survey of current occupational therapy practice. British Journal of Occupational Therapy 66 (6), 263–268.

World Health Organization, 2001. International Classification of Functioning, Health and Disability. World Health Organization, Geneva.

World Health Organization, 2002. The World Health Report: 2002: Reducing Risks, Promoting Healthy Life. World Health Organization, Geneva.

Wulf, G., Shea, C., Lethwaite, R., 2010. Motor skill learning and performance: a review of influential factors. Medical education 44, 75–84.

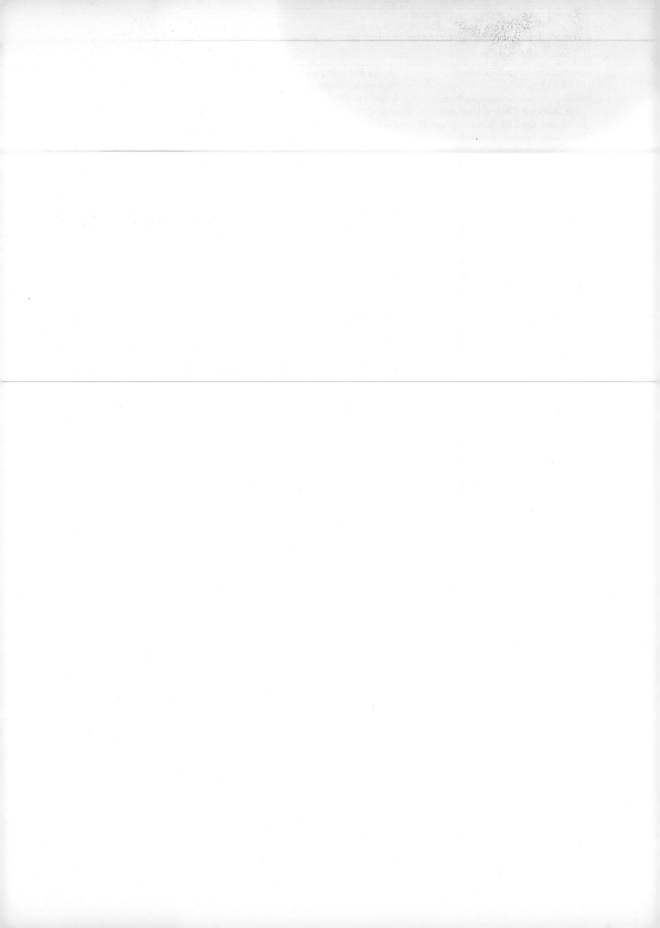

Section 4

Evolving areas of knowledge

The evolving theory of clinical reasoning

16

Carolyn A. Unsworth

OVERVIEW

This chapter explores clinical reasoning in occupational therapy. It provides an overview of the development of clinical reasoning in occupational therapy, definitions of the different types of clinical reasoning, and explains how acquisition of expertise is promoted through clinical reasoning. A major review of clinical reasoning research is then presented. While it has long been established that clinical reasoning enables therapists to integrate theory into practice, the final section of the chapter examines the process of theory development and maps this against developments and research growth in the area of clinical reasoning in occupational therapy. Hence, this chapter builds an argument that clinical reasoning is developing into a theory.

Key points

- Clinical reasoning has been studied by occupational therapy researchers since 1982. Clinical reasoning is distinct from clinical decision-making.
- Many types or modes of clinical reasoning have been identified and described, including narrative, procedural, interactive, conditional, ethical and pragmatic reasoning.
- One of the hallmarks of expertise is the therapist's ability to reason rapidly and intuitively. The clinical reasoning of an expert is deeply internalized, and the therapist can draw appropriately on relevant ideas, solutions or information from an extensive knowledge bank and range of experiences.
- There have been over 30 empirical studies conducted to investigate the clinical reasoning of occupational therapists. Qualitative and quantitative findings from

Key points—cont'd

this research are slowly building a picture of occupational therapy reasoning.
- Clinical reasoning is evolving into a theory in its own right. Research evidence to support the evolving theory of clinical reasoning is slowly assembling. Further studies that build on existing work, organize this phenomenon into a conceptual framework and empirically test this framework are urgently required.

Introduction

In 1983, Schön (p.42) penned the following analogy:

> In the varied topography of professional practice, there is a *high hard ground* in which practitioners can make effective use of the research-based theory and technique. Moreover, there is the *swampy lowland* in which situations are confusing 'messes' incapable of technical solution. The difficulty is that the problems of the high hard ground, however great their technical interest, are often relatively unimportant to clients or to the larger society, whereas in the swamp, the problems of greatest human concern are found.

This chapter welcomes you to the swamp!

The way we think and reason, in essence, makes us who we are as individuals. Furthermore, groups of people who come together for specific purposes often share patterns, modes and constellations of thinking and reasoning. As a professional group, occupational therapists share a mode of thinking and reasoning that is quite particular and quite different from that of other health professionals. Of course, many elements and aspects of this thinking are shared with other clinicians, but it is the way the thinking is constructed and how this reasoning enables our theories of human occupation to be practised that is unique. Writing about clinical reasoning in occupational therapy today is commonplace, and all of the introductory texts and compendia in the profession include material on clinical reasoning. Furthermore, I would guess that all occupational therapy education programmes internationally include some training or exposure to the idea of clinical reasoning. However, clinical reasoning has only been described in our profession over the past 25 years or so. Although the idea was first brought to the attention of therapists by Rogers (1982) and Rogers and Masagatani (1982) and Rogers' Eleanor Clarke Slagle lectureship the following year (1983), it was not till the *American Journal of Occupational Therapy* released its special edition on clinical reasoning in November 1991, and Mattingly and Fleming published their text, *Clinical Reasoning: Forms of Inquiry in a Therapeutic Practice*, in 1994 that the idea of clinical reasoning entered mainstream practice and became the buzz word of the early 1990s. News of this concept spread rapidly around the occupational therapy world, and there was an 'ah-ha' moment as the profession collectively recognized clinical reasoning as a way of naming and explaining all the hidden elements of practice that were so essential in the art (as opposed to the science) of occupational therapy practice. Early scholarly activities investigating clinical reasoning revealed that our thinking was indeed special and unique, and construction of a language to describe the tacit as well as overt elements of practice commenced. But what exactly is clinical reasoning? How does a therapist do it? What can make a therapist better at it? Some ideas to answer these questions are provided in this chapter, commencing with the first section, which provides an overview of what clinical reasoning is.

What is clinical reasoning?

Issues in arriving at a definition

It is not easy to put forth a simple definition of clinical reasoning, since this is quite a complex construct. To start, we must acknowledge that clinical reasoning is also described in the occupational therapy literature as 'therapeutic reasoning' (Kielhofner & Forsyth 2002), 'professional reasoning' (Schell & Schell 2008) and 'occupational reasoning' (Rogers 2010). All of these are also excellent terms. The terms 'professional reasoning' and 'therapeutic reasoning' acknowledge that occupational therapy practice is not confined to the clinic. Using the term 'occupational reasoning' ensures that our thinking is targeted to the 'systematic method of thinking about the occupational engagement of humans that supports the occupational therapy process' (Rogers 2010, p.57). But renaming the clinical reasoning rose does not make it smell any sweeter. Therefore, while this chapter adopts the traditional term that is so easily recognized, the reader is asked to consider that other terms can also be used.

The second issue to raise, before a definition is offered, concerns the intertwined nature of clinical reasoning and clinical decision-making. In discussing reasoning and decision-making in occupational therapy practice, Harries and Duncan (2009) observed that, in the occupational therapy literature, clinical reasoning tends to be used to cover all the thinking processes that involve reasoning, problem-solving judgement and decision-making. These authors go on to present material on two theories of judgement and decision-making from cognitive psychology, cognitive continuum theory (Hammond & Brehmer 1973) and dual-processing theory (Stanovich & West 2000), and show how these theories can further our understanding of occupational therapy practice. Harries and Duncan describe how, within dual-processing theory, two thinking systems are outlined that have been shown to be neurologically different (Goel et al 2000). The S1 system, as it is called, is a fast automatic form of processing. Through the S1 system, judgements are largely tacit. On the other hand, the slower and more deliberate S2 system is more analytical, focuses on one task at a time, and considers the outcome of different decisions from a more objective basis. The S1 system is more focused on the art of clinical reasoning, and the S2 on the science of objective decision-making. Ideally, we need both these elements in a successful clinical practice, and we need to explore both literatures to gain an understanding of what these approaches offer us. However, it is beyond the size and introductory nature of this chapter to explore both these concepts. This chapter focuses on the more context-dependent, phenomenologically grounded clinical reasoning. Texts that delve deeper into clinical reasoning in the allied health literature include those by Schell and Schell (2008) and Higgs et al (2008). The chapter will refer to, but not describe, decision-making in any detail. To gain an appreciation of the full complexity of the science of judgement and decision-making, the reader is referred to Klein et al (1993), Dowie and Elstein (1988) or Hardman (2009).

Definition of clinical reasoning

It is hard to be succinct when defining clinical reasoning. The *Oxford Dictionary* defines reasoning as 'the intellectual faculty by which conclusions are drawn from premises . . . [and] to reach conclusions by connected thought' (Thompson 1995, p.1144). But this definition does not convey the scope or complexity of clinical reasoning in occupational therapy. Higgs and Jones (2000, p.11) define clinical reasoning as 'a process in which the clinician, interacting with significant others (client, caregivers, healthcare team members), structures meaning, goals and health management strategies based on clinical data, client choices, and professional judgment and knowledge'. In occupational therapy, clinical reasoning can be defined as the reflexive thinking associated with engaging in a client-centred professional practice. This includes the thinking when planning to be with the client (and their caregivers and other health professionals), when the therapist is with the client and afterwards when reflecting on time with the client. Clinical reasoning draws on empathy, intuition, judgement and common sense. Clinical reasoning is constantly changing in response to a multitude of hidden and overt influences and contextual factors, which may be inhibitory or enabling. Clinical reasoning plays out in the occupational therapist's mind in narratives and images (adapted from Unsworth 1999). Within the clinical reasoning construct, many modes or types of reasoning have been identified. These are described in the next section of the chapter.

A language to describe the modes of clinical reasoning

Cheryl Mattingly (a medical anthropologist) and Maureen Fleming (an occupational therapist) worked with a large team of experts, including Gilette, Schön and Cohen, to conduct the first large-scale enquiry into the clinical reasoning of occupational therapists. The American Occupational Therapy Foundation funded a study between 1986 and 1988 involving 14 therapists at a 900-bed acute care facility in a large city in the USA. The two major findings of the study were an understanding of the practice cultures that occupational therapists work within and the beginnings of a language to describe the modes of reasoning used by occupational therapists (Mattingly & Fleming 1994). Many refinements and additions have been made to this framework, but the fundamental ideas laid out in Mattingly and Fleming's text provide the foundation for understanding clinical reasoning in occupational therapy. The language that has now developed in occupational therapy in the field of clinical reasoning has been drawn from medicine, philosophy, anthropology and sociology.

An overview of these different modes of clinical reasoning and related terminology used in the field are provided below, and Table 16.1 provides a detailed examination of the language of clinical reasoning in occupational therapy. The third column in the table provides an example of how this language might be used in clinical practice in the narrative (first-person) form. The use of narrative examples to illustrate how therapists reason is now quite popular in occupational therapy texts. Mattingly and Fleming's text came to life through the use of these narratives, and several occupational therapy writers have since adopted this approach to illustrate texts with both what and how a therapist thinks (see, for example, Unsworth 1999, Kielhofner 2008, Crepeau et al 2009). This approach helps students and novice therapists to learn both what a particular therapy technique is, and, very importantly, what a therapist thinks as they engage in practice.

Narrative reasoning and chart talk

Mattingly documented how occupational therapy was a profession that sat comfortably between two practice cultures, and therefore described occupational therapy as a 'two body practice' (1994, p.37). On the one hand, occupational therapists work within a biomedical framework. Even when therapists do not work in a medical setting, our profession is primarily concerned about the relationship between health, occupation and well-being. Therefore, our concern with health connects us to medicine and a biomechanical understanding. Occupational therapists also have their own professional practice culture, which operates in the social,

Table 16.1 Types/modes of clinical reasoning in occupational therapy and other related constructs

Mode of thinking	Description (and examples of researchers who coined/use this term)	Clinical example
Narrative reasoning	The use of storytelling and creation to explore therapy. Used when therapists work in a more phenomenological practice sphere where the emphasis is on the meaning of the client's illness and illness experience (Mattingly & Fleming 1994)	Robyn enters the hospital's allied health staff lunch room and flops into a chair. Her colleagues, Dana, Matty and Pip, are already there. Pip observes that Robyn looks exhausted. Robyn replies: 'I've just been working with the new lad. He's only four, but he spent the whole session wailing for his mum. The puppets caught his attention for a few minutes and I made a start but that was about it. His leg muscles are so tight, but I'm sure the [tendon release] surgery will make a huge difference in the long run . . . I just need to find what will turn on the light and get him interested and motivated. I'm going to try and call his mum later and get some more information from her . . .'
Scientific reasoning	The process of hypothesis generation and testing that generally is referred to as hypothetico-deductive reasoning. Used to make a diagnosis of the client's medical condition. Although more concerned with identifying the client's occupational problems rather than the medical diagnosis, therapists do draw on the ideas of scientific reasoning when reasoning procedurally (Schell & Cervero 1993)	Saran reports on her initial assessment of 73-year-old Peter at the team meeting. 'I assessed the new client, Peter, yesterday in terms of ability to complete personal ADLs. I found him to be independent with verbal supervision for all tasks such as toileting, showering, dressing and grooming. He plans to return to his home without any support and use public transport to get to the shops, visit his doctor and do his banking. Given what I observed yesterday, I doubt he will be independent in all these activities by next week. I will commence an IADL assessment today, and intervention will aim at facilitating his independence and also putting local community supports in place.'
Diagnostic reasoning	Used to identify underlying impairments or occupational performance issues, define desired outcomes, set goals, develop intervention/solutions (Rogers & Holm 1991)	Brian has been working in acute care for only a few months and has used a hypothesis testing approach (Unsworth 1999) to determine the underlying cognitive impairments that are limiting his client's ability to make a cup of tea. 'He presents as really confused, and so I was very cautious in putting everything out on the bench and I didn't have the water in the kettle any hotter than tap water. He started by breaking open the teabag and tipping the tea into the cup. Then he tipped in half the sugar from the sugar pot, played around with this for a while and then filled the cup with milk. Before the session, I was wondering what was going on and whether he had some complex perceptual problems. But over the session it became clear that he has ideational apraxia. This hypothesis fits with the fact that he has left brain damage as a result of the stroke and has quite severe receptive aphasia as well.'
Procedural reasoning	The thinking associated with the procedural aspects of therapy, such as the evaluations and interventions to be used with the client, and how the client is performing. Procedural reasoning represents the more scientific components of practice, which	Alex works on a stroke ward. His new client has cognitive and perceptual problems. 'So I did a dressing assessment with Mr P this morning and the hypotheses were just flying around my head. He has so many cognitive and perceptual problems but hardly any physical ones . . . so I just watched him and tried a few things as we went. He looks as

(Continued)

Table 16.1 Types/modes of clinical reasoning in occupational therapy and other related constructs—cont'd

Mode of thinking	Description (and examples of researchers who coined/use this term)	Clinical example
	include systematic data collection, hypothesis formation and testing (Mattingly & Fleming 1994)	if he has a unilateral neglect and some short-term memory problems, as well as complex perceptual problems . . . but I've got to check for homonymous hemianopia too. So I'm just trying to work out which standardized assessments to do . . . maybe the RPAB [Rivermead Perceptual Assessment Battery] or LOTCA [Lowenstein Occupational Therapy Cognitive Assessment] and the BIT [Behavioural Inattention Test] . . . but I probably don't have enough time for all three, so maybe just the LOTCA and some confrontation testing to check for neglect versus homonymous hemianopia versus both.'
Interactive reasoning	Concerned with how the therapist interacts with the client. Referred to as the underground practice by Mattingly and Fleming, since the therapists they studied were able to describe what they had done with the client but generally not their interactions. Therapists use interactive reasoning to engage the client in therapy, and consider the best approach to communicate with the client, to understand the client as a person, understand the client's problems from the client's point of view, individualize therapy, convey a sense of acceptance/trust/hope to the client, break tension through the use of humour, build a shared language of actions and meanings, and monitor how the treatment session is going (Mattingly & Fleming 1994)	Dana describes to her fieldwork student some of her interactive reasoning as she gets to know her clients during an initial interview. As Dana will get to know these clients over several months, she reasons that she has this time to use the initial interview to 'go deep'. 'So what I do is just start off with the initial interview structure but explore any directions the client's responses take me in. I don't want to limit this opportunity to get to know the client by sticking to the form, as the sooner I can get my head around understanding who this person is and what makes them tick, the better the therapy plans we make will be. I try to keep it light and friendly so the client feels at ease and that it's an open and sharing environment. If there is an opportunity to share a joke I will . . . or if the client becomes upset or distressed, then I take time to support them through this and slowly we move on. I guess what I'm aiming for is to get the clients to see me as someone who is going to be useful in their recovery and someone they can trust.'
Conditional reasoning	Takes into account the whole of the client's condition, as the therapist considers the client's temporal contexts (past, present and future) and their personal, cultural and social contexts. Hence, this type of reasoning is used when trying to understand what is meaningful to the client in their world by imagining what their life was like before the illness or disability, what it is like now and what it could be like in the future (Mattingly & Fleming 1994)	Maryella is reflecting on a session with Joseph, a 5-year-old boy with developmental delay. She started by interviewing Joseph and then undertook Ayres Clinical Observation to examine his motor skills. She completed this assessment about 12 months ago as well. 'So I did this assessment last year and I haven't seen Joseph for over 6 months since his family moved away for his Dad's work. Now they're back so I'm just checking on where Joseph is up to with school and socially, and how he feels about coming home and so on. So we've had a chat and I can really tell he's made a lot of good gains. He's a bit anxious about starting back at his old school, so I've been reassuring him about that and now I'm just using Ayres Clinical Obs assessment to run through his current performance. He's made some nice gains over the time he's been away; he has more core trunk stability and I can really see changes compared with the last time I saw him in terms of balance, righting reactions and even fine motor coordination. I think we can work on some more advanced goals now with him, such as . . .'

(Continued)

Table 16.1 Types/modes of clinical reasoning in occupational therapy and other related constructs—cont'd

Mode of thinking	Description (and examples of researchers who coined/use this term)	Clinical example
Ethical reasoning	The thinking that accompanies analysis of a moral dilemma where one moral conviction or action conflicts with another, and then generating possible solutions and selecting action to be taken (Rogers 1983, Barnitt & Partridge 1997)	Alan had a head injury and attends a day therapy programme as an outpatient. His therapist, Kate, reflects on the fact that Alan takes illegal drugs (Unsworth 2004b): 'So Alan still lives in his parents' house, but he can't stay there much longer, and they want him out. Alan takes drugs and I find it a real dilemma. I have to help him find other housing, but he shares his drugs around, and I'm really worried that if I help him find a group home, then he could be putting other people at risk. I also feel really disappointed because he's made such amazing gains in therapy and he could do so much, but when he takes drugs he just loses all his cognition, basically. He just sits there and misses out on therapy, and it's a real shame. Sometimes I think the therapy I provide is going to waste ... should I spend less time with him and more with my other clients who seem to make more gains? I try not to dwell on it but it's a bit disappointing, as if he didn't do drugs, then he could easily be living in a good home and making fantastic progress towards independent living and getting some part-time voluntary work. Anyway, it's his life and I try not to judge him. But I have to think some more about what kind of place he can live in so he doesn't put others at risk as well.'
Generalization reasoning	Within the forms of procedural, interactive, conditional and pragmatic reasoning, therapists use generalization reasoning to draw on past experience or knowledge to assist them in making sense of a current situation or client circumstance. The kind of reasoning in force when a therapist thinks about a particular issue or scenario with a client, then reflects on their general experiences or knowledge (i.e. making generalizations) related to the situation, and then refocuses the reasoning back on the client (Unsworth 2005)	Max works in a short-stay residential facility, helping adolescents with intellectual disability to become more independent. 'So Kate is making some good gains with her goal of grooming, which includes managing her long hair and doing some basic make-up. So often these kids have a kind of learned helplessness since their parents have often done everything for them. So with Kate, she asks for help all the time but really she can do it. So I think it's more about reassurance and just reinforcing what a great job she's doing. So that's what I'm focusing on with Kate in this session, supporting and reassuring her that she can do her hair and so on and that she's doing a great job.'
Pragmatic reasoning/ management reasoning	Concerned with the therapist's practice and personal contexts. The practice context includes organizational, political environments and economic influences, such as resources and reimbursement. Personal context includes the reasoning surrounding the therapist's own motivation, negotiation skills, repertoire of therapy skills, ability to read the practice culture, and what Törnebohm (1991) described as life	Xui Sing works in community health with elderly clients living at home. 'I really want to be able to provide my client, Mrs Beller, with an adjustable over-toilet frame, as I know her husband is having hip replacement surgery in 6 weeks and he's a lot bigger than her. So if I get an adjustable one, they can both use it. But our centre has just had a major policy change in equipment allocation, and I think I can only provide a seat that is a fixed height and suitable for her. Maybe they can afford to buy an adjustable one now, or maybe we'll have to worry about Mr Beller later when he has his surgery? I'll have to work

(Continued)

Table 16.1 Types/modes of clinical reasoning in occupational therapy and other related constructs—cont'd

Mode of thinking	Description (and examples of researchers who coined/use this term)	Clinical example
	knowledge and assumptions (Schell & Cervero 1993, Barris 1987, Neuhaus 1988, Fondiller et al 1990). Lyons and Crepeau (2001) labelled pragmatic (practice context) reasoning as management reasoning	out the best solution based on their needs now, their budget and what my centre can provide.'
Embodiment	Our bodies, as well as our minds, gather a great deal of information as we work with clients. For example, we can smell if the client has not washed or if a wound is not healing well, and we use our sensation to feel the client's muscles and how their body moves. This is referred to as embodied knowledge and it is not always possible to put this knowledge into words. Although therapists have long recognized the importance of information from our bodies about our clients, the embodied nature of clinical reasoning is a relatively new area for research in occupational therapy (Schell & Harris 2008)	Helen describes how she knows when an autistic child begins to relax and settle into an activity. 'Well, if I describe a typical client, then I could tell you about Paul. So let's say I've started with a warm-up activity outside climbing the rope ladder and swinging on the bars, so it's a gross motor activity using major muscle groups. And that's really helpful, so that when he comes inside I might then start with a large weighted floor puzzle. This kind of "heavy work", with lots of joint compression seems to help kids like Paul to relax. And as he's moving the puzzle, I can see his whole body kind of slows and I can place my hands over his back or at his hips, and feel the tension releasing and his muscles relaxing.'
Worldview	Defined in philosophy as 'a global outlook on life and the world' (Wolters 1989, p.15, Hooper 1997). Worldview is the *influence* of the therapist's personal context *on* clinical reasoning. While some writers describe pragmatic reasoning as incorporating this personal context (e.g. Schell & Cervero 1993), others view this as a separate factor which has an impact on reasoning rather than being a separate form of reasoning (e.g. Unsworth 2004a)	Asher describes his worldview. 'Well, I suppose my worldview makes me who I am, and I guess it colours everything I think and do. It's about my faith and what values I hold and my sense of right and wrong. Sometimes I'm aware of it but mostly I'm not. I guess I have to think about what my worldview is, when I'm confronted with it being different from the client's. It's times like these I really have to work at not making judgements about the client but try to see it from their point of view or try to accept that it's OK to have that particular worldview. When I have OT fieldwork students, they find this hard at times. Often you can't solve the dilemma for them, but at least you make them aware of what the problem is — in other words, you can at least look at it objectively for what the problem is, and also see that it's normal to have to work at understanding these issues and resolving or making peace with these differences.'
Intuition	Defined as the 'knowledge of a fact or truth, as a whole; immediate possession of knowledge; and knowledge independent of the linear reasoning process' (Rew 1986, p.23). Within Cognitive Continuum Theory, Hammond (1996) posits that cognition can	Fiona reflects on the development of her intuition and its value in her practice. 'When I first started in mental health, working with depressed clients, I would have done A, B and C as I was taught and expected to do by others in the team. But now I'm 8 years on, and I do so many things differently based on that experience. And I'm really

(Continued)

Table 16.1 Types/modes of clinical reasoning in occupational therapy and other related constructs—cont'd

Mode of thinking	Description (and examples of researchers who coined/use this term)	Clinical example
	be ordered on a continuum from intuition to analysis	comfortable with what the A, B, C is, and I can see where it will work and where it will need to be changed. And I just trust my intuition. When I was new at this job, I didn't have the same "feel" or gut instinct for clients that I have now. But now I can just sense when something isn't quite right or when the client is going downhill … even if that isn't what they're telling me. And I trust this intuition.'
Reflection	Involves reviewing performance and examining it in detail by relating it to past knowledge and experiences and relating it to future action, to enhance understanding. There are several types of reflection, including reflection about past experiences (reflection on action), reflecting in the present (reflection in action) and looking forward or anticipatory reflection (reflection for action). Reflection is a bridge to link theory and practice (Schön 1983, Alsop & Ryan 1996, McKay 2009)	Akhmed describes the value in setting aside time for reflection in his practice. 'Each week I try to put some time aside on Friday to go back over the week and identify the highlights and low points, and I reflect on what worked well and the problems … both working with clients and with other staff. I don't keep a journal but some of my colleagues do. But I try to make some notes about events and feelings, and use this time to think about doing things differently or better. Then I also have professional supervision once a month, and I identify something from these "Friday reflections" to really go into more detail … and I find these sessions really useful. My mentor really pushes me to think about the issue from so many different angles and I use her approach when I'm thinking back over the week on my own.'

cultural and psychological sphere that is concerned with the client's experience of the illness and the meaning of the illness (Mattingly 1994). Usually, a biomechanical or scientific approach (the body as a machine) does not sit well alongside the more phenomenological sphere (the lived body). However, in occupational therapy, these two seem to make perfect sense. As Mattingly (1994) notes, occupational therapists seemed to have the ability to shift rapidly and easily between thinking about the client and the disease process and resulting occupational performance issues (for example), and developing an understanding of the person and the client's experience of the illness.

When therapists are thinking and working in a biomechanical sphere, they use chart talk to present information on the client and discuss evaluation and intervention issues. Hence, chart talk is generally used when the occupational therapist is talking about the client's medical problem, or writing case notes using brief and factual language. This kind of communication fits well in the biomedical world. However, when

working in the more phenomenological practice sphere, occupational therapists use narrative reasoning to tell the story of therapy (Mattingly 1994, Unsworth 2004a). Storytelling is never static. Stories can be told of the past and of the present and created for the future. Stories can be rewritten and changed midstream. Hence, thinking in narratives fits perfectly with the ever-changing therapy environment.

The therapist with the three-track mind

While narrative reasoning may be described as a core form of reasoning, Fleming (1994) went on to develop the idea of 'the therapist with the three-track mind' (p.119). The therapist with the three-track mind describes three dominant modes of reasoning found in the clinical reasoning study and confirmed in more recent research (Alnervik & Sviden 1996, Unsworth 2004a). Fleming argued that therapists use these different kinds of reasoning when working in the different practice spheres. Therefore, procedural reasoning, which is similar to the problem-solving or hypothetico-deductive approach used in medical enquiry, fits well in the biomechanical sphere. The other forms of reasoning described by Fleming, interactive reasoning and conditional reasoning, fit more readily in the phenomenological or meaning making practice sphere (Fleming 1994). These forms of reasoning are all defined and described in Table 16.1. However, it is important to note how intertwined these are throughout the therapy process. Mattingly and Fleming (1994) described how the perspective gained from reasoning in one track might inform reasoning in another. This idea, that the different forms of reasoning interact and overlap, has been supported in subsequent clinical reasoning research (Unsworth 2004a).

Other modes of clinical reasoning and related terms

Early clinical reasoning researchers, such as Rogers and Masagatani (1982) and Barris (1987), as well as researchers following in the footsteps of Mattingly and Fleming, have also contributed terms to describe modes of clinical reasoning, or to describe constructs that fit with clinical reasoning. Some of these terms, such as ethical, scientific, pragmatic, generalization and diagnostic reasoning, and related constructs such as intuition, embodiment, world-view and reflection, are defined and illustrated in Table 16.1. It is important to note that some of these terms, such as procedural, interactive, conditional and pragmatic reasoning, fit better within an S1 or reasoning approach to understanding thinking processes. Other terms, such as scientific and diagnostic reasoning, fit better with an S2 approach.

Clinical reasoning and expertise

Differences between the clinical reasoning of novice and expert therapists

Research in occupational therapy on novice–expert differences has often portrayed this construct as a dichotomy. However, as described by Dreyfus and Dreyfus (1980) in their work on chess players and airline pilots, and then adapted for use in the health sciences by nursing researcher Benner (1984), expertise occurs on a continuum. It is now widely accepted that there are five phases one passes through on the journey from novice to expert, and these are novice, advanced beginner, competent, proficient and expert. It is also widely documented that increasing years of experience do not always equate with increasing expertise; some therapists never reach expert status but remain stuck at the level of competent or proficient practice (Benner et al 1996, Gibson et al 2000, Unsworth 2001). There have been several occupational therapy studies on the differences between novice and expert therapists (Hallin & Sviden 1995, Strong et al 1995, Robertson 1996, Gibson et al 2000, Unsworth 2001, Mitchell & Unsworth 2005). One of the consistent findings from these studies and from studies of other health professionals is that experts think and reason differently from novices; experts know how (non-propositional or tacit knowledge) rather than know what (propositional or factual book-learned knowledge), their knowledge is embedded in action and experience, and much of their knowledge is automatic and intuitive (Dreyfus & Dreyfus 1980, 1986). Occupational therapy research in this area has revealed that, while novice and expert differences may be readily apparent, the differences between the other levels of expertise are not so apparent. Further research is required to help us identify the hallmarks and key reasoning patterns at each of the three mid-phases (advanced beginner, competent, proficient) so we can aid therapists who are 'stuck' at a particular level to move forward on their journey to expertise.

One of the goals of an occupational therapy educational programme is to ensure that students exit with the skills, tools, behaviours, attitudes and reasoning abilities needed to be excellent occupational therapists. Therefore, educators use novice–expert research findings to help students and novices to gain insights into expert thinking so they may hasten their journey on this continuum. However, expertise is not a point of arrival but rather a lifelong quest. This is because expertise is heavily context-dependent and a clinician who excels in one field of practice, such as psychiatry, may have novice skills only in working with clients who are recovering from stroke. In addition, clinicians who have attained expert status in a particular context must continue to expand and hone skills on their quest for professional excellence. Hence, novices and experts alike can benefit from undertaking an activity that has been shown as a key to enhancing clinical reasoning, and that is reflection.

Enhancing clinical reasoning skills through reflection

Reflection, as described in Table 16.1, is concerned with reviewing one's performance and examining it in detail by relating it to past knowledge and experiences and relating it to future action, to enhance understanding. Reflection is often referred to as the bridge that links theory and practice (Schön 1983, Alsop & Ryan 1996, McKay 2009). It is essential that all therapists, novices as well as experts, have the time and opportunity to reflect on practice both alone and with a supervisor or mentor. Reflective activities designed to enhance clinical reasoning include storytelling, pre-briefing and debriefing, reflective questions after working with a client, reflective journal writing, reviewing critical incidents with a mentor, participation in discussion groups, and videotaping and viewing sessions with clients. Additionally, activities with a reflective partner can also be helpful; together therapists can note significant similarities and differences between clients with similar disease processes or occupational performance issues and consider how these differences can influence treatment (Alsop & Ryan 1996, McKay 2009). Therapists who take the time to reflect nurture their clinical reasoning skills, thus promoting excellent practice.

A review of empirical research on clinical reasoning in occupational therapy, 1982–2009

There have been over 100 journal articles, book chapters and books on clinical reasoning in occupational therapy written over the past 25 years. The sheer quantity of musings and research in this area reflects the value that our profession places on clinical reasoning and the commitment made to exploring and understanding it. While the reflective discussions and information presented in a lot of the writing on clinical reasoning provide a raft of ideas

for research, this section of the chapter details the evidence or the empirical research published on clinical reasoning in occupational therapy. Occupational therapy practice requires a sound evidence base (Holm 2000). Evidence-based practice may be defined as the judicious use of evidence to make sound decisions about practice. Therefore, decision-making, thinking and reasoning are at the heart of putting evidence into practice. Occupational therapy urgently needs more empirical studies on clinical reasoning, so we are confident that we are judicious in putting the best evidence into practice. Hence, research into clinical reasoning where data were collected with occupational therapists and analysed in some way, either qualitatively or quantitatively, is summarized below. As a result of this process, we can more easily identify where work has been done, and clearly see how this can be built upon as we continue the mammoth task of exploring and understanding clinical reasoning in occupational therapy.

The literature between 1983 and 2009 was searched using the following databases: Medline, CINAHL, AMED and OTDBASE. The key terms used were 'clinical reasoning' or 'reasoning' or 'thinking' combined with 'occupational therapy'. Reference lists of articles retrieved and many of the recent books or book chapters on clinical reasoning in the health professions were then searched by hand. Articles were included in the review if they met the following criteria:

1. They researched an element of clinical reasoning and hence the words clinical reasoning were included in either the title or abstract.
2. They were published in a peer-reviewed journal.
3. They included a sample that involved at least one occupational therapist.
4. Data analysis was undertaken.
5. Results were presented and a discussion on the findings was included.

Furthermore, articles were excluded if:

1. They focused on how to teach clinical reasoning to students.
2. They researched reasoning used or required in a particular area of practice and where the focus was on the area of practice.
3. They researched clinical decision-making rather than reasoning processes.

Hence, several of the articles by Maureen Neistadt on teaching clinical reasoning (see, for example, Neistadt 1987, Neistadt & Atkins 1996) were excluded, while studies such as McKay and Ryan's (1995) work on the clinical reasoning used by students on fieldwork was included. Research examining the scientific decision-making processes of occupational therapists (S2 rather than S1 reasoning) was excluded, such as my own work (e.g. Unsworth et al 1995, Unsworth & Thomas 1993, Unsworth et al 1997, Unsworth 2007), and research by Priscilla Harries (e.g. Harries & Harries 2001, Harries & Gilhooly 2006) and Medhi Rassafiani (Rassafiani et al 2006, 2008). Research examining how clinical reasoning can be used to manage a particular area of practice was also excluded (e.g. Fortune & Ryan 1996). The empirical studies that met the selection criteria are presented in Table 16.2.

The table reveals that there have been relatively few (31) published empirical studies on clinical reasoning in occupational therapy. It is particularly notable that there are very few researchers who have published multiple or related papers. It also seems that the research does not seem to build on what has come before, but is rather fragmented. Hopefully, this will change as a new wave of international researchers and doctoral students publish their findings.

Building a theory of clinical reasoning through scholarship of practice

One of the central aims of the clinical reasoning study funded by the American Occupational Therapy Foundation was to discover the practical theories-in-use of the occupational therapy profession so that this tacit knowledge could be documented and passed on. Mattingly and Fleming (1994) were able to realize this goal because their research adopted a participatory action research approach within an ethnographic framework. The occupational therapists were not studied from a distance, but rather they became part of the research team as they examined their own practice, working with the researchers in what Schön (1983) refers to as a 'scholarship of practice'. This term can be defined as 'delivering and generating evidence for practice through a partnership between academia and practice' (Melton et al 2009, p.13).

This approach to describing how theory can be generated from practice is quite distinct from the traditional basic science view that theory is generated prior to its application in the field. Over the past 15 years, many occupational therapy writers have identified how occupational therapists do seem to have a problem with integrating theory into practice (Duncan 2006, Kielhofner 2009, Melton et al 2009). It appears that therapists are somewhat disillusioned with the relevance of theory in daily practice. Therefore, the scholarship of practice approach has been identified as a way of growing relevant theory from within practice, to support and promote that practice (Argyris & Schön 1974, Schön 1983, Creek & Ormston 1996). This section of the chapter examines how theories evolve, and proposes that clinical reasoning is actually developing into a theory itself through scholarship of practice.

In Chapter 5 of this text and the previous edition (2006), Duncan describes not only the value and importance of having theory to underpin practice, but also the complexities surrounding our use and misuse of theory terms such as paradigm, conceptual practice model, frame of reference and approach. Since the idea that clinical reasoning in occupational therapy is developing into a theory in its own right is relatively new (Unsworth & Schell 2006, Schell et al 2008), it is too early map out its structure, function and relationships to the core beliefs of the occupational therapy profession. It may transpire that clinical reasoning becomes incorporated into an existing occupational therapy theory, or it may become known as a frame of reference, since frames of reference link theory to practice and reasoning is often described in this way. Since it is premature to use any particular label at this stage, for the purposes of this chapter, the term 'theory' of clinical reasoning will be adopted and used in its broadest sense.

Theories may be defined as connected sets of ideas that form a base for practice or action. Theories attempt to explain and predict phenomena (Walker & Ludwig 2004), and help us to recognize what we know and to organize what we do (Mitcham 2003). Differing opinions concerning how theory is generated have also been proposed. In occupational therapy, Mitcham (2003) describes the process of theory generation as involving six sequential steps, starting with observation and ending with tested theory.

Table 16.2 Review of empirical research on clinical reasoning in occupational therapy 1983–2009

Year	Author Journal	Aim Setting	Sample of OTs Country	Main finding
1982	Rogers & Masagatani OTJR	To describe the clinical reasoning used to decide client problem area and treatment goals. Acute care physical setting. Focus on Assessment Physical rehabilitation	n = 10 USA	Data were analysed qualitatively and a six stage model was developed to describe the therapists' reasoning processes: 1. search for medical information, 2. select standard assessments, 3. implement assessment plan, 4. define client problems, 5. specify treatment objectives, and 6. evaluate the assessment process. Noted that therapists found it difficult to articulate their thinking
1987	Barris OTJR	To explore and describe the assessment processes used by therapists Mental health	n = 19 USA	Initial assessments varied between therapists in terms of format and content. There is a great deal of routinization in decisions made
1990	Fondiller et al OTJR	To identify values that influence clinical reasoning in occupational therapy using qualitative research methods Recognized experts from a variety of settings	n = 9 USA	Participants answered a series of open-ended questions in response to a case study. Eighteen value statements were reported that influence clinical reasoning and these were placed in two groups: therapist-related statements and treatment-related statements. Concluded that the pervasive presence of values in clinical reasoning must be acknowledged
1991	Fleming AJOT	To answer the question of what is clinical reasoning in occupational therapy Acute care physical setting	N = 14 USA	Identified the two-bodied practice of occupational therapy: the 'lived body' or phenomenological approach vs. the 'body as a machine' or biomechanical approach to working with clients. Developed a language for clinical reasoning, including the therapist with the three-track mind: procedural, interactive and conditional reasoning
1993	Sviden & Saljo AJOT	To examine the ways in which professional education affects occupational therapy students' perceptions and descriptions of patients' non-verbal behaviour Educational setting	n = 13 Sweden	Students found it difficult to discuss individual cases in relation to newly acquired theoretical knowledge. It was concluded that students would benefit more from increased opportunity to analyse individual cases by means of theoretical knowledge, rather than increased instruction in theory
1995	McKay & Ryan BJOT	To investigate the use of narrative reasoning by an occupational therapy student and an experienced therapist No information provided	n = 2 UK	The expert and novice told different narrative stories; however, it was found that the student's story could be enhanced to include more narrative by asking probing and reflective questions
	Sviden OTRJ	To examine the different methods in which occupational therapy students report how they would respond to patients' non-verbal communication of affect Educational setting	n = 13 Sweden	Students' comments showed evidence of change after 1.5 years of occupational therapy education, when compared with the beginning of their course. The change may be regarded as cognitive in nature because comments became more differentiated and organized

(Continued)

Table 16.2 Review of empirical research on clinical reasoning in occupational therapy 1983–2009—cont'd

Year	Author Journal	Aim Setting	Sample of OTs Country	Main finding
	Creighton et al AJOT	To investigate experienced occupational therapists' clinical reasoning as they presented and modified therapeutic activities to treat their clients Spinal cord injury	n = 4 USA	Consistent with previous research, the therapists demonstrated multilayered thinking. However, hierarchical structuring of knowledge also emerged unexpectedly as a dominant theme in their reasoning
	Strong et al BJOT	To use nominal group techniques to ascertain the differences between novice and expert therapist reasoning Mixed settings, including hospitals, schools, paediatric care and psychiatry	n = 19 Australia	The study revealed that, when making clinical decisions, a wider range of factors was considered by experts than by students. Clinical reasoning was also rated to be at a higher level by experts than by students. The factors identified by the experts as important in clinical reasoning were derived from both the scientific and narrative domains. Students identified the most important factors from the pragmatic and narrative domains, as well as one factor from the scientific domain
	Hallin & Sviden SJOT	To explore the differences in the way that expert occupational therapists reflect on practice. This study asked the experts to describe their impressions after viewing a videotape of a patient in three different scenarios Neurological rehabilitation	n = 6 Sweden	Five qualitatively different types of comment were revealed: confident, tentative, generalized, teaching and understanding. The extent to which individuals used these types of comment differed, which in turn varied in relation to the three different scenarios
1996	Roberts BJOT	To examine the content and process of occupational therapists' reasoning when given a referral letter. The study approached reasoning from the cognitive sciences, based on what is known about human cognition and information-processing theories Therapists were entering postgraduate study and came from a variety of settings	n = 38 UK	The content of therapists' reasoning focused on gathering information about the client and suggesting intervention. The processes of thinking were found to be similar to those observed in studies of medical problem-solving, and there was an element of hypothetico-deductive reasoning, as has been observed in medicine. The process included problem-sensing, cue acquisition, problem formulation and problem solution
	Hagedorn BJOT	To examine experienced occupational therapists' clinical reasoning and decision-making processes when making a decision regarding the first intervention in a familiar type of case Physical rehabilitation	n = 6 UK	Occupational therapists used schematic processing to speed identification of problems and find solutions. Hagedorn found that theory had become so embedded in practice that therapists were no longer conscious of it. Schematic models representing therapists' mental problem space were developed
	Alnervik & Sviden OTJR	To examine whether descriptions of treatment sessions conducted by occupational therapists differed cognitively, depending on whether they were involved in storytelling or reflection practice. Also to examine the frequency	n = 5 Sweden	Procedural reasoning (focused on treatment interventions) was found to predominate in both storytelling and reflection using both quantitative and qualitative analysis. Accounts of reflection on practice did not contain any features distinguishing them from storytelling. A much

(Continued)

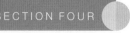

Table 16.2 Review of empirical research on clinical reasoning in occupational therapy 1983–2009—cont'd

Year	Author Journal	Aim Setting	Sample of OTs Country	Main finding
		with which different types of reasoning were used in these practices Medical and neurological rehabilitation, hand surgery and rheumatology		smaller number of comments were also categorized as conditional or interactive reasoning
	Mew & Fossey AOTJ	To explore the client-centred aspects of the clinical reasoning of an occupational therapist when using the Canadian Occupational Performance Measure Physical rehabilitation	n = 1 Australia	Three aspects of client-centred reasoning were discussed: collaboration to define problems and determine the goals of therapy; the therapist's acknowledgement of the client's feelings; and the therapist's understanding of the client
	Munroe BJOT	To investigate the scope and nature of clinical reasoning which required occupational therapists to describe the content and meaning of their thinking during routine interventions with clients and carers living in their own homes Community setting	n = 30 UK	Patterns of reasoning consisted of three elements: reflection, reasoning and decision-making. Reflection in action was commonplace during the home visits. Reasoning was found to be relativistic or pragmatic in response to contextual influences. The therapists tended to use coded meaning when explaining their thinking, which may in part account for the difficulties in articulating the reasoning that underpins clinical action. Decision-making was found to be concerned more with interactive as opposed to technical or procedural issues
	Robertson BJOT	To explore the differences in clinical reasoning in occupational therapy between student and clinicians No information provided	n = 67 New Zealand	Internal representations of clinical problems are changed by practical experience. Clinicians and students have access to the same information but this is more clearly defined and organized in the case of the clinician
1997	Hooper AJOT	To explore the worldview of an occupational therapist and how her beliefs influence the delivery of service Physical setting	n = 1 USA	A therapist's worldview frames clinical practice and shapes delivery of service. The therapist's view of reality can be categorized into four areas: '(a) what she believes about ultimate reality; (b) what she believes about life, death, and eternity; (c) what she believes about human nature; and (d) what she believes about the nature of knowing' (Hooper 1997, p.328). This worldview shapes the therapist's practice
	Crabtree & Lyons BJOT	A single case study exploring an occupational therapist's clinical reasoning as they worked in a large public hospital Acute care setting	n = 1 Australia	The therapist demonstrated a range of clinical reasoning strategies, as outlined in previous literature. These strategies operated in harmony and conflicted at different times. The view that clinical reasoning is an extremely complex process was reinforced
	Barnitt & Partridge PRI	To describe qualitatively and then compare ethical dilemmas reported by eight occupational therapists and eight	n = 8 UK	Occupational therapists were found to use a narrative style when describing ethical reasoning. Dealing with ethical dilemmas was found to be a

(Continued)

Table 16.2 Review of empirical research on clinical reasoning in occupational therapy 1983–2009—cont'd

Year	Author Journal	Aim Setting	Sample of OTs Country	Main finding
		physiotherapists Variety of physical and mental health settings		stressful but positive experience. Factors that influenced capacity to deal with the dilemma included previous experience, time for reflection and support from peers
1999	Sviden & Hallin SJOT	To explore whether therapists' clinical reasoning varied depending on their field of practice (rheumatology and neurology) Physical rehabilitation	n = 12 Sweden	Differences between these two groups of therapists were found, and it was proposed that differences in clinical reasoning may influence patient–therapist interaction. The analysis focused on the way the occupational therapists reasoned in order to make sense of the situation. Five qualitatively different groups of comment were identified: confident, tentative, understanding, generalized and teaching
2000	Gibson et al OTHC	To compare the clinical reasoning process of a novice and an experienced occupational therapist Inpatient hospital with a rehabilitation unit	n = 2 USA	Emerging themes included definitions of clinical reasoning, factors influencing clinical reasoning, sources used when reasoning, ability to prioritize, patient viewed as an individual, patients' role in treatment, and clinical reasoning as an evolving process. Both similarities and differences between the therapists were also found
2001	Unsworth SJOT	To examine qualitatively and quantitatively the differences in clinical reasoning of novice and expert occupational therapists Physical rehabilitation	n = 5 Australia	Three expert and two novice occupational therapists working in rehabilitation settings wore a head-mounted video camera while completing assessment, treatment and discharge planning sessions. Differences were found between novices and experts in both the amounts and types of clinical reasoning used. The findings suggest that novice therapists could benefit from spending more time reflecting on the therapy process and discussing their therapy with expert colleagues
2003	Doumanov & Rugg IJTR	To explore clinical reasoning and compare the factors that influence it in qualified occupational therapists and support staff Community rehabilitation teams for older clients	n = 20 UK	Occupational therapists were more likely to take a holistic view to client care. Support staff followed the treatment plans developed by the occupational therapy staff, and sought approval from the therapist prior to making any treatment decision. Concluded that the thinking of these two groups of staff is necessarily different (owing to education rather than experience) and that support staff cannot be expected to perform the same duties as occupational therapists in community rehabilitation settings
	Ward AJOT	To investigate the clinical reasoning of occupational therapists in group practice Mental health	n = 1 USA	Clinical reasoning used by the therapists in psychosocial task groups included interactive, narrative, conditional and pragmatic reasoning.

(Continued)

Table 16.2 Review of empirical research on clinical reasoning in occupational therapy 1983–2009—cont'd

Year	Author Journal	Aim Setting	Sample of OTs Country	Main finding
				The gestalt of their practice was uncovered through therapists' descriptions of the multiple levels of consciousness used in the therapy environment and larger environmental context
2004	Mitchell & Unsworth AOTJ	To present the findings of a survey that intended firstly to provide an overview of the occupational therapy role in community health centre settings, and secondly to gather some basic data on the nature of the clinical reasoning processes used during occupational therapy practice in this field Community healthcare	n = 36 Australia	Community health occupational therapists were mature in age and widely experienced. They undertook a wide range of roles. The expert therapists were confident of their skills in client-related tasks and were strongly client-centred in their reasoning. In general, the experts agreed on the reasoning needed for the case scenarios given
2004a	Unsworth BJOT	To examine the relationship between client-centred practice and clinical reasoning, explore the concept of pragmatic reasoning and present a diagrammatic conceptualization of current knowledge of clinical reasoning Physical rehabilitation	n = 13 Australia	A diagram was presented to illustrate the results, which included the overlapping nature of the types of reasoning, that a reciprocal relationship seems to exist between client-centred practice and interactive reasoning, that pragmatic reasoning was only related to the therapist's practice context, and that all forms of reasoning were influenced by the therapist's worldview
2005	Mitchell & Unsworth BJOT	To examine the clinical reasoning of five expert and five novice occupational therapists when conducting home visits Community health care	n = 10 Australia	Differences were found in the amounts and types of clinical reasoning used by novices versus experts; novices used more procedural reasoning, whereas experts used more conditional and mixes of different reasoning types. Qualitative results illustrated the smooth flow of the home visits conducted by experts, whereas novices depended on external structure such as assessment forms to guide the process. Expert reasoning was more confident and clear, while novices were more awkward and self-conscious
	Unsworth AJOT	To use a head-mounted video camera and debriefing interview to explore current conceptualizations of clinical reasoning in occupational therapy Physical rehabilitation	n = 13 Australia	The dominant forms of reasoning used were procedural, interactive and conditional. Therapists were also seen to be using aspects of pragmatic reasoning and used a newly identified form of reasoning termed generalization reasoning to draw on past experience or knowledge to assist them in making sense of a current situation or client circumstance
2007	Nikopoulou-Smyrni & Nikopoulos DR	To develop and collect preliminary data on the application of 'Anadysis' (a new integrated clinical reasoning model), involving patients suffering from stroke or	n = 4 UK	Used pretest and post-test design, the reasoning of participants using the current reasoning model of their discipline and the new Anadysis model (n = 12, including 4 occupational therapists).

(Continued)

Table 16.2 Review of empirical research on clinical reasoning in occupational therapy 1983–2009—cont'd

Year	Author Journal	Aim Setting	Sample of OTs Country	Main finding
		transient ischaemic attack. This approach was compared with a current clinical reasoning model Physical rehabilitation		Results revealed substantially higher median percentages of 'correct' responses in clinical reasoning among clinicians using the new integrated model when compared with the control group
2008	Kuipers & Grice AOTJ	To describe the repertory grid technique, to investigate the clinical reasoning of an experienced occupational therapist working in the area of upper limb hypertonia following brain injury Physical rehabilitation	n = 1 Australia	Qualitative results were presented in themes, including importance of clinical expertise and theoretical frameworks to guide practice, and the difference between 'broad' and 'specific' aspects of practice, as well as differentiation between 'therapist and client-related' aspects of the clinical situation. Quantitative analysis after the interview indicated that clinical reasoning was structured in terms of upper limb performance and client-centred aspects of the therapy process
2009	Kuipers & Grice AOTJ	To examine the impact of a protocol on the clinical reasoning of novice and expert occupational therapists when working with clients who have upper limb hypertonia following brain injury Physical rehabilitation	n = 21 Australia	Novice participants changed their reasoning after exposure to a protocol on treatment for upper limb hypertonia. Prior to exposure, novices relied on therapy tasks, the problem-solving process, environmental factors and standard practice to structure their reasoning. Following exposure, novices' clinical reasoning changed to reflect more closely experts' reasoning, which was a more collaborative model of care

Key
AJOT = American Journal of Occupational Therapy; AOTJ = Australian Occupational Therapy Journal; BJOT = British Journal of Occupational Therapy; DR = Disability and Rehabilitation; FOHPE = Focus on Health Professional Education; IJTR = International Journal of Therapy and Rehabilitation; OTJR = Occupational Therapy Journal of Research; OTHC = Occupational Therapy in Health Care; PRI = Physiotherapy Research International; SJOT = Scandinavian Journal of Occupational Therapy
AUS = Australia; CAN = Canada; NZ = New Zealand; SA = South Africa; UK = United Kingdom

Steps of theory development

1. Observation of the phenomena over time.
2. Recognition that phenomena present themselves in certain ways.
3. Organization of the phenomena into a conceptual framework.
4. Empirical testing of the propositions and concepts that hold the conceptual framework together.
5. Refinement and retesting propositions and concepts.
6. Acceptance of the new theory (adapted from Mitcham 2003).

This description of theory development implies a coordinated, concerted approach to theory generation. What we know from the definitions of modes of clinical reasoning as presented in Table 16.1, and the research undertaken and summarized in Table 16.2, is that the approach to researching and understanding clinical reasoning has been far from coordinated. However, these stages of theory development do fit well with our understanding of clinical reasoning as a contextualized phenomenon that alters depending on the circumstances. In mapping the development of clinical reasoning as a theory against these steps, it is also important to note that the approach adopted here is to build on the foundation of clinical reasoning, as laid by Mattingly and Fleming (1994), rather than fragment research in this area by seeking out new interpretations of this phenomenon (Unsworth 2004a).

The first step in theory development is to observe the phenomena over time and recognize how clinical reasoning presents itself. The occupational therapy literature is rich with descriptive observations and explorations of clinical reasoning and how it is an interactive phenomenon that varies depending on the practice context and the broader social, cultural and political environment. What is required now is more directed effort to organize clinical reasoning into a conceptual framework for occupational therapy practice. Towards this end, models of clinical reasoning can be seen as emerging from the literature. Models describe a phenomenon in a familiar way so as to increase our understanding (Young & Quinn 1992).

Five models are presented here to explain the phenomenon of clinical/professional reasoning:

- the linear model, as developed by Dewey (1929, 1934) and described by Ryan (1998)
- Mattingly and Fleming's foundation research on clinical reasoning
- the model presented by Higgs et al (2000, 2008)
- Schell's ecological model of professional reasoning (Schell 2009)
- Unsworth's updated conceptualization of clinical reasoning (2004a, 2005; see Fig. 16.1).

Although Ryan (1998) also describes a narrative model of clinical reasoning, there is insufficient information on its components and definitions to describe it in any detail. Each of these models is outlined below. In these descriptions, note is taken of whether the model has an S1 focus (clinical reasoning), and also an S2 element (decision-making). Models reflecting an S2-only approach have not been included in this chapter.

Dewey (1929, 1934): linear model of clinical reasoning (S1 and S2)

This is a classic description of general reasoning (Ryan 1998). It has many similarities to the hypothetico-deductive model of reasoning used in early medical research. This linear model consists of five stages, including reflecting on ideas, formulating hypotheses, evaluating hypotheses for truths, determining a course of action, and formulating a verbal statement to represent the hypothesis (Ryan 1998). The linear model has been widely adopted in medicine, as it fits well with the problem-solving approach required for medical diagnosis.

Mattingly and Fleming (1994): two-bodied practice and the therapist with the three-track mind (S1)

Although not articulated as a model, the documentation of the two-bodied practice and the therapist with the three-track mind none the less contributes to a developing model of clinical reasoning in occupational therapy. The eloquent description of the two-bodied practice (1994) reassures and supports occupational therapists in the belief that their practice is indeed complex, as it spans both the biomedical culture (in which we use chart talk) and the social, cultural and psychological issues surrounding the meaning of the illness (in which we use narrative reasoning). The notion of the therapist with the three-track mind provides an excellent description of three core modes of reasoning: procedural, interactive and conditional reasoning.

Higgs et al (2000, 2008): contextualized model of clinical reasoning (S1 and S2)

Higgs and Jones (2000) described an integrated, patient-centred model of clinical reasoning. They depicted an expanding spiral that reflected the clinician's growing understanding of the client and the clinical problem. At the beginning of the spiral was the clinician's encounter with the client and at the end was the final outcome. The tubing of the spiral represented the interaction of the six elements that make up the model: cognition, metacognition, the clinical problem, knowledge, the environment and the client's input. In the third edition of their text, Higgs et al (2008) describe clinical reasoning as a contextualized phenomenon, and add four meta-skills to the model, including the ability to derive knowledge and practise wisdom from reasoning and practice, the location of reasoning as relating to the selected practice model, the reflexive ability to promote personal growth in clients and self, and the use of critical creative conversations to make clinical decisions.

Schell et al 2008, Schell 2009: the ecological model of professional reasoning (S1)

Schell describes professional reasoning and the resulting therapy action as the interface of the therapist, the client and the practice context. Each practitioner brings to the therapy situation knowledge and skills that are grounded in life experiences, including personal characteristics such as physical capacities, sensory profile, personality and intelligence profile, as well as enculturated factors such as values, beliefs and preferences. These form a *personal self*, which is an inescapable lens through which the therapist frames the therapy encounter. Layered over or entwined with this personal self is the *professional self*, which includes the therapist's professional knowledge from education, experiences from prior clients, and therapy beliefs, along with knowledge of specific technical skills and therapy routines available for use in the practice context (Fondiller et al 1990, Törnebohm 1991, Mattingly & Fleming 1994, Burke 1997). The personal and professional selves act in concert to respond to various problems of practice. Clients also come to therapy with their own life experiences and contexts, which also shape the therapeutic encounter.

Unsworth (2004a, 2005, Fig. 16.1): Occupational Therapy Model of Clinical Reasoning (S1)

Based on the research foundation laid by Mattingly and Fleming (1994), Schön (1983, 1988), Barris (1987), Hooper (1997), Schell and Cervero (1993), Unsworth (2004a) proposed a three-tier structure to depict clinical reasoning. At the top of Unsworth's model is worldview (moral beliefs and socio-cultural perspective) (Wolters 1989), which influences and modifies all other modes of reasoning. The middle level of the diagram contains the three main forms of reasoning: procedural, interactive and conditional. The fact that therapists also seemed to use two or three forms of procedural/interactive/conditional reasoning simultaneously is presented by the use of a Venn diagram, and generalization reasoning is included in each of these modes. The last level of the diagram contains pragmatic reasoning (dealing with what can be achieved, given the practical constraints or benefits of the environment). The arrows flow around the model to indicate that these modes of reasoning or influences on reasoning all have an impact on each other. In Unsworth (2004a), it was stated that this model operates in the client-centred practice of occupational therapy. This model is expanded here in Figure 16.1 to incorporate the practice and contextual elements that also influence clinical reasoning. This updated model includes the client, acknowledging that reasoning is shaped by the interactive nature of the clinical encounter. The client's reasoning is also shaped by their worldview, their thoughts about health status and expectations of what occupational therapy has to offer. Clients also have many practical issues to consider that affect their therapy, such as their finances and family politics. This kind of pragmatic thinking is influenced by the client's life environment, which exists for both clients and therapists. Life environment is concerned with the social, cultural and political systems in which we live. However, a great deal more research is required to test, modify and expand this model into a conceptual framework.

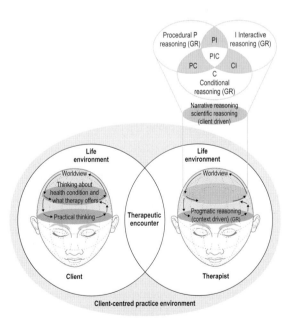

Fig. 16.1 • The Occupational Therapy Model of Clinical Reasoning. This model is based on an earlier version (Unsworth 2004a), and attempts to draw in elements from the other models to work towards building a conceptual framework.

Directions for further research in clinical reasoning

The Occupational Therapy Model of Clinical Reasoning, as illustrated in Figure 16.1, attempts to bring together some of the concepts articulated in the other models in a more integrated fashion to begin work on the third step of theory-building, which is to organize the phenomena into a conceptual framework. Research to build this framework is required in the spirit of scholarship of practice. As proposed by Nixon and Creek (2006), we need to construct theory by 'developing collaborative models of thoughtful practice that challenge assumptions and suggest new lines of inquiry'. Areas for research on the model include exploration of the relationship between pragmatic reasoning and worldview. Embodied knowledge is also not explicitly included in the model, and research is required to examine how a therapist reasons with their whole body.

Research is also required to test empirically if the components of the model are sound and hold true across different environments and over time. Finally, there is a need for further longitudinal studies of clinical reasoning. Most of the research undertaken by occupational therapists provides snapshots of practice, and what we need now are studies that track therapists reasoning, and, importantly, shifts in reasoning, over time. We need to have a better understanding of the patterns of reasoning that promote the best therapy outcomes and gain further insights into how to share these patterns with novice therapists.

Summary

When visiting clinics around the world, I see occupational therapists striving to provide the best evidence-based therapy possible. This commitment and aspiration to achieve excellence are supported by clinical reasoning. Therefore, it is crucial in our profession that we continue to research and write about clinical reasoning. The clinical reasoning of occupational therapists is a multifaceted process and forms part of the central framework of the profession. In daily practice, clinical reasoning results from the complex interactions between the therapist's own worldview, modes of reasoning and life environment, as well as the worldview, life environment and reasoning of the client. This chapter has explored the concept of clinical reasoning in occupational therapy and related factors such as intuition, worldview, expertise and reflection. It is proposed that occupational therapy researchers and writers in the area of clinical reasoning are slowly contributing to the construction of a theory of clinical reasoning. The challenge now is to ensure that the theory is built using a systematic framework and that research undertaken benefits from a scholarship of practice approach.

> **Reflective learning**
>
> - Use your own words to describe what clinical reasoning is, and differentiate clinical reasoning from clinical decision-making.
> - Describe two of the most common modes of clinical reasoning you use in practice (or you used in your last fieldwork). Reflect on why you selected these two. Consider what other reasoning modes you might use to enhance your practice in the future.
> - Many of the factors that shape our pragmatic reasoning have the potential to impact negatively on what we can do or offer clients. Can you think of an example or scenario that could lead to the kind of pragmatic reasoning that limits delivery of an ideal therapy service? What could you do to counteract the forces that lead to this kind of pragmatic reasoning?
> - Identify an episode in your career (or while doing fieldwork) that has been difficult due to discordance between your worldview and something happening in the clinic or with a client. What happened, why, and what would you do differently next time?
> - Models of clinical reasoning contributing to a theory of clinical reasoning are presented in the text. Describe a research study that you think might add to our understanding of clinical reasoning in occupational therapy and contribute to theory development in this field.

Acknowledgements

Many thanks to my research assistant, Adrian Kamer, for assistance in compiling the information presented in Table 16.2.

References

Alnervik, A., Sviden, G., 1996. On clinical reasoning: patterns of reflection on practice. Occupational Therapy Journal of Research 16 (2), 98–110.

Alsop, A., Ryan, S.E., 1996. Making the Most of Fieldwork Education: a Practical Approach. Stanley Thornes, Cheltenham.

Argyris, C., Schön, D.A., 1974. Theory in Practice: Increasing Professional Effectiveness. Jossey-Bass, San Francisco.

Barnitt, R., Partridge, C., 1997. Ethical reasoning in physical therapy and occupational therapy. Physiotherapy Research International 2, 178–194.

Barris, R., 1987. Clinical reasoning in psychosocial occupational therapy: the evaluation process. Occupational Therapy Journal of Research 7, 147–162.

Benner, P., 1984. From Novice to Expert. Excellence and Power in Clinical Nursing Practice. Addison–Wesley, Menlo Park, CA.

Benner, P.E., Tanner, C.A., Chesla, C.A., 1996. Expertise in Nursing Practice: Caring, Clinical Judgement and Ethics. Springer, New York.

Burke, J.P., 1997. Frames of meaning: An analysis of occupational therapy evaluations of young children. Dissertation Abstracts International 58 (03), 644.

Crabtree, M., Lyons, M., 1997. Focal points and relationships: a study of clinical reasoning. British Journal of Occupational Therapy 60 (2), 57–64.

Creek, J., Ormston, C., 1996. The essential elements of professional motivation. British Journal of Occupational Therapy 59, 7–10.

Creighton, C., Dijkers, M., Bennett, N., Brown, K., 1995. Reasoning and the art of therapy for spinal cord injury. American Journal of Occupational Therapy 49, 311–317.

Crepeau, E.B., Cohn, E.S., Boyt Schell, B.A. (Eds.), 2009. Willard and Spackman's Occupational Therapy, eleventh ed. Lippincott Williams & Wilkins, Baltimore.

Dewey, J., 1929. Experience and Nature. WW Norton, New York.

Dewey, J., 1934. Art as Experience. Minton & Balch, New York.

Doumanov, P., Rugg, S., 2003. Clinical reasoning skills of occupational therapists and support staff: a comparison. International Journal of Therapy and Rehabilitation 10, (5), 195–203.

Dowie, J., Elstein, A., 1988. Professional Judgement: a Reader in Clinical Decision Making. Cambridge University Press, Cambridge.

Dreyfus, H.L., Dreyfus, S.E., 1986. Mind Over Machine: The Power of Human Intuition and Expertise in the Era of the Computer. Free Press, New York.

Dreyfus, S.E., Dreyfus, H.L., 1980. A Five-Stage Model of the Mental Activities Involved in Directed Skill Acquisition. Unpublished report supported by the Air Force Office of Scientific Research (AFSC). USAF (Contract F49620-79-C-0063), University of California at Berkeley, Berkeley.

Duncan, E.A.S., 2006. An introduction to conceptual models of practice and frames of reference. In: Duncan, E.A.S. (Ed.), Foundations for Practice in Occupational Therapy. Elsevier, Edinburgh.

Fleming, M.H., 1991. The therapist with the three-track mind. American Journal of Occupational Therapy 45, 1007–1014.

Fleming, M.H., 1994. The therapist with the three track mind. In: Mattingly, C., Fleming, M.H. (Eds.), Clinical Reasoning: Forms of Inquiry in a Therapeutic Practice. FA Davis, Philadelphia, pp. 119–136.

Fondiller, E.L., Rosage, L.J., Neuhaus, B.E., 1990. Values Influencing Clinical Reasoning in Occupational Therapy: An Exploratory Study. Occupational Therapy Journal of Research 10, 41–55.

Fortune, T., Ryan, S., 1996. Applying Clinical Reasoning: a Caseload Management System for Community Occupational Therapists. British Journal of Occupational Therapy 59 (5), 207–211.

Gibson, D.B., Velde, B., Hoff, T., et al., 2000. Clinical reasoning of a novice versus an experienced occupational therapist: a qualitative study. Occupational Therapy in Health Care 12 (4), 15–31.

Goel, V., Buchel, C., Frith, C., et al., 2000. Dissociation of mechanisms underlying syllogistic reasoning. NeuroImage 12 (5), 504–514.

Hagedorn, R., 1996. Clinical decision making in familiar cases: a model of the process and implications for practice. British Journal of Occupational Therapy 59 (5), 217–222.

Hallin, M., Sviden, G., 1995. On expert occupational therapists' reflection-on-practice. Scandinavian Journal of Occupational Therapy 2, 69–75.

Hammond, K.R., 1996. Human Judgment and Social Policy: Irreducible Uncertainty, Inevitable Error, Unavoidable Injustice. Oxford University Press, New York.

Hammond, K.R., Brehmer, B., 1973. Quasi rationality and distrust: implications for international conflict. In: Summers, D., Rappoport, L. (Eds.), Human Judgement and Social Interaction. Holt, Rinehart & Wonston, New York, pp. 338–391.

Hardman, D., 2009. Judgment and Decision Making: Psychological Perspectives. BPS Blackwell, Chichester.

Harries, P., Duncan, E.A.S., 2009. Judgement and decision-making skills for practice. In: Duncan, E.A.S. (Ed.), Skills for Practice in Occupational Therapy. Elsevier, Edinburgh, pp. 25–39.

Harries, P., Gilhooly, K., 2006. Identifying occupational therapists' referral priorities in community health. Occupational Therapy International 10 (2), 150–164.

Harries, P., Harries, C., 2001. Studying clinical reasoning, Part 2: Applying social judgment theory. British Journal of Occupational Therapy 64 (6), 285–292.

Higgs, J., Jones, M., 2000. Clinical Reasoning in the Health Professions, second ed. Butterworth–Heinemann, Melbourne.

Higgs, J., Jones, M., Loftus, S.L., et al., 2008. Clinical Reasoning in the Health Professions, third ed. Butterworth–Heinemann, Melbourne.

Holm, M.B., 2000. Our mandate for the new millennium: evidence-based practice. American Journal of Occupational Therapy 54, 575–585.

Hooper, B., 1997. The relationship between pretheoretical assumptions and clinical reasoning. American Journal of Occupational Therapy 51 (5), 328–338.

Kielhofner, G., 2008. Model of Human occupation: Theory and Application, fourth ed. Lippincott Williams & Wilkins, Baltimore.

Kielhofner, G., 2009. Conceptual Foundations of Occupational Therapy, fourth ed. FA Davis, Philadelphia.

Kielhofner, G., Forsyth, K., 2002. Thinking with theory: a framework for therapeutic reasoning. In: Kielhofner, G. (Ed.), Model of Human Occupation: Theory and Application, third ed. Lippincott Williams & Wilkins, Baltimore, pp. 162–178.

Klein, G.A., Orasanu, J., Calderwoon, R., et al., 1993. Decision Making in Action: Models and Methods. Ablex, Norwood, NJ.

Kuipers, K., Grice, J.W., 2008. Clinical reasoning in neurology: use of the repertory grid technique to investigate the reasoning of an experienced occupational therapist. Australian Occupational Therapy Journal 56 (4), 275–284.

Kuipers, K., Grice, J.W., 2009. The structure of novice and expert occupational therapists' clinical reasoning before and after exposure to a domain-specific protocol. Australian Occupational Therapy Journal 56 (6), 418–427.

Lyons, K.D., Crepeau, E.B., 2001. The clinical reasoning of an occupational therapy assistant. American Journal of Occupational Therapy 55, 577–581.

Mattingly, C., 1994. Occupational therapy as a two-body practice: the body as machine. In: Mattingly, C., Fleming, M.H. (Eds.), Clinical Reasoning: Forms of Inquiry in a Therapeutic Practice. FA Davis, Philadelphia, pp. 37–63.

Mattingly, C., Fleming, M.H., 1994. Clinical Reasoning: Forms of Inquiry in a Therapeutic Practice. FA Davis, Philadelphia.

McKay, E.A., 2009. Reflective practice: doing, being and becoming a reflective practitioner. In: Duncan, E.A.S. (Ed.), Skills for Practice in Occupational Therapy. Churchill Livingstone, Edinburgh, pp. 55–72.

McKay, E.A., Ryan, S., 1995. Clinical reasoning through story telling: examining a student's case story on a fieldwork placement. British Journal of Occupational Therapy 58 (6), 234–238.

Melton, J., Forsyth, K., Freeth, D., 2009. Using theory in practice. In: Duncan, E.A.S. (Ed.), Skills for Practice in Occupational Therapy. Churchill Livingstone, Edinburgh, pp. 9–24.

Mew, M.M., Fossey, E., 1996. Client-centred aspects of clinical reasoning during an initial assessment using the Canadian Occupational Performance Measure. Australian Occupational Therapy Journal 43, 155–166.

Mitcham, M.D., 2003. Integrating theory and practice: using theory creatively to enhance professional practice. In: Brown, G., Esdaile, S.A., Ryan, S.E. (Eds.), Becoming an Advanced Healthcare Practitioner. Butterworth–Heinemann, New York, pp. 64–89.

Mitchell, R., Unsworth, C.A., 2004. Role perceptions and clinical reasoning of community health occupational therapists undertaking home visits. Australian Occupational Therapy Journal 51 (1), 13–24.

Mitchell, R., Unsworth, C.A., 2005. Clinical reasoning during community health home visits: expert and novice differences. British Journal of Occupational Therapy 68 (5), 215–223.

Munroe, H., 1996. Clinical reasoning in community occupational therapy. British Journal of Occupational Therapy 59 (5), 196–202.

Neistadt, M.E., 1987. Classroom as clinic: a model of teaching clinical reasoning in occupational therapy education. American Journal of Occupational Therapy 41, 631–637.

Neistadt, M.E., Atkins, A., 1996. Analysis of the orthopedic content in an occupational therapy curriculum from a clinical reasoning perspective.

American Journal of Occupational Therapy 50, 669–675.

Neuhaus, B.E., 1988. Ethical considerations in clinical reasoning: the impact of technology and cost containment. American Journal of Occupational Therapy 42, 288–294.

Nikopoulou-Smyrni, P., Nikopoulos, C.K., 2007. A new integrated model of clinical reasoning: development, description and preliminary assessment in patients with stroke. Disability and Rehabilitation 29 (14), 1129–1138.

Nixon, J., Creek, J., 2006. Towards a theory of practice. British Journal of Occupational Therapy 69 (2), 77–80.

Rassafiani, M., Ziviani, J., Rodger, S., et al., 2006. Managing upper limb hypertonicity: factors influencing therapists' decisions. British Journal of Occupational Therapy 69 (8), 373–378.

Rassafiani, M., Ziviani, J., Rodger, S., et al., 2008. Occupational therapists' decision-making in the management of clients with upper limb hypertonicity. Scandinavian Journal of Occupational Therapy 15 (2), 105–115.

Rew, L., 1986. Intuition: concept analysis of a group phenomenon. Advances in Nursing Science 8 (2), 21–28.

Roberts, A.E., 1996. Clinical reasoning in occupational therapy: idiosyncrasies in content and process. British Journal of Occupational Therapy 59 (8), 372–376.

Robertson, L., 1996. Clinical reasoning, Part 2: Novice/expert differences. British Journal of Occupational Therapy 59 (5), 212–216.

Rogers, J.C., 1983. Clinical reasoning: the ethics, science, and art. American Journal of Occupational Therapy 37, 601–616.

Rogers, J.C., 2010. Occupational reasoning. In: Curtin, M., Molineux, M., Supyk-Mellson, J. (Eds.), Occupational Therapy and Physical Dysfunction. Enabling Occupation. Churchill Livingstone, Sydney, pp. 57–65.

Rogers, J.C., Holm, M.B., 1991. Occupational therapy diagnostic reasoning: a component of clinical reasoning. American Journal of Occupational Therapy 45, 1045–1053.

Rogers, J.C., Masagatani, G., 1982. Clinical reasoning of occupational

therapists during initial assessment of physically disabled patients. Occupational Therapy Journal of Research 2, 195–219.

Rogers, J.C., 1982. Teaching Clinical Reasoning in Practice in Geriatrics. Physical and Occupational Therapy in Geriatrics 1 (3), 29–37.

Ryan, S., 1998. Influences that shape our reasoning. In: Creek, J. (Ed.), Occupational Therapy New Perspectives. Whurr, London, pp. 47–65.

Schell, B.A.B., 2009. Professional reasoning in practice. In: Crepeau, E.B., Cohn, E., Schell, B.A.B. (Eds.), Willard and Spackman's Occupational Therapy. Wolters Kluwer, Philadelphia, pp. 314–327.

Schell, B.A.B., Cervero, R.M., 1993. Clinical reasoning in occupational therapy: an integrative review. American Journal of Occupational Therapy 47, 605–610.

Schell, B.A.B., Harris, D., 2008. Embodiment: reasoning with the whole body. In: Schell, B.A.B., Schell, J.W. (Eds.), Clinical and Professional Reasoning in Occupational Therapy. Lippincott Williams & Wilkins, Philadelphia, pp. 69–87.

Schell, B.A.B., Schell, J.W. (Eds.), 2008. Clinical and Professional Reasoning in Occupational Therapy. Wolters Kluwer, Philadelphia.

Schell, B.A.B., Unsworth, C.A., Schell, J.W., 2008. Theory and practice: new directions for research in professional reasoning. In: Schell, B.A.B., Schell, J.W. (Eds.), Clinical and Professional Reasoning in Occupational Therapy. Lippincott Williams & Wilkins, Philadelphia, pp. 401–431.

Schön, D.A., 1983. The Reflective Practitioner: How Professionals Think in Action. Basic, New York.

Schön, D.A., 1988. Educating the Reflective Practitioner. Jossey-Bass, San Francisco.

Stanovich, K.E., West, R.W., 2000. Individual differences in reasoning: implications for the rationality debate? Behavioral and Brain Sciences 23 (5), 645–726.

Strong, J., Gilbert, J., Cassidy, S., et al., 1995. Expert clinicians' and students' views on clinical reasoning in occupational therapy. British Journal of Occupational Therapy 58 (3), 119–123.

Sviden, G., 1995. Responding to patients' nonverbal communication of affect. Occupational Therapy Journal of Research 15 (2), 85–102.

Sviden, G., Hallin, M., 1999. Differences in clinical reasoning between occupational therapists working in rheumatology and neurology. Scandinavian Journal of Occupational Therapy 6, 63–69.

Sviden, G., Saljo, R., 1993. perceiving patients and their nonverbal reactions. American Journal of Occupational Therapy 47 (6), 491–497.

Thompson, D. (Ed.), 1995. Concise Oxford Dictionary, ninth ed. Oxford Clarendon, Oxford.

Törnebohm, H., 1991. What is worth knowing in occupational therapy? American Journal of Occupational Therapy 45, 451–454.

Unsworth, C.A., 1999. Cognitive and Perceptual Disorders: A Clinical Reasoning Approach to Evaluation and Intervention. FA Davis, Philadelphia.

Unsworth, C.A., 2001. The clinical reasoning of novice and expert occupational therapists. Scandinavian Journal of Occupational Therapy 8, 163–173.

Unsworth, C.A., 2004a. Clinical reasoning: how do worldview, pragmatic reasoning and client-centredness fit? British Journal of Occupational Therapy 67, 10–19.

Unsworth, C.A., 2004b. How therapists think: Exploring therapists' reasoning when working with patients who have cognitive and perceptual problems following stroke. In: Gillen, G., Burkhardt, A. (Eds.), Stroke Rehabilitation: A Function-Based Approach, second ed. Mosby, St Louis, pp. 358–375.

Unsworth, C.A., 2005. Using a head-mounted video camera to explore current conceptualizations of clinical reasoning in occupational therapy. American Journal of Occupational Therapy 59, 31–40.

Unsworth, C.A., 2007. Using social judgment theory to study occupational therapists' use of information when making licensing recommendations to older and functionally impaired drivers. American Journal of Occupational Therapy 61 (5), 493–502.

Unsworth, C.A., Schell, B.A., 2006. Clinical Reasoning: Development of a Theory-in-use. In: Proceedings of the 14th International Congress of the World Federation of Occupational Therapists, Sydney 24–28 July.

Unsworth, C.A., Thomas, S.A., 1993. Information use in discharge accommodation recommendations for stroke patients. Clinical Rehabilitation 7, 181–188.

Unsworth, C.A., Thomas, S.A., Greenwood, K.M., 1995.

Rehabilitation team decisions concerning discharge housing for stroke patients. Archives of Physical Medicine and Rehabilitation 76, 331–340.

Unsworth, C.A., Osberg, J.S., Graham, A., 1997. Admitting pediatric trauma patients to rehabilitation following acute care: decision making practices in the U.S.A. and Australia. Journal of Pediatric Rehabilitation 1, 207–218.

Walker, K.F., Ludwig, F.M., 2004. Perspectives on Theory for the Practice of Occupational Therapy, third ed. Pro-ed, Austin, TX.

Ward, J.D., 2003. The nature of clinical reasoning with groups: a phenomenological study of an occupational therapist in community mental health. American Journal of Occupational Therapy 57 (6), 625–634.

Wolters, A.M., 1989. On the idea of worldview and its relationship to philosophy. In: Marshall, P.A., Griffioen, S., Mouw, R. (Eds.), Stained Glass: Worldviews and Social Science. University Press of America, New York, pp. 14–26.

Young, M.E., Quinn, E., 1992. Theories and Principles of Occupational Therapy. Churchill Livingstone, London.

Community-based rehabilitation

17

Rachel Thibeault   Michèle Hébert

OVERVIEW

This chapter provides an overview of community-based rehabilitation (CBR), its history, its philosophical tenets, its goals and its process. From the Independent Living Movement of the 1960s to the recent impetus provided by the Convention on the Rights of People with Disabilities, the history of CBR is reviewed with a special focus on social justice. This historical overview leads to the presentation of a current definition of CBR with its core values highlighted, including empowerment, enablement, equality, dignity for all, participation and integration. The goals of CBR are then explored, among them access to adequate rehabilitation services, elimination/reduction of environmental barriers, promotion of the human rights of people with disabilities, social integration and community participation, and equitable political and legal representation. A description of a typical CBR participative process follows, based on the World Health Organization (WHO) CBR matrix. The overview of CBR concludes with an analysis of its strengths and limitations; issues of power, sustainability, coordination, inclusion, relevance and expectations are discussed. Finally, the chapter reflects on the similarities between CBR and occupational therapy, and its official endorsement by the World Federation of Occupational Therapists (WFOT).

Key points

- CBR and occupational therapy both stem from historical needs for greater social justice.
- CBR, like occupational therapy, fosters empowerment, enablement and better quality of life for people with disabilities.

Key points—cont'd

- CBR offers flexible, local, low-cost, non-institutional answers to the needs of people with disabilities through local resources and equitable access.
- The WHO defines CBR as the model of choice for community development for people with disabilities.
- WFOT supports occupational therapists working within a CBR framework.

Introduction

Although barely mentioned in mainstream media, 3 May 2008 was nevertheless a moving, historic day. Human rights agencies had been preparing feverishly for the official announcement and people with disabilities worldwide were massed around giant TV screens or in community halls, finally witnessing the entry into force of the first human rights convention of the 21st century: the United Nations Convention on the Rights of Persons with Disabilities (CRPD). At last, not only would the needs of over 650 million people with disabilities be taken into account, but the traditional perception of disability as a curse or burden was also being challenged on the world stage. Boldly shedding the dominant medical–social welfare model, the CRPD called for full participation of people with disabilities and anti-discrimination legislation with a special focus on capability to counteract the enduring inability stigma.

The Convention has been deemed revolutionary, a long-awaited victory for the world's largest minority (Convention on the Rights of Persons with Disabilities 2009). And, to whoever might wonder why the Convention represents such a watershed moment, the United Nations' data on disability provide clear answers. Currently, people with disabilities constitute over 10% of the world's population, a number that steadily increases along with population growth, average life expectancy and the range of medical resources to prolong or protect life (World Health Organization 2009a). Most of them, over 80%, reside in the southern hemisphere, and 20% of the 'bottom billion', the poorest people on Earth, live with a disability. People with disabilities are chronically and vastly under-represented in all social systems, including education and employment (Werner 1998, Wiman et al 2002), and United Nations Children's Fund (UNICEF) studies also indicate that 30% of street children struggle with a disability (Convention on the Rights of Persons with Disabilities 2009).

Since only 45 countries have so far embedded legislation aimed at protecting the rights of people with disabilities in their legal framework (Turmusani et al 2002), these rights have remained largely ignored (Boyce & Lysack 1997, Thibeault 2008). People with disabilities are routinely perceived as second-class citizens incapable of making their own decisions and are often treated as wards of the state. Recognition of their rights was and is still a precarious affair, but it gained considerable momentum in the early 1970s with the advent of primary healthcare (PHC) (Périquet 1984). This new concept called for true community consultation, participation and education in healthcare and it appealed greatly to people with disabilities. Quickly percolating through their ranks, it gave rise shortly thereafter to a budding movement by and for people with disabilities called community-based rehabilitation (CBR) (Boyce & Lysack 1997, Willig-Levy 2009). Through a series of grassroots initiatives mostly taking place in the southern hemisphere, CBR gradually established itself, but with numerous glitches along the way. Perceptions softened slowly, with government agencies still leaning towards patronizing attitudes and top-down decisions imposed without consultation with people with disabilities. The first major breakthrough occurred in 1978, at the Alma Ata conference on primary healthcare, held under the aegis of the World Health Organization (WHO). In Alma Ata, health was defined as a prerequisite to socially and economically productive lives. Burden of disease and disability, and its associated costs, were then identified as major obstacles on the road to economic self-sufficiency for the southern hemisphere. It was imperative to resolve the issue for the economy to

run smoothly and, to do so, two main strategies were proposed. The first was called Disability Prevention through Impairment Reduction. This strategy implied that all social sectors needed to be mobilized in order either to prevent disability or to adapt to existing disabilities. The onus of full social participation shifted from the individual to society, and the confining of people with disabilities to institutions or lives of stigma and ostracism was no longer seen as acceptable. The second strategy, Rehabilitation Delivery, entailed the design of community-based services with an appropriate system of supervision and referral. Together, these two initial strategies articulated CBR core values and gave a more definite shape to the emerging movement. CBR was officially born (Périquet 1984).

The philosophical tenets behind CBR

Over time, the two initial strategies of Disability Prevention through Impairment Reduction and Rehabilitation Delivery expanded into more complex conceptual horizons. New notions and paradigms were integrated, fleshing out the original philosophical nucleus. These notions or paradigms were not specific to the context of disability, but were inserted into the growing CBR framework for their relevance to any vulnerable population. Among them, the following have exercised the greatest influence on CBR's evolution.

In the 1960s and 1970s, the concept of *empowerment* nearly became a household name, thanks to the Independent Living Movement that spread through the USA and beyond (Willig-Levy 2009), bringing independence for people with disabilities into the realm of the possible. It was defined as 'the multidimensional social process that helps people gain control over their own lives . . . and that fosters power in people for use in their own lives, their communities and in their society, by acting on issues they define as important' (Page & Czuba 2009, p.1).

Empowerment meant that people with disabilities could and should be involved in all decisions concerning them. This was especially contentious at the time since, in CBR, the word disability applies just as much to the psychological as to the physical, and ostracism of those with mental disabilities was even more prevalent then than it is today.

The concept of *enablement* was coined shortly thereafter and could be described as the operational application of empowerment. While empowerment aims to ascertain the legitimacy of making choices, enablement provides the means to actualize decisions. Going beyond the notion of power, it encompasses 'the adequate power, means, opportunity, or authority (to do something), to make (something) possible' (Reverso 2009, p.1). When implemented correctly, enablement should translate into full participation, facilitation and self-advocacy (Helander 1999).

As means and opportunities are closely linked to resources, which are often quite scarce in the southern hemisphere, new ways of addressing the challenges faced by people with disabilities had to be explored. These included the creative provision of low-cost services and, because professionals are too costly to offer and monitor services continually on site, the responsibility of day-to-day service delivery was passed on to local communities. Two principles were then added: a commitment to low-cost services and a clear recognition of the local communities' responsibility for their CBR programmes (Gautron 1999).

Finally, in the early 1990s, the Disability Action Group, a unit within the United Nations Development Programme (PNUD), embedded CBR within the WHO structure and anchored its foundations in five guiding principles: equality, social justice, solidarity, integration and dignity for all persons with disabilities (ILO et al 2004). This is why, in many ways, CBR is considered more of a social movement than a rehabilitation approach. And, as with any social movement, its main purpose is to change mentalities.

CBR's goals and objectives

The scope of the required social change was too broad and could not be tackled in its entirety. So, to make dignity for all a reality, priorities had to be established. In the 1990s, five key objectives were selected by the WHO. These were:

- access to adequate rehabilitation services
- elimination/reduction of environmental barriers
- promotion of the human rights of people with disabilities
- social integration and community participation
- equitable political and legal representation (Helander 1999, World Health Organization 2009b).

These goals ebbed and flowed over the years and a 2004 joint task force on CBR involving the International Labour Organization (ILO), the United Nations Educational, Scientific and Cultural Organization (UNESCO) and WHO reoriented CBR on rehabilitation, equalization of opportunity, poverty reduction and social inclusion of people with disabilities (ILO et al 2004).

CBR's current definition and scope

This repositioning led to the current definition of CBR:

> CBR focuses on enhancing the quality of life for people with disabilities and their families, meeting basic needs and ensuring inclusion and participation. CBR is a multisectoral approach, comprises 5 major elements: health, education, livelihood, social justice and empowerment . . . and uses predominantly local resources. (World Health Organization 2009b, p.1)

The goals of CBR are to ensure the benefits of the Convention on Rights of Persons with Disabilities reach the majority by:

1. supporting people with disabilities to maximize their physical and mental abilities, to access regular services and opportunities, and to become active contributors to the community and society at large;
2. activating communities to promote and protect the human rights of people with disabilities, for example by removing barriers to participation;
3. facilitating capacity building, empowerment and community mobilization of people with disabilities and their families. (WHO 2009b, p.1)

In short, CBR has come back to its roots with a renewed and explicit emphasis on programme sustainability, partnerships, and sensitivity to gender and special needs.

The CBR structure

The 2004 joint task force presented CBR as:

> a strategy within general community development . . . [that] is implemented through the combined efforts of people with disabilities themselves, their families, organizations and communities, and the relevant governmental and non-governmental health, education, vocational, social and other services. (ILO 2004, p.6)

Despite apparent clarity, significant debate has occurred over the structure of CBR. Initially meant as a purely bottom-up rather than top-down approach (Werner 1988, 1998, Peat 1997), it did not deliver on its promises of yielding purely grass-roots rehabilitation systems. The original vision revolved around communities that would spontaneously initiate the request for rehabilitation services and involved six major groups that would join forces to provide a continuum of care (Helander 1999); people with disabilities, at the centre of the process, would define their needs and be assisted by volunteer family trainers, local CBR agents and local stakeholders, who together constitute the local CBR committee. In turn, whenever needed, this local CBR committee would call upon personnel in referral facilities and national specialists to tackle issues too complex for local means. However, this ideal scenario remained elusive; people with disabilities frequently lacked the necessary awareness and self-confidence to launch the projects, and the impetus for the creation of CBR programmes came mostly from the outside. 'Hybrid' CBR programmes have thus emerged that bring together a wide range of players wielding varying degrees of influence (Kuipers et al 2003, Finkenflügel et al 2008).

Currently, there are over 10 different configurations that would still qualify as CBR programmes (Finkenflügel et al 2008). Their common, defining CBR features lie in keeping the needs and quality of life of people with disabilities as the main focus, remaining rooted in the local community and promoting equal opportunities. Since the 2004 joint paper, efforts have been made to introduce within the general CBR agenda the issues of human rights, poverty, inclusive communities accessible for all, and a more active role for organizations of people with disabilities.

The most common CBR settings

Although some CBR programmes have taken hold in the developed nations, most occur in the southern hemisphere in poor urban or rural settings. In the northern hemisphere, except for the Canadian Arctic (Thibeault & Forget 1997), CBR programmes have been developed by relatively affluent subgroups such as farmers with disabilities or ethnic minorities wishing to ensure delivery of community rehabilitation services in their mother tongue (Peat 1997). Although these are still the exception, several analysts and healthcare providers advocate the use of CBR in wealthier economies as well (Peat 1997, Lindsay et al 2008, Hirsch 2009).

The CBR process

CBR usually unfolds according to a 15-step process but, given the diversity of CBR formats (Finkenflügel et al 2008), these steps only reflect general guidelines and not cast-in-stone directions. Moreover, the steps do not necessarily always follow this sequence in a linear fashion.

Initiating CBR

As previously mentioned, CBR programmes are mostly initiated by ministries, non-governmental organizations (NGOs) or other external bodies, but no programme will be developed unless the community becomes the principal stakeholder and participant. Public and private consultations are held to assess community willingness and, if there is sufficient interest, a CBR management team is created and proceeds to the first needs and strengths assessment (ILO et al 2004).

The CBR management team oversees the process on behalf of the initiator and is composed of one or several representatives of the initiating body, representatives of the local community (for example, people with disabilities, relatives, influential persons, political or religious leaders and so on) and experts, as it is deemed appropriate. Experience has demonstrated that early involvement of influential persons is crucial for future success. The CBR management team, more removed from immediate CBR activities, should not be confused with the local CBR committee described below, which is responsible for the actual carrying out of the CBR activities.

Assessing the community: needs, strengths and existing services

The assessment includes several core features necessary to determine the nature and scope of future activities:

- number of people with disabilities within a given area
- demographic data, such as age and gender
- types of disability
- work histories
- community resources that could be mobilized to support people with disabilities
- potential grants

- influential people already sensitized to the situation of people with disabilities, and so on.

Existing services have to be identified, defined and understood, creating a conceptual map of local service delivery, in order to grasp the eventual position of the budding CBR programme relative to other providers and avoiding duplication. This assessment may be completed via surveys, door-to-door interviews and key informants. While completing the assessment, two major pitfalls must be carefully avoided. Firstly, surveys might create expectations among people with disabilities and the evaluators need be very transparent. The purpose and impact of the survey should be clearly separated from any financial losses or gains. Indeed, it is common for people with disabilities in the southern hemisphere to associate surveys with two opposite realities: the expectation of receiving money, and being asked for money. Consequently, the assessment process should be framed as a dialogue, meant to reach mutual understanding and allowed to unfold fairly slowly. As a rule, the establishment of a CBR programme is done incrementally, in an organic and gradual fashion.

Sensitizing the broader community and stimulating participation

This stage may take many forms. These include community get-togethers, with food and beverages being served in a festive atmosphere where people without disabilities mingle with people with disabilities. Minimally competitive games are designed to highlight the competence of people with disabilities and to allow people without disabilities to experience some basic simulations of impaired hearing, impaired sight and motor limitations. The games and mingling are intended to reduce prejudice and enable networking between both groups.

Others means of sensitization include raffles (draws), bingo and talent nights, and other similar activities used to create an informal platform for community sensitization around disability. Continuing education workshops for local professionals or policy-makers may also be organized on topics relating to disability, autonomy and dignity.

Creating a local CBR committee

If, following the sensitization stage, there is firm motivation on the part of the main stakeholders, a local CBR committee is created. It draws from the same pool used for the CBR management committee: people with disabilities, relatives, influential persons, political or religious leaders, schoolteachers and so on. The local CBR committee's mandate differs from that of the CBR management committee. The local CBR committee's function is to participate in the design, implementation and monitoring of CBR activities and to constitute an essential bridge between the CBR programmes and its community. It also counts one extra member: the CBR agent. Depending on the setting, CBR agents have normally received between 3 and 18 months' training that spans basic knowledge in occupational therapy, physical therapy and programme management. Together with the people with disabilities, CBR agents are the chief facilitators, the local driving force behind programmes. In some instances, they are paid workers, an aspect that contradicts the original CBR concepts that called for an almost entirely voluntary structure.

Mobilizing financial resources

Ensuring financial viability is obviously paramount for the success of any CBR programme. Projects must have some source of funding. The three main ones are income-generating activities, sponsorship and grants. Of the three, income-generating activities have been associated with the most sustainable CBR programmes. Income-generating activities can be divided into two categories: intermittent events (such as fund-raising, baking sales, concerts, etc.) and permanent microfinance projects (such as peanut butter production, vegetable gardens, day care services, etc.). It is the latter that contribute the most to sustainability.

Designing the management structure

Each local CBR committee has to select a management format adapted to its needs. These generally entail four components:

- *the programme component*, dealing with the identification of target populations, goals, objectives and definition of procedures
- *the personnel component*, dealing with required expertise and respective roles and responsibilities
- *the financial component*, dealing with budgetary management and provisions

- *the monitoring and evaluation component*, dealing with all data collection necessary for answering sponsors' requirements and improving services.

Training the local CBR committee members

The world of disability is usually unknown to the people without disability. Since all committee members work as a team, they, with and without disability alike, must cultivate a set of shared assumptions and goals. Initial training deals with the recognition of disability and its consequences, the refusal to equate disability with inability, and the development of a collective strength-based vision.

Training the volunteers

Volunteers are people who agree to support CBR activities in their communities. Quite often, family members or neighbours of people with disabilities, they assist them on a regular basis, sometimes daily. They generally receive some brief initial training from the CBR agent, followed by ongoing training as specific situations arise. They learn, for example, how to enable activities of daily living, facilitate mobility or foster socializing. If therapeutic exercises have to be practised, it is with the help of the volunteers.

Promoting local leadership and disabled persons' organizations (DPOs); linking with other CBR programmes

CBR programme managers often overlook one very useful contribution they can make: connecting all interested people in their area within the field of disability and beyond. This includes organizations of people with disabilities (still labelled DPOs in most settings). CBR programmes can run joint leadership training courses and awareness campaigns with DPOs; they can share relevant information, strengthen networks and press for new avenues for people with disabilities with agencies such as cooperatives or credit unions.

Moreover, CBR programmes are encouraged to connect with other CBR initiatives to rationalize resources whenever possible and share learning. This can often be facilitated through the creation of a

CBR resource centre. Such a centre might offer timely advice, training activities, learning materials for the members, and information on the programmes for external agencies. It increases CBR's social exposure and legitimacy, and quickly becomes a hub for informal communication and support.

Involving public authorities

Without necessarily having them as sitting members on the local CBR committee, CBR projects can gain significantly from having open lines of communication with public authorities and keeping them informed of their activities and the obstacles they encounter. Through de facto sensitization, close collaborations with officials can promote faster and broader change that is beneficial to people with disabilities in the public sphere and provide channels conducive to quicker resolution of issues stemming from current public policies.

Tackling gender equality and inclusion of all age groups

Prior to empowering people with disabilities and starting activities, CBR projects must undergo an internal audit to ensure that the foundations are built on equitable grounds. This assessment focuses not only on member representation, but also on resource allocation and burden of care. It asks questions such as whether or not all age groups will benefit from the same or equivalent advantages, and whether the burden of care of the most severely disabled members will be equitably distributed among male and female volunteers.

Sensitizing the members to mental health issues

Even within CBR programmes, stigma towards mental disabilities is strong. To maximize communication, normalize rapport and equalize opportunities, an internal formal education process must take place involving all members.

Empowering people with disabilities

Many CBR projects include educational programmes in their activities. These focus on human rights, the new UN CRPD, and on women's and children's rights. Special attention is paid to national legislation concerning people with disabilities, specifically regarding employment, healthcare, education and transport. Leadership and advocacy training is also offered, most often in an experiential, non-didactic format.

Implementing activities

Before launching CBR activities, a careful analysis must be performed. This can be summarized into five key points:

- What are the main needs observed?
- Which among those can initially be tackled most successfully?
- What activities would answer those needs?
- Where are the best points of entry in the CBR matrix (Fig. 17.1)?
- What strategies would be best?

Once the priority needs have been identified, the local CBR committee must decide on the strategy, using the CBR matrix. The CBR matrix maps the different CBR possibilities and can be entered at any point, depending on the issue at hand. Are work and income generation the pressing problems? Then action will first be planned along the livelihood axis. If it is access to school, then the education axis will be used, and so on.

Next, specific strategies and activities are defined. For example, a CBR committee might decide to lobby to make the local school accessible to children with disabilities through a series of sensitization workshops with stakeholders from the education and health sectors, followed shortly thereafter by negotiation sessions. If they succeed, volunteers would then make regular visits to the school to assist the children with disabilities and enable integration. Reports would be made to the committee and the next step might be to request modifications to the curriculum to include skills training suited to the needs of children with disabilities. The most successful CBR projects develop gradually, building on incremental gains.

Monitoring and evaluation

Ideally, monitoring and evaluation should address community participation, ownership, equity, process, impacts and unforeseen outcomes. A 360-degree format gathers the most useful information if carried out in a way that is respectful of the community's customs. Written surveys should not be used in a culture based on oral tradition. Transparent sharing of evaluation data among all stakeholders is also more in line with CBR's philosophy.

Strengths and weaknesses of CBR

At the community level, CBR undeniably fosters greater sensitization and improves social perceptions around disability (Gautron 1999). It offers flexible, local, low-cost, non-institutional answers

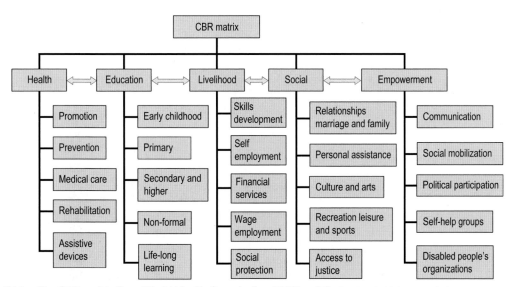

Fig. 17.1 • The CBR matrix (from World Health Organization 2009b p.57). Reprinted with kind permission.

to the needs of people with disabilities and methodologies adapted to their context and future growth (Kuipers et al 2008, Finkenflügel 2009). It aims to reach the greater number of people with disabilities in a holistic, participative way while simultaneously linking them to national policy- and decision-makers (Kuipers et al 2008). Unfortunately, CBR projects are still too often planned for and not with people with disabilities (Werner 1998, International Consultation to Review Community-Based Rehabilitation 2009). The CBR programme is then seen as being imposed from the outside and users with disabilities become disenfranchised. As a rule, a condescending approach tends to translate into poor fit and lack of ownership and engagement on the community's part.

Sustainability also poses a major challenge, given the high turnover observed among volunteers and CBR agents (Gautron 1999, Kuipers et al 2008). Volunteers generally follow two main scenarios. They leave because the brief training they have received allows them to find paid employment elsewhere or, despite repeated messages throughout the selection process, they harbour the continued hope of eventually being hired as an employee, become disillusioned when this does not occur, and quit. With the rise of HIV/AIDS, a third scenario is also becoming more prevalent. Volunteers engage in CBR activities to support their relatives living with disabilities secondary to HIV/AIDS, but they themselves eventually have to leave as the disease claims their energy and health. With CBR agents, turnover is mostly linked to better vocational opportunities in the private sector, as their broad and versatile training makes them attractive recruits for local industry.

Lack of coordination also threatens the survival of many CBR programmes. Historically, people with disabilities have faced systematic abuse and rejection and, as a result, have grown distrustful of official services and agencies. CBR programmes frequently function in a vacuum divorced from national and international resources and policies (International Consultation to Review Community-Based Rehabilitation 2009). Multi-sectoral collaboration is, therefore, a key ingredient in any successful programme, and the earlier a range of stakeholders is involved, the more positive the outcome.

Paradoxically, CBR programmes often tend to overlook one of their own core values: namely, inclusion. Research has shown (International Consultation to Review Community-Based Rehabilitation 2009) that some programmes neglect the needs of women and children, with a strong priority being given to adult males. In some instances, CBR programme managers advocate for men only, stating that female members should not aspire to full citizenship and that children have no human rights. To overcome this, a clear commitment to equity, solidarity and human rights for all needs be entrenched at all levels of the organization from the earliest stages. This lack of inclusion also applies to people with mental health conditions and other non-visible disabilities (Chatterjee et al 2009, International Consultation to Review Community-Based Rehabilitation 2009). The bulk of CBR activities and resources end up being focused on physical disabilities to the detriment of less obvious issues. A regular, systematic review of each member's needs is therefore required to highlight specific needs and ensure equity.

Unrealistic expectations constitute a fairly common pitfall in CBR. Over time, as the magnitude of people's needs becomes apparent, communities might develop unattainable goals. This can undermine morale, create conflict and jeopardize team work. Another weakness of CBR is that agents' and volunteers' needs can remain unmet, as they often struggle with their basic training, which is insufficient for them to carry out their duties properly relating to service delivery, general management and evaluation (Kuipers et al 2008).

Finally, another hazardous trend lies in the widespread lack of distinction that exists between home-based and community-based modes. By definition, CBR is more than home-based services; it is a strategy for equalization of opportunities that is community-owned and driven (Gautron 1999). To the untrained eye, service delivery may nevertheless look equivalent in both cases. However, CBR has a broader mandate, which is underlined by a strong philosophy of social justice, a philosophy at risk of being eroded in the absence of explicit recognition.

In short, CBR has many challenges, but these should not overshadow the remarkable gains that it has made. CBR has unquestionably contributed very significantly to the well-being of people with disabilities and is now seen as a critical tool for reducing poverty (International Consultation to Review Community-Based Rehabilitation 2009).

New avenues are now opening up. CBR can play a key role in the rebuilding of civil society in post-conflict settings (Boyce et al 2002) and there is new emphasis on its potential for enhancing quality of life and strengthening human rights (Finkenflügel 2009).

CBR and occupational therapy

Although CBR practice is not restricted to occupational therapists and includes professionals from all fields related to disability, its intrinsic worth is readily acknowledged by occupational therapists. As enablers, occupational therapists share fundamental CBR values. The WFOT defines occupational therapy as follows:

> Occupational therapy is a profession concerned with promoting health and well being through occupation. The primary goal of occupational therapy is to enable people to participate in the activities of everyday life. Occupational therapists achieve this outcome by enabling people to do things that will enhance their ability to participate or by modifying the environment to better support participation. (World Federation of Occupational Therapists 2009a, p.1)

There is a significant overlap between this definition and the definition of CBR offered above. Occupational therapy and CBR both foster empowerment, enablement and better quality of life for people with disabilities. They also stem from similar conceptual roots, which include social justice and full citizen participation. In both cases, social justice and personal choice lie at the core of the process. It is unsurprising, therefore, that the WFOT endorsed CBR in its official position paper on the issue:

> WFOT recognizes that occupational therapists have contributed to making a difference in the lives of people with disabilities and their families through community based rehabilitation (CBR). WFOT supports and promotes the development and dissemination of CBR programs and the human rights of people with disabilities. WFOT supports the design and implementation of integrated occupational therapy practice-research-education projects in CBR.

> This position implies that occupational therapists engage in coalitions with people who experience disabilities, their families and communities, advocating with them and for their issues, sharing individual experiences and enabling professional organizations to support people with

disabilities' needs and rights of dignity and inclusion, in both developing and developed societies. (World Federation of Occupational Therapists 2009b, p.1)

Summary

CBR and occupational therapy share a strong philosophical kinship. They both arose from significant social struggles that marked the 20th century; occupational therapy came into being as an answer to the plight of soldiers wounded in the First World War, while CBR was the brainchild of the Independent Living Movement. Vulnerable groups of people with disabilities were seeking more equitable ways to reclaim full citizenship, and both CBR and occupational therapy have constituted valuable tools towards that goal. So, the close conceptual ties between CBR and occupational therapy are expressed not only in intangible mission statements, but also in a commonality of very concrete goals and methods. CBR and occupational therapy both acknowledge the need for greater social justice and aim to promote the well-being and rights of people with disability through empowerment, enablement and participation. Their methods are client- or community-centred and focus on what is meaningful for the clients, be they individuals or groups. They give power and voice to people with disabilities on the long road to equality.

Reflective learning

- Conceptually, what would be potential areas of conflict between CBR and occupational therapy?
- How does power sharing with people with disabilities currently differ between more institutional occupational therapy and CBR?
- What would you include in the occupational therapy role within a CBR project?
- How would you structure monitoring and evaluation within a CBR framework?
- What other new avenues for CBR could you identify where occupational therapy could play a key role?

References

Boyce, W., Lysack, C., 1997. Understanding the community in Canadian CBR: critical lessons from abroad. Canadian Journal of Rehabilitation 10 (4), 261–272.

Boyce, W., Koros, M., Hodgson, J., 2002. Community based rehabilitation:

a strategy for peace-building. BMC International Health and Human Rights 2, 6. Available from: http://www.biomedcentral.com/1472-698X/2/6.

Chatterjee, S., Pillai, A., Jain, S., et al., 2009. Outcomes of people

with psychotic disorders in a community-based rehabilitation programme in rural India. British Journal of Psychiatry 195, 433–439. Available from: http://bjp.rcpsych.org/cgi/content/abstract/195/5/433.

Convention on the Rights of Persons with Disabilities, 2009. United Nations. Available from: http://www.un.org/disabilities/convention/facts.shtml (accessed 18.11.09).

Finkenflügel, H., 2009. Prospects for community-based rehabilitation in the new millennium. In: Møller, V., Huschka, D. (Eds.), Quality of Life and the Millennium Challenge: Advances in Quality-of-Life Studies, Theory and Research. Springer, Amsterdam, pp. 265–274.

Finkenflügel, H., Cornielje, H., Velema, J., 2008. The use of classification models in the evaluation of CBR programmes. Disability and Rehabilitation 30 (5), 348–354.

Gautron, B., 1999. La Réadaptation à Base Communautaire. IDC, Paris.

Helander, E., 1999. Prejudice and Dignity: An Introduction to Community-based Rehabilitation, second ed. UNDP, New York.

Hirsch, M., 2009. Community-based rehabilitation for Parkinson's disease: from neurons to neighborhoods. Parkinsonism and Related Disorders 15, S114–S117.

ILO, UNESCO, WHO, CBR, 2004. A Strategy for Rehabilitation, Equalization of Opportunities, Poverty Reduction and Social Inclusion of People with Disabilities. Joint Position Paper. WHO. Available from: http://whqlibdoc.who.int/publications/2004/9241592389_eng.pdf (accessed 02.11.09).

International Consultation to Review Community-Based Rehabilitation (CBR), 2009. WHO. Available from: http://www.aifo.it/english/resources/online/books/cbr/reviewofcbr/Report.Helsinki.CBR.May.pdf (accessed 21.10.09).

Kuipers, P., Kuipers, K., Mongkolsrisawat, S., et al., 2003. Categorising CBR service delivery: the roi-et classification. Asia Pacific Disability Rehabilitation Journal 14 (2), 128–137.

Kuipers, P., Wirz, S., Hartley, S., 2008. Systematic synthesis of community-based rehabilitation (CBR) project evaluation reports for evidence-based policy: a proof-of-concept study. BMC International Health and Human Rights 8, 3. Available from: http://ukpmc.ac.uk/articlerender.cgi?artid=1404189.

Lindsay, P., Bayley, M., Hellings, C., et al., 2008. Stroke rehabilitation and community reintegration. Outpatient and community-based rehabilitation. In: Canadian Best Practice Recommendations for Stroke Care, CMAJ 179 (12 Suppl.), E58–E61.

Page, N., Czuba, C.E., 2009. Empowerment: What Is It? Journal of Extension Available from: http://www.joe.org/joe/1999october/comm1.php (accessed 20.11.09).

Peat, M., 1997. Community Based Rehabilitation. WB Saunders, London.

Périquet, A.O., 1984. Community-based rehabilitation services: the experience of Bacolod, Philippines and the Asia/Pacific Region. World Rehabilitation Fund Information Exchange 26, 1–63.

Reverso. 2009. Reverso Dictionary. Available from: http://dictionary.reverso.net/englishdefinition/enablement (accessed 3.10.09).

Thibeault, R., 2008. Les grands défis de la santé internationale. In: Beaudet, P., Hassam, P., Schaffer, J. (Eds.), Introduction au Développement International. Presses de l'Université d'Ottawa, Ottawa, pp. 300–317.

Thibeault, R., Forget, A., 1997. From snow to sand: community-based rehabilitation perspectives from the Arctic and Africa. Canadian Journal of Rehabilitation 10 (4), 315–328.

Turmusani, M., Vreede, A., Wirz, S.L., 2002. Some ethical issues in community-based rehabilitation initiatives in developing countries. Disability and Rehabilitation 24 (10), 558–567.

Werner, D., 1988. Disabled Village Children. Hesperian Foundation, Palo Alto.

Werner, D., 1998. Nothing About Us Without Us. Healthwrights, Palo Alto.

Willig-Levy, C., 2009. A People's History of the Independent Living Movement. Independent Living Institute. Available from: http://www.independentliving.org/docs5/ILhistory.html#anchor2 (accessed 4.12.09).

Wiman, R., Helander, E., Westland, J., 2002. Meeting the Needs of People with Disabilities — New Approaches in the Health Sector. World Bank, Washington.

World Federation of Occupational Therapists, 2009a. What is Occupational Therapy?. Available from: http://www.wfot.org/information.asp (accessed 5.10.09).

World Federation of Occupational Therapists, 2009b. Position Paper on CBR. Available from: http://www.wfot.org/office_files/CBRposition%20Final%20CM2004%281%29.pdf (accessed 11.12.09).

World Health Organization, 2009a. Projections of Mortality and Burden of Disease, 2004–2030. Available from: http://www.who.int/healthinfo/global_burden_disease/projections/en/index.html (accessed 17.10.09).

World Health Organization, 2009b. Community-based Rehabilitation. United Nations. Available from: http://www.who.int/disabilities/cbr/en/index.html (accessed 7.12.09).

Occupational science: genesis, evolution and future contribution

18

Matthew Molineux   Gail E. Whiteford

OVERVIEW

Throughout its history, occupational therapy has had distinct periods of conceptual and theoretical development that had an impact on the emergence of subsequent models of practice and the implementation of distinct intervention strategies. Considered retrospectively, some of these developments may now be regarded as having had net negative outcomes, such as the influence of reductionist medicine, which led to instrumentally focused occupational therapy. In this chapter, the authors chart the development of occupational science as one of the most distinct developments the profession has witnessed. The chapter presents an overview of the genesis of occupational science alongside a discussion of some of the attendant issues and tensions associated with its subsequent development. Consideration of the value and contribution of occupational science in informing both the epistemological and practice foundations of the profession is covered, prior to a presentation of a research agenda for occupational science in the future. In essence, it is hoped that the reader will gain a clearer sense of how and why occupational science developed; what it has meant to the profession to date; and, finally, what it may contribute to understandings of the complex phenomenon of human occupation through a coherent and focused research agenda.

Key points

- Effective occupational therapy practice is founded on an understanding of occupation and its impact on health.

Key points—cont'd

- Occupational therapists must have a thorough understanding of humans as occupational beings and of the relationship between occupation and health.
- Occupational science has been one of the most significant developments in the history of occupational therapy.
- The future of occupational science rests on its ability to generate new and useful knowledge, as judged by its stakeholders.
- A research agenda for occupational science, which covers all the levels at which occupation is organized, is one way to ensure appropriate knowledge generation and application.

Introduction

How new knowledge is generated, tested and then infused into practice is a key concern in all disciplines. Whilst information is abundant in our age, how we make sense of it is especially challenging. Like other disciplines, then, occupational therapy finds itself in a historic moment in which the need to develop the epistemological foundations upon which it is based is of central concern. Unlike other disciplines, though, occupational therapy has experienced particular tensions with respect to the relationship between its central philosophical premise: that is, there is a dynamic interaction between occupation and health, and how this is addressed in practice. Specifically, this tension may be attributed to the conceptual and methodological inconsistencies between the biomedical and human/social science paradigms, which both inform occupational therapy curricula, practice and research.

To this end, the development of occupational science may be seen as a cogent response, one that has already had significant positive impacts on the practice terrain of occupational therapy and promises to play an even more important role in the next several decades. In this chapter, we chart the genesis, or development, of occupational science and how it has evolved over time. We also posit some suggestions as to how its research agenda can inform the contribution of occupational therapy in a range of practice contexts in the future.

History and development

Occupational science was first named by Yerxa and colleagues (1989, p.6) as 'the study of the human as an occupational being including the need for and capacity to engage in and orchestrate daily occupations in the environment over the lifespan'. The naming of occupational science in the late 1980s was the culmination of a period of work by occupational therapy academics at the University of Southern California, who were developing a proposal for a doctoral programme. In doing so, they gave much thought to the focus of that programme, and felt that the profession of occupational therapy would be usefully served by scholars in a science of occupation. The commencement of that PhD programme and the publication of the first paper that proposed occupational science marked the formal recognition of the new discipline. However, examination of the history of occupational therapy reveals that the naming of occupational science was merely the climax of a slow but steady movement within the profession. For this reason, it has been said that occupational science is not merely a chance happening (Clark & Larson 1993).

A science of occupation was first mooted by the National Society for the Promotion of Occupational Therapy in 1917 (Wilcock 2001, 2003, Larson et al 2003). The initial objectives of that organization, which later became the American Occupational Therapy Association, proposed that it should concentrate on 'the advancement of occupation as a therapeutic measure, the study of the effects of occupation upon the human being, and the dissemination of scientific knowledge of this subject' (Dunton et al 1917). As the profession grew, only the therapeutic use of occupation received much attention (Wilcock 2003), despite continued calls for theoretical unity within the profession, which

was consistent with the history and philosophy of early occupational therapy (Clark & Larson 1993). Prominent figures such as Meyer, Slagle, Reilly and Ayres had proposed that such unity would be provided by a basic science that focused on occupation (Yerxa et al 1989).

Although occupational science grew out of occupational therapy, when it was formally proposed in the late 1980s it was represented as a distinct entity. The difference between the two, as outlined at that time, rested in the type of science they embodied. Occupational science was seen as a basic science: that is, one that dealt with 'universal issues about occupation without concern for their immediate application' (Yerxa et al 1989, p.4). Occupational therapy, on the other hand, was seen as being concerned with the application of knowledge about occupation for therapeutic ends (Clark et al 1991). Furthermore, it has been stressed throughout the history of occupational science that it is not a model or frame of reference, but a social science or field of enquiry (Clark & Larson 1993, Clark 1997, Wilcock 2001, Larson et al 2003). Given the complexity of occupation and its relationship with health, occupational science has always been seen as an interdisciplinary field (Yerxa et al 1989).

The history of occupational science has been characterized by simultaneous acceptance and controversy. No overview of occupational science would be complete without an acknowledgement of this paradox. Although occupational science is still developing, it has made significant steps towards becoming a well-established discipline (Clark 2006). Some of the milestones and achievements include regular occupational science symposia in countries around the world, including the USA, UK, Canada, Australasia and Japan. A research conference dedicated to occupational science is now well established in the USA. The *Journal of Occupational Science* has been in publication since 1993, and a growing number of books exist that focus explicitly on occupational science, on occupation or on understanding humans as occupational beings (Zemke & Clark 1996, Wilcock 1998, Kramer et al 2003, Pierce 2003, Molineux 2004, Watson & Swartz 2004, Whiteford & Wright-St Clair 2005, Christiansen & Townsend 2010). Occupational science has also featured in occupational therapy journals for several decades now, and many journals have published entire issues devoted specifically to the field (see, for example, Johnson & Yerxa 1990, Molineux 2000b, Zemke 2000, Clark 2001). Furthermore, occupational science is now embedded in the international standards for occupational therapy education (World Federation of Occupational Therapists 2002).

The emergence and continued development of occupational science has been a cause of concern for some occupational therapists. While Mosey (1992) saw that occupational science might prove useful for occupational therapy, she did argue for complete partition of the two. She proposed that separation would allow for a clear distinction to be made regarding the focus and form of enquiry in each field. Her suggestion was that occupational science should concentrate on theory development (focus) through basic research (form), while occupational therapy should concern itself with the testing and refinement of frames of reference through applied research. Her concerns were that, if complete partition did not occur, then an unhealthy co-dependence would develop, it would be unclear what was a discipline and what was a profession, and the research which took place would be poorly focused. Given that she viewed both forms of enquiry as valuable, she encouraged each field to concentrate on the type of research most applicable to its domain of concern (Mosey 1993). In response, Clark and colleagues (1993) from the University of Southern California argued that the differentiation between basic and applied research was not dichotomous, as Mosey (1992) proposed, and so to categorize occupational science and occupational therapy was inappropriate. This was an interesting assertion, given that only a few years earlier the same authors, with others, had proposed occupational science as a basic science (Yerxa et al 1989). Clark and colleagues now saw that such rigid categorization would unnecessarily limit research and stifle potentially useful work (Clark et al 1993, Carlson & Dunlea 1995).

Issues of basic and applied sciences have featured heavily in other debates about occupational science. There has been some question, for example, as to whether or not a basic science of occupation is necessary at all, given that an abundance of knowledge about occupation exists in other disciplines (Kielhofner 2002). What is clear, however, is that, while other fields may address issues that might usefully inform an understanding of occupation, these fields do not use the concept of occupation as the focus of enquiry (Clark et al 1993, Carlson & Dunlea 1995, Zemke & Clark 1996, Haggard 2002, Polatajko 2004). As a result, 'the concept of occupation as an organiser of theory and research falls outside the domain of traditional disciplines' (Clark et al 1991, p.305).

The relationship between basic and applied forms of research has also stimulated wider debates around approaches to knowledge generation. Although this was first raised by Mosey (1992), it has been more fully examined recently, in particular by proponents of the Model of Human Occupation. Their concern is with the way that knowledge informs practice. They contrast approaches to knowledge generation, which include, from the outset, concern for how that knowledge can be used by practitioners, and those whose concern is knowledge generation without guidance on how to use that in practice. It is argued that using a conceptual model of practice (as defined by Kielhofner 1992, 1997) and related methods, such as the scholarship of practice (Braveman et al 2001, Kielhofner 2005), ensures that the dialectic which exists between theory and practice is preserved. This ensures that any knowledge generated not only addresses the concerns of practitioners but also has clear guidance on how that knowledge can be used in practice (Kielhofner 1997, 2002, Taylor et al 2002). This approach can be contrasted with occupational science, which informs practice but may not necessarily provide specific tools or methods to be utilized by occupational therapy practitioners (Clark 1997, Forsyth 2001a,b, Molineux 2001).

It can be seen, then, that occupational science and occupational therapy are closely linked, and that in fact the former emerged from the latter. Indeed, it could be said that they were not initially two distinct entities, as the National Society for the Promotion of Occupational Therapy recognized the need to understand occupation and the dynamic relationship between occupation and health, and that this sat comfortably alongside the therapeutic use of occupation. However, it is worth noting that occupational science was formally labelled just over 20 years ago and it continues to develop and negotiate relationships with occupational therapy and other fields. Despite its youth, occupational science has much to offer and this will be discussed in the next section of this chapter.

The value and contribution of occupational science

Although there has been much debate about occupational science and related issues, such as approaches to knowledge generation and the relationship between theory and practice, even those who have raised concerns about the new discipline have also seen its potential (Mosey 1992, 1993, Kielhofner 1997, Forsyth 2001a, Rey 2001, Hinojosa 2003). The value of occupational science has been well documented and includes (Yerxa et al 1989, Clark et al 1991, 1998, 2004, Clark & Larson 1993, Carlson & Dunlea 1995, Zemke & Clark 1996, Molineux 2000a, Yerxa 2000, Larson et al 2003, Wilcock 2003):

- providing support for what occupational therapists do in practice
- improving current services to clients and developing new approaches for therapy
- understanding humans as occupational beings
- explicating the relationship between occupation and health
- differentiating occupational therapy from other professions
- enhancing services outside of traditional health and social care boundaries

Of course, the real test of occupational science will be whether or not it stands the test of time and can make a place for itself alongside other academic disciplines. There is little doubt that the debates and discussion will continue and it will be worth examining those debates in order to understand their foundation. One such examination (Molke et al 2004) has noted that, while the number of occupational science publications in 2000 was much greater than in 1990, the articles were still being published in the occupational therapy or occupational science literature and not in other fields. While not growing outside of occupational therapy, that same analysis revealed that occupational science has grown within the international occupational therapy community.

It is this growing base of evidence as to both the power and the potential of occupation that has been one of the most significant contributions of occupational science to date. Whereas generations of occupational therapy researchers had been focusing on the efficacy of specific treatment regimes aimed at reducing impairment, occupational science has re-focused attention on the more fundamental concern of the relationship between doing and well-being. Significantly, there has been a very important outcome of this focus on doing and well-being that has subsequently had a subtle but profound impact on occupational therapy practice. This has been the centralization of the person.

Centralization of the person refers to a conceptual and philosophical shift to an appreciation of the client of occupational therapy services as being both the expert with respect to their own occupational history and *the most* significant agent of change. Correspondingly, the role of the professional is re-cast as a facilitator, coach, resource conduit and advocate, hence equalizing the power relationship. Viewed thus, we can see that this has represented a shift away from the dominance of biomedicine as a guiding paradigm: a paradigm in which the locus of expertise and authority (and, some would argue, meaning) resided with the professional. Inevitably, such a shift has created some tensions. Specifically, these tensions are experienced most overtly by occupational therapists working in acute care settings where the milieu is one in which a truly person-centred approach becomes not just philosophically challenging but pragmatically almost untenable (Wilding & Whiteford 2009).

Whilst a full examination of this particular issue is beyond the scope of this chapter, a paradigm tension such as that described above does have implications for what sorts of research question should become prioritized in occupational science. Accordingly, the next section presents an exploration of what should be incorporated into a coherent research agenda for the future, alongside a critical examination of some of the philosophical underpinnings of what constitutes valid research.

The research agenda of occupational science

As has been suggested in the previous section, one of the features that characterizes occupation is complexity; indeed, some authors have advocated that complexity theory itself should be the basis for developing understandings of occupation as a multidimensional human phenomenon (Creek 2003, Whiteford et al 2005). Such complexity represents a two-edged sword when it comes to research, however. On the one hand, the complex features of occupation make it a rich field of enquiry. On the other hand, the complexity of occupation requires careful consideration of methodological strategies employed to comprehend it best.

Methodologically, discussions and developments in occupational science research to date have highlighted the importance of narrative approaches in understanding occupation. As numerous authors have argued over time, the dynamism of occupation cannot be captured through traditional experimental means. Indeed, because of its context dependence, occupation cannot be reduced to sets of variables that are controlled or manipulated. It is precisely the random and sometimes chaotic environmental interactions that are the everyday fabric of occupational engagement as lived experience. Narrative approaches have been identified as being a more ontologically appropriate means through which to understand how meaning through occupation is developed over a life course (Frank 1996, Molineux & Rickard 2003, Wicks & Whiteford 2003), the significance of occupational 'motifs' (Clark et al 1996), the relationship between occupation and gender (Wicks & Whiteford 2005), and that between occupation and identity (Christiansen 2004). Additionally, and very importantly for the future, a narrative approach to understanding occupation or 'doing' has also been identified as being more consistent with indigenous knowledge paradigms (Yalmambirra 2000, Ratima & Ratima 2004).

As may be evident, the case for narrative ways of knowing and understanding occupation as a situated phenomenon have been well argued and are generally well accepted. There is, however, a broader methodological discussion that still needs to take place with respect to diversity. Understanding occupation in different contexts and at the different levels at which it occurs (micro though macro) requires a conscious adoption of methodological pluralism. Such pluralism allows diverse research methods and approaches to be utilized, depending on the nature of the research focus or question. For example, understanding the impacts of living with a chronic illness on patterns and meanings of occupational engagement may predicate a narrative approach, whilst understanding patterns of occupational engagement nationally would require population-level statistical information. Alternatively, attempting to illuminate impacts of, for example, a new industrial development on the occupations of a specific community would require a multi-method orientation utilizing approaches such as focus groups, surveys, time use instruments and individual interviews. Clearly, whilst this is an arena in which there is still much debate and dialogue to be had, it is of central importance to the ongoing development of occupational science and its research foci. But what are these foci and how do they relate to an overarching research agenda? Whilst we do not have the space in this chapter to discuss these in any great depth, we will start with a brief description

of the current and future research agenda of occupation science as a segue into a presentation of what we, the authors, consider to be the specific foci for future enquiry.

In essence, the future of occupational science, and indeed its potential to inform and guide occupational therapy, lie in its ability to generate new and useful knowledge as judged by its stakeholders. Relevancy has overwhelmingly become the concern of not just stakeholders but funders, academics and practitioners alike when they discuss research. This represents a timely and appropriate response when, at worst, many abuses of intellectual and human rights have historically occurred in the name of research and, at best, research has been compromised in its usefulness by a lack of regard for application in real-world contexts. The notion of research as praxis, eloquently argued some time ago by feminist Patti Lather (1986), is based on a requirement for research to be focused on generating knowledge that leads to changes in practice in order to empower people. And that is exactly what a research agenda in occupational science needs to do. When we consider occupation and its centrality not only in people's lives but in society per se, a research agenda to understand it further must necessarily address those *structural* issues that enable or preclude people from engaging in occupation, as well as individual ones. This means including consideration of the historic, political and economic factors shaping access and participation for whole groups of people and the discursive traditions that influence policy development. As described, then, it is an ambitious agenda. Accordingly, and in order to stand as a discipline alongside others, the enactment of this pluralistic research agenda must also be systematic, rigorous and defensible.

As to the specific foci of occupational science research, they are best articulated within a structural framework relating to the levels at which occupation occurs and is organized. These levels are (from micro through macro): the individual, the family, society, and population. Such a construction differs from that developed by Polatajko (2004), which focused on six areas of enquiry relating to the who, how, when where and so on of occupation and occupational engagement.

The rationale for the approach adopted by the authors in this chapter is that focusing on the structural elements that enable and constrain occupation provides us with a more powerful appreciation of causation as it relates to occupation. That is, it allows us to understand that what people *do* never occurs in a vacuum. Rather, all human occupation is *situated*, an essential characteristic that has been described as follows:

> All occupation takes place in a context. That is, no human action is independent of the social, cultural, political and economic contexts in which it occurs. These contextual forces, to a greater or lesser extent, shape the form and performance of the occupation as well as the meaning ascribed to it by an individual or group. (Whiteford et al 2005, p.10)

Developing understandings of this complex rubric within which occupation takes place and the causal relationships that exist and exert a powerful influence not only on form and performance but also on legitimacy and opportunity obviously represents a significant challenge. Such a challenge will not be met though an ad hoc programme of enquiry, which to some extent may be a criticism levelled at occupational science research in the past. One of the areas that has been explored relatively rigorously, however, has been that of individual determinants of occupation.

Level: the individual

There are several reasons why research into human occupation has largely been focused at the level of the individual. The first relates to the specific professional history of occupational therapy (where, to date, most occupational science researchers have come from) as being shaped by biomedical concerns with human systems and structures. The second reason is that such an orientation reflects the dominance of traditional Western epistemological concerns with the individual, rather than the collective. This orientation has been criticized as representing a barrier to more culturally diverse ways of knowing and understanding occupation, with suggestions that the claiming of the theoretical basis of occupation as an essentially Western tradition alienates others through claiming an authority that is 'further canonised when coded into a exclusive set of concepts and language that favour a particular social and cultural context' (Iwama 2005, p.252).

Such criticisms are valid and point strongly to the need for adoption of more inclusive epistemologies, a notion supported by the authors and one of the reasons for creating a schema for research that addresses multiple levels (including collective) through which to understand occupation. This fact

notwithstanding, however, the research to date that has focused on occupational development across the lifespan, mind/brain/body and occupational performance, occupation and time use, and individual constructions of meaning relative to occupational engagement have provided some rich understandings. Although such understandings may have limited cultural generalizability, they have enabled a more informed articulation of the centrality of occupation in the lives of people and the relationship to sense of self. In turn, this has led to clearer understandings of the impacts of disruption to forming established and projected patterns of occupational engagement. Given current social trends, however, some of the areas of future concern at the level of the individual should necessarily include:

- an exploration of the relationship between occupation, choice and mental health
- leisure occupations and their contribution to efficacy and identity
- the impact of new technologies on occupational capacities.

Level: the family

Families may be viewed as a primary vehicle for the development of value systems with respect to chosen and obligatory occupations; it is through people's experiences in families of origin that they learn about what is valuable, important and discretionary (Whiteford 2010). All of us have either experienced or observed family members condone or reject certain occupations and occupational behaviours. From the occupation of paid employment to the more subtle arena of leisure occupations, the influence of family values on choices made by individuals is sometimes overt, sometimes subtle, but usually pervasive. Indeed, in real terms, the value accorded to occupations in family groups influences the mobilization of human and non-human resources. Of course, family values are also reflective of the social and cultural context in which they occur; the time and effort required by a family to support an Olympic athlete or concert pianist in the making need also to be viewed as relative to the societal value associated with each.

Given the significant influence of families on occupational development, then, it is surprising that relatively little research with an occupational focus has taken place to date. Some of the major foci to date have revolved around co-occupations in family units, parenting as an occupation, and patterns of occupational engagement in families who have a child with a disability. Certainly, though, a stronger orientation to diversity must inform the research agenda of the future in this area. This is especially true in a context in which what defines a family unit has changed dramatically over time (Stagnitti 2005), gender roles have been revised, and families experience increasing levels of stress. Accordingly, research in the future would be well served by addressing, for instance, time use patterns in families (Zuzanek 2009), occupational stressors on families, occupational development of children in families living in resource-poor settings and jobless households, and families with sole- or same-sex couple parents.

Level: community/society

Because what constitutes a community has changed in recent times with the emergence of *virtual* communities, a definition at the outset seems prudent in this section. Perhaps one of the best descriptions comes from Christiansen and Townsend (2004, p.142), who have attempted to analyse communities critically from an occupational perspective:

> Human communities consist of groups of people who do things together and individually. People participate collectively through reflection, communication or action in occupations such as labour, sports, intellectual pursuits or home building. Bonds that draw and keep people thinking about each other and occupied together may include shared beliefs, shared geography, shared interests, shared experiences or shared kinship.

As is evident from the above definition, the emphasis is on the element of what is common, or shared, between people. However, exactly what it is that is shared will influence the types and forms of occupation that people in communities will be engaged in together. A case in point, for example, is the erosion of geographic communities as a site of common occupations, as evidenced in contemporary cities around the globe. Whereas, previously, living near someone meant some commonality in terms of interest or lifestyle, this is no longer the case. Indeed, many people fall into the category of finding that they spend more time occupationally engaged with people halfway around the globe than with people who live within a 10-kilometre radius. Clearly, if we think about the dependence of traditional communities located in geographic space, and about the input of those members to build community capacity

in some form (for example, through participating in a neighbourhood watch programme or for a working bee in a local playground), then the implications of this development are serious. Who participates in and who gets left out of what people 'do' together in any type of community becomes a key issue. Despite the demographic and technological shifts influencing what constitutes a community and how it is experienced, people do still have an innate sense of belonging and identity relative to space (Mackay 2007), an issue that needs to inform public policy globally.

To date, these issues and others addressing broader political and economic influences on communities have been tentatively explored in the occupational science literature. Specific foci have included, for example, patterns of occupational engagement in communities, social and cultural influences on occupation and occupational role development, political and legislative influences on occupational participation of community members, and occupational alienation and deprivation. If we are to serve society best, however, the research agenda in this area must be referenced to the broader discourse of social inclusion, which is the specifically stated orientation of many countries. Social inclusion developed in Europe and the UK as a response to greater migrant worker mobility, increased population diversity and inadequate welfare supports (Wotherspoon 2002). In essence, social inclusion is concerned with ensuring that 'people have the resources, opportunities and capabilities they need to learn, work, engage and have a voice' (Australian Social Inclusion Board 2010, p.15). Clearly, these are areas that are (or should be) of interest to occupational scientists, who may focus on, for example, the impacts made on communities by people such as asylum-seekers, who have been occupationally deprived, understanding whether work creation schemes have an effect and why/why not, and identifying how governments can best build occupation/community capacity to enhance civic engagement.

Level: population

If you can imagine the levels we have identified here as a lens, starting with the closest focus on the individual, then this is the lens zoomed right out to the broadest level at which we can understand, and hopefully capture, human occupation. It is also perhaps the most contentious, as enquiry into population-related phenomena has traditionally been the province of economists, epidemiologists and statisticians. Whilst this may be so, Wilcock (2003) argued that, in fact, occupational therapists, prior to their inculcation into a biomedical belief system, were largely oriented to addressing the root causes of population ill health. Historical antecedents notwithstanding, bringing an occupational perspective to how we make sense of the many dimensions of population well-being is both cogent and timely when we face a projected population globally of 9.3 billion in 2050.

To date, this relatively small area of enquiry has been concerned with issues relating to population policy, population health status indicators and economic/employment status indicators. Whilst these foci need all remain on the agenda, the future should also include deepening our understandings of phenomena that are causally more complex but have an underlying occupational dimension — e.g. childhood obesity, ill health as a result of loneliness and isolation, and the impact of globalization upon occupational participation rates in developing countries.

In summary, this section has been a presentation and exploration of the research agenda of occupational science. It is not exhaustive, and needs to be read and understood in relation to the ongoing development of occupational science. Nevertheless, it has been presented here because understanding occupation from different perspectives and at different levels is crucial to the development of new knowledge. Such new knowledge has the potential to inform not only the development of relevant and appropriate occupational therapy services, but government policy and resource allocation. This, however, will not be a passive process. Rather it must be one in which researchers, educators, practitioners, managers and diverse community groups enact a willingness to discuss and debate key philosophical and conceptual issues in order to ensure change in social practices. Central to this process must be a commitment to highlighting occupation as a unique, guiding paradigm. Such a commitment must come from all parties.

Summary

This chapter has provided an overview of the genesis of occupational science and its evolution to date. It has demonstrated that, although the discipline was only formally named in the late 1980s, the seeds were sown at the foundation of the occupational therapy profession. Although occupational science has undergone much development to date, it is worth remembering that it is still emerging. As such, the precise boundaries of the field continue to be tested and negotiated. That occupational science continues to be refined makes this period in the history of the science and therapy of occupation most exciting, with more stimulating debates to come. One of these must be the relationship between occupational science and other disciplines. Occupational science has always been purported to be multidisciplinary, but it remains the case that most (but not all) occupational scientists are occupational therapists. An issue that occupational therapists must wrestle with further is the nature of knowledge generation in the profession and the relationship between knowledge and practice. For example, while models of practice are undoubtedly useful, it would be worth considering further whether or not they are the only way of translating knowledge into practice.

Occupational science is concerned with furthering our understanding of humans as occupational beings and the relationship between occupation and health. This chapter has provided a brief overview of the research agenda of the field, organized within a framework relating to the levels at which occupation occurs and is organized. These included research into occupation at the level of the individual, the family, communities and whole populations. Although this framework is not inconsistent with occupational therapy, it challenges therapists to maintain an occupational focus, and to take a broader view of their contribution to the health of humans. Occupational science continues to provide useful insights into the factors that facilitate and inhibit the ability of individuals to achieve and maintain health through occupation. In addition, occupational science is explicating new concepts, such as social inclusion and occupational justice, which require further scholarly development as to how they can most powerfully inform practice (Whiteford & Townsend 2010). This new direction is one of the most exciting results of the development of occupational science. It remains unclear, however, how willing occupational therapists are to respond to the challenge to move outside their comfort zone and utilize their expertise with diverse groups of people in different settings and in new ways.

Reflective learning

- Consider the nature of contemporary occupational therapy practice, locally and globally. To what extent do you see an occupational perspective of humans and health enacted in practice?
- To what extent do you think occupational therapy literature supports an occupation-based approach to occupational therapy practice?
- How do you, and other occupational therapists you know, incorporate occupational science into practice?

- What do you think are the key research priorities for occupational therapy, if the profession is to contribute to the health of individuals, groups and societies?
- What research methods are appropriate for addressing the proposed research agenda for occupational science?

References

Australian Social Inclusion Board, 2010. Social Inclusion in Australia: How Australia is Faring. Commonwealth of Australia, Canberra.

Braveman, B., Helfrich, C., Fisher, G., 2001. Developing and maintaining community partnerships within 'A Scholarship of Practice'. Occupational Therapy in Health Care 15 (1/2), 109–125.

Carlson, M., Dunlea, M., 1995. Further thoughts on the pitfalls of partition: a response to Mosey. American Journal of Occupational Therapy 49 (1), 73–81.

Christiansen, C., 2004. Occupation and identity: becoming who we are through what we do. In: Christiansen, C., Townsend, E. (Eds.), Introduction to Occupation: The Art and Science of Living. Prentice Hall, Upper Saddle River, pp. 121–139.

Christiansen, C., Townsend, E., 2004. The occupational nature of communities. In: Christiansen, C., Townsend, E. (Eds.), Introduction to Occupation: The Art and Science of Living. Prentice Hall, Upper Saddle River, pp. 141–172.

Christiansen, C., Townsend, E. (Eds.), 2010. Introduction to Occupation: The Art and Science of Living, second ed. Prentice Hall, Upper Saddle River.

Clark, F., 1997. Overview of theoretical models: occupational science. In: Crist, P., Royeen, C., Schkade, J. (Eds.), Infusing Occupation into Practice. American Occupational Therapy Association, Bethesda, pp. 13–17.

Clark, F., 2001. Occupational science: the foundation for new models of practice [special issue]. Scandinavian Journal of Occupational Therapy 8 (1).

Clark, F., 2006. One person's thoughts on the future of occupational science. Journal of Occupational Science 13 (3), 167–179.

Clark, F., Larson, E., 1993. Developing an academic discipline: the science of occupation. In: Hopkins, H., Smith, H. (Eds.), Willard and Spackman's Occupational Therapy. JB Lippincott, Philadelphia, pp. 44–57.

Clark, F., Parham, D., Carlson, M., et al., 1991. Occupational science: academic innovation in the service of occupational therapy's future. American Journal of Occupational Therapy 45 (4), 300–310.

Clark, F., Zemke, R., Frank, G., et al., 1993. Dangers inherent in the partition of occupational therapy and occupational science. American Journal of Occupational Therapy 47 (2), 184–186.

Clark, F., Ennevor, B., Richardson, P., 1996. A grounded theory of techniques for occupational storytelling and occupational story making. In: Zemke, R., Clark, F. (Eds.), Occupational Science: The Evolving Discipline. FA Davis, Philadelphia, pp. 373–392.

Clark, F., Wood, W., Larson, E., 1998. Occupational science: occupational therapy's legacy for the 21st century. In: Neistadt, M., Crepeau, E. (Eds.), Willard and Spackman's Occupational Therapy. JB Lippincott, Philadelphia, pp. 13–21.

Clark, F., Jackson, J., Carlson, M., 2004. Occupational science, occupational therapy and evidence based practice: what the Well Elderly Study has taught us. In: Molineux, M. (Ed.), Occupation for Occupational Therapists. Blackwell, Oxford, pp. 200–218.

Creek, J., 2003. Occupational Therapy Defined as a Complex Intervention. College of Occupational Therapists, London.

Dunton, W.R., 1917. History of occupational therapy. Modern Hospital 8, 60.

Forsyth, K., 2001a. Occupational science as a selected research priority [letter]. British Journal of Occupational Therapy 64 (8), 420.

Forsyth, K., 2001b. What kind of knowledge will most benefit practice? [letter]. British Journal of Occupational Therapy 64 (12), 619–620.

Frank, G., 1996. The concept of adaptation as a foundation for occupational science research. In: Zemke, R., Clark, F. (Eds.), Occupational Science: The Evolving Discipline. FA Davis, Philadelphia, pp. 47–55.

Haggard, L., 2002. Broadening horizons [letter]. British Journal of Occupational Therapy 65 (2), 98–99.

Hinojosa, J., 2003. Therapist or scientist — how do these roles differ? American Journal of Occupational Therapy 57 (2), 225–226.

Iwama, M., 2005. Occupation as a cross-cultural construct. In:

Whiteford, G., Wright-St Clair, V. (Eds.), Occupation and Practice in Context. Churchill Livingstone, Sydney, pp. 242–253.

Johnson, J., Yerxa, E., 1990. Occupational science [special issue]. Occupational Therapy in Health Care 6 (4).

Kielhofner, G., 1992. Conceptual Foundations of Occupational Therapy. FA Davis, Philadelphia.

Kielhofner, G., 1997. Conceptual Foundations of Occupational Therapy, second ed. FA Davis, Philadelphia.

Kielhofner, G., 2002. Challenges and Directions for the Future of Occupational Therapy. World Federation of Occupational Therapists, 13th World Congress, Stockholm, Sweden.

Kielhofner, G., 2005. Scholarship and practice: bridging the divide. Am. J. Occup. Ther. 59 (2), 231–239.

Kramer, P., Hinojosa, J., Royeen, C. (Eds.), 2003. Perspectives in Human Occupation: Participation in Life. Lippincott Williams & Wilkins, Baltimore.

Larson, E., Wood, W., Clark, F., 2003. Occupational science: building the science and practice of occupation through an academic discipline. In: Crepeau, E., Cohn, E., Schell, B. (Eds.), Willard and Spackman's Occupational Therapy. tenth ed. Lippincott Williams & Wilkins, Philadelphia, pp. 15–26.

Lather, P., 1986. Research as praxis. Harvard Educational Review 56 (3), 257–275.

Mackay, H., 2007. Advance Australia Where? Hachette, Sydney.

Molineux, M., 2000a. Another step in the right direction [editorial]. British Journal of Occupational Therapy 63 (5), 191.

Molineux, M., 2000b. Occupational science [special issue]. British Journal of Occupational Therapy 65 (5).

Molineux, M., 2001. Being clear about what is being debated [letter]. British Journal of Occupational Therapy 64 (10), 519–520.

Molineux, M. (Ed.), 2004. Occupation for Occupational Therapists. Blackwell, Oxford.

Molineux, M., Rickard, W., 2003. Storied approaches to understanding occupation. Journal of Occupational Science 10 (1), 52–60.

Molke, D., Polatajko, H., Laliberte Rudman, D., 2004. The promise of occupational science: a developmental assessment of an emerging academic discipline. Canadian Journal of Occupational Therapy 71 (5), 269–280.

Mosey, A.C., 1992. Partition of occupational science and occupational therapy. Am. J. Occup. Ther. 46 (7), 851–853.

Mosey, A.C., 1993. Partition of occupational science and occupational therapy: sorting out some issues. Am. J. Occup. Ther. 47 (8), 751–754.

Pierce, D., 2003. Occupation by Design: Building Therapeutic Power. FA Davis, Philadelphia.

Polatajko, H., 2004. The study of occupation. In: Christiansen, C., Townsend, E. (Eds.), Introduction to Occupation: The Art and Science of Living. Prentice Hall, Upper Saddle River, pp. 29–46.

Ratima, M., Ratima, M., 2004. Practice in an indigenous context. In: Whiteford, G., Wright-St Clair, V. (Eds.), Occupation and Practice in Context. Churchill Livingstone, Sydney, pp. 230–241.

Rey, D., 2001. Resources and research priorities [letter]. British Journal of Occupational Therapy 64 (10), 518–519.

Stagnitti, K., 2005. The family unit in post modern society. In: Whiteford, G., Wright-St Clair, V. (Eds.), Occupation and Practice in Context. Churchill Livingstone, Sydney, pp. 213–229.

Taylor, R., Braveman, B., Forsyth, K., 2002. Occupational science and the scholarship of practice: implications for practitioners. New Zealand Journal of Occupational Therapy 49 (2), 37–40.

Watson, R., Swartz, L. (Eds.), 2004. Transformation through Occupation. Whurr, London.

Whiteford, G., 2010. Occupation in context. In: Curtin, M., Molineux, M., Supyk Mellson, J. (Eds.), Occupational Therapy and Physical Dysfunction. Churchill Livingstone, London, pp. 135–151.

Whiteford, G., Townsend, E., 2010. A participatory occupational justice framework. In: Kronenberg, F.,

Pollard, N. (Eds.), Occupational Therapies without Borders - Volume 2 Towards an ecology of occupation-based practices. Elsevier, London.

Whiteford, G., Wright-St Clair, V. (Eds.), 2005. Occupation and Practice in Context. Churchill Livingstone, Sydney.

Whiteford, G., Klomp, N., Wright-St Clair, V., 2005. Complexity theory: understanding occupation, practice and context. In: Whiteford, G., Wright-St Clair, V. (Eds.), Occupation and Practice in Context. Churchill Livingstone, Sydney, pp. 3–15.

Wicks, A., Whiteford, G., 2003. The use of life histories in understanding occupation across the life span. Australian Occupational Therapy Journal 44 (1), 126–138.

Wicks, A., Whiteford, G., 2005. Gender, occupation and participation. In: Whiteford, G., Wright-St Clair, V. (Eds.), Occupation and Practice in Context. Churchill Livingstone, Sydney, pp. 197–212.

Wilcock, A., 1998. An Occupational Perspective of Health. Slack, Thorofare, NJ.

Wilcock, A., 2001. Occupational science: the key to broadening horizons. British Journal of Occupational Therapy 64 (8), 412–417.

Wilcock, A., 2003. Occupational science: the study of humans as occupational beings. In: Kramer, P., Hinojosa, J., Royeen, C. (Eds.), Perspectives in Human Occupation: Participation in Life. Lippincott Williams & Wilkins, Baltimore, pp. 156–180.

Wilding, C., Whiteford, G., 2009. practice to praxis: reconnecting moral vision with philosophical underpinnings. British Journal of Occupational Therapy 72 (10), 434–440.

World Federation of Occupational Therapists, 2002. Revised Minimum Standards for the Education of Occupational Therapists. World Federation of Occupational Therapists, Forrestfield.

Wotherspoon, T., 2002. The dynamics of social inclusion. Perspectives on Social Inclusion working paper series. Laidlaw Foundation, Toronto.

Yalmambirra, 2000. Black time, white time: your time, my time. Journal of Occupational Science 7 (3), 133–137.

Yerxa, E., 2000. Occupational science: a renaissance of service to humankind through knowledge. Occup. Ther. Int. 7 (2), 87–98.

Yerxa, E., Clark, F., Jackson, J., et al., 1989. An introduction to occupational science: a foundation for occupational therapy in the 21st century. Occupational Therapy in Health Care 6 (4), 1–17.

Zemke, R., 2000. Occupational science [special issue]. Occup. Ther. Int. 7 (2).

Zemke, R., Clark, F. (Eds.), 1996. Occupational Science: The Evolving Discipline. FA Davis, Philadelphia.

Zuzanek, J., 2009. Time use imbalance: developmental and emotional costs. In: Matuska, K., Christiansen, C. (Eds.), Life Balance. Slack, Thorofare NJ, pp. 207–222.

Index

Notes:
As the subject of this book concerns occupational therapy, entries under this term have been kept to a minimum. Readers are advised to look for more specific terms. Page numbers suffixed by 'b', 'f', or 't' refer to boxes, figures or tables respectively.

To save space in the index, the following abbreviations have been used:
CBR, Community-Based Rehabilitation; CMOP, Canadian Model of Occupational Performance; MOHO, Model of Human Occupation; PEOP, Person-Environment-Occupational Performance model.

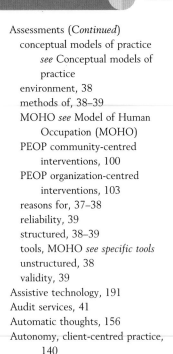